Praise for *Mastering Patient and Family Education*

"This book is packed with practical strategies and tips about essential topics, including technology, tele-health, language barriers, and health literacy. It is a must-read for those who care about improving outcomes for their patients and families."

–Glenn Flores, MD, FAAP
Professor of Pediatrics, Clinical Sciences, and Public Health
...ved Chair in Pediatrics
...ation Health Research
...l Pediatrics Fellowship
...on Diversity (RAPID)
...Health System of Texas

"Engagement and em... ...gnized cornerstones of good paediatric hea... ...a comprehensive, systematic, and evider... ...ctrum and in vari-ous healthcare settings... ...and respective orga-nizations in masterin... ...re. But, importantly, their model is nurse-l...

...BS, MHA, DSc, AM
...Professor of Paediatrics
...South Wales, Australia

"Marshall and collea... ...proach to educating nurses on... ...egivers in self-managing health cor... ...mpowering, thought-provoking,...

...i, PhD, ANP, FAAN
...ties, Associate Dean
Distinguished Pro... ...l Co-Director of the
for Research, Audrie... ...Fellowship Program
...s School of Nursing

"A contemporary, e... ...ring patient and family education. C... ...althcare team ap-proach and emphas... ...cators, clinicians, and students."

...RN, FACN, FAAN
...gy, Sydney, Australia
...isation Collaborating
...rsing and Midwifery

Mastering Patient & Family Education

A Healthcare Handbook for Success

Lori C. Marshall, PhD, MSN, RN

Sigma Theta Tau International
Honor Society of Nursing®

The Honor Society of Nursing, Sigma Theta Tau International (STTI) is a nonprofit organization whose mission is to support the learning, knowledge, and professional development of nurses committed to making a difference in health worldwide. Founded in 1922, STTI has 130,000 members in 86 countries. Members include practicing nurses, instructors, researchers, policymakers, entrepreneurs and others. STTI's 499 chapters are located at 698 institutions of higher education throughout Australia, Botswana, Brazil, Canada, Colombia, Ghana, Hong Kong, Japan, Kenya, Malawi, Mexico, the Netherlands, Pakistan, Singapore, South Africa, South Korea, Swaziland, Sweden, Taiwan, Tanzania, the United States, and Wales. More information about STTI can be found online at www.nursingsociety.org.

Sigma Theta Tau International
550 West North Street
Indianapolis, IN, USA 46202

To order additional books, buy in bulk, or order for corporate use, contact Nursing Knowledge International at 888.NKI.4YOU (888.654.4968/US and Canada) or +1.317.634.8171 (outside US and Canada).

To request a review copy for course adoption, e-mail solutions@nursingknowledge.org or call 888.NKI.4YOU (888.654.4968/US and Canada) or +1.317.634.8171 (outside US and Canada).

To request author information, or for speaker or other media requests, contact Marketing, Honor Society of Nursing, Sigma Theta Tau International at 888.634.7575 (US and Canada) or +1.317.634.8171 (outside US and Canada).

ISBN: 9781940446301
EPUB ISBN: 9781940446318
PDF ISBN: 9781940446325
MOBI ISBN: 9781940446332

Library of Congress Cataloging-in-Publication Data

Marshall, Lori C. (Lori Carmel), 1962- , author.
  Mastering patient and family education : a healthcare handbook for success / Lori C. Marshall.
    p. ; cm.
  Includes bibliographical references.
  ISBN 978-1-940446-30-1 (alk. paper) -- ISBN 978-1-940446-31-8 (epub) -- ISBN 978-1-940446-32-5 (pdf) -- ISBN 978-1-940446-33-2 (mobi)
  I. Sigma Theta Tau International, issuing body. II. Title.
  [DNLM: 1. Inpatients--education. 2. Patient Education as Topic. 3. Nurse's Role. 4. Nurse-Patient Relations. 5. Professional-Family Relations. WX 158.5]
  RT90
  613--dc23
                          2015026012

First Printing, 2015

Publisher: Dustin Sullivan
Acquisitions Editor: Emily Hatch
Editorial Coordinator: Paula Jeffers
Cover Designer: Michael Tanamachi
Indexer: Joy Dean Lee

Principal Book Editor: Carla Hall
Development and Project Editor: Kezia Endsley
Copy Editor: Erin Geile
Proofreader: Todd Lothery
Interior Design and Page Composition: Rebecca Batchelor

Dedication

To Mary Dee Hacker, RN, MBA, FAAN, who advocates for patient self-determination with vision and passion and reminds us all that interprofessional collaboration is everything if we are to improve the health and wellbeing of our patients.

To my nursing and healthcare colleagues from around the globe: Thank you for enriching my knowledge and expanding my worldview beyond California.

And finally, to my mother, Filomena Spina Marshall, a nurse since 1950 and the reason I am proud to say I am a nursing professional today.
I love you, Mom.

–Lori C. Marshall

Acknowledgments

This book would not be possible without the help of a few key people. I believed Emily Hatch enough to say yes when she said she'd be there to support me through this process. Without her confident and calming presence, this book would be "in process" forever. My thanks to her and the entire publishing team at Sigma Theta Tau International.

I need to thank my friends Sandie Hoffman Middlestaat, Sandy Jordan Bailey, and Theresa Furtado for helping me rest my brain in between words.

This book would not be possible without the expert contributors who took the time to write down their knowledge to share with the world.

I also want to acknowledge the staff (Alma, Luis, Evan), Family Advisory member Sharilee Hayden, and nurses (Majella Doughty, Sharon Chinn, et al.) who work in, teach in, plus support the Family Resource Center at Children's Hospital Los Angeles. You live this book with passion and commitment every day. I cannot thank you enough for all you've done for patients and families.

About the Author

Lori C. Marshall, PhD, MSN, RN

Administrator, Patient Family Education and Resources, Children's Hospital Los Angeles; Assistant Adjunct Professor, School of Nursing, University of California, Los Angeles; Assistant Professor, Price School of Public Policy and Keck School of Medicine, University of Southern California

Marshall has worked at Children's Hospital Los Angeles since 1998, serving in a variety of roles. Currently she is the administrator, Patient Family Education and Resources. Aside from her role at CHLA, she is an assistant adjunct professor at the University of California, Los Angeles School of Nursing and assistant professor in the Division of Pediatrics at Keck School of Medicine. She is on the teaching faculty for the Master of Health Administration Program at the Sol Price School of Public Policy, USC, and taught in the Master of Academic Medicine Program at USC from 2008 to 2014. Marshall has over 39 years of experience in healthcare, with 28 years of that focused in leadership and education roles. These experiences go beyond the hospital setting, serving as the director of nursing for a home-health agency in Southern California and an education specialist for the outpatient clinics at Children's Hospital of Orange County. She has presented as an invited speaker in the United States, Italy, and Australia on the subjects of teams, teamwork, quality, and patient and family education.

Marshall obtained her bachelor of science degree in nursing at California State University, Fullerton; her master of science in nursing degree with an emphasis in education and administration at California State University, Dominguez Hills; and her PhD in education with an emphasis on educational psychology and human performance from the University of Southern California.

Contributing Authors

Linda Alexander, BSN, MBA, RN, CCM

Chief Clinical Officer, Total Health Care

Considered one of the most talented, results-driven executives in healthcare today, Linda Alexander embraces the philosophy that collaborative, inspiring leadership cuts across traditional boundaries. Alexander, chief clinical officer of Total Health Care, is responsible for clinical operations and population health management of 120,000 members. She leads the managed care organization's care management strategies to deliver optimum services in the era of healthcare reform. She is sought after by state and national organizations to speak on care integration and population health management strategies.

Alexander has nearly 20 years of proven healthcare leadership with an emphasis on care management/utilization management, physician alignment, operational efficiency, strategic planning, and quality/performance improvement. The Detroit native earned a bachelor of science in nursing from the University of Detroit-Mercy and a master of business administration-organizational development from Wayne State University in Detroit. She is the mother of three sons.

Amal Al-Hasawi, BSChem, BSN, RN

Head Nurse of Endoscopy & Day Procedure Unit
King Fahad Specialist Hospital–Dammam

Amal Al-Hasawi is a head nurse of Endoscopy and Day Procedure Unit at King Fahad Specialist Hospital in Dammam. She earned the spot as head nurse after 7 years of experience as registered nurse. She participated as speaker at the Saudi Health Conference 2013, Saudi Arabia. Al-Hasawi obtained her first bachelor's degree in chemistry from College of Sciences, Dammam University, Saudi Arabia. After that she decided it was time for a change of career. She opted to study and obtained the bachelor's degree in nursing from King Saud Bin Abdulaziz University for Health Sciences, Riyadh, Saudi Arabia. Added to her ongoing scholarly achievements, she is in the process of completing her executive master of science in the Health Administration program at the University of Alabama at Birmingham.
Al-Hasawi's professional transformation from a competent bedside nurse to a confident head nurse has proven her motivation and dedication to advocate for patients and their families.

Rita Anderson, DNP, RN, FACHE

Executive Director, Nursing Services
King Fahad Specialist Hospital–Dammam

Rita Anderson is executive director of nursing services at King Fahad Specialist Hospital in Dammam. She has held senior leadership positions for over 25 years. She has spoken at several international conferences and has been published in several professional peer-reviewed journals. Anderson obtained her bachelor's degree in nursing and her master's degree in nursing administration from The Ohio State University. She received her doctorate of nursing practice in executive leadership with American Sentinel University. She is actively involved in national and international professional organizations including Sigma Theta Tau International, the American Nurses Association, and the American Organization of Nurse Executives. She also achieved Fellow status with the American College of Healthcare Executives. Anderson has been working internationally for much of her career with a very culturally diverse workforce from over 30 different countries, many of whom do not speak the language of the patients being served. This has posed many challenges for ensuring adequate patient engagement and education. Various strategies have been put in place to facilitate the process, but more innovations are being sought.

Andrew Bielat, BS, BA

Manager, Language Access
CyraCom, Inc.

Andrew Bielat is a manager in the Language Access department at CyraCom, an international interpreter company that specializes in phone and video interpretation. He has been in the language services industry for the last 5 years, focusing on helping facilities reduce the cost of language access, improving adoption across all staff members, and ultimately providing better quality of care to LEP patients. Bielat coordinates language access roundtables around the country and is responsible for CyraCom's annual Healthcare Language Services Summit. He graduated from the University of Arizona with a bachelor's degree in business administration, marketing focus, and a Spanish minor.

Ana C. Chávez, BS, CHI

Language & Cultural Specialist II, CHI Certified Healthcare Interpreter
Children's Hospital Los Angeles

Ana C. Chávez has worked at Children's Hospital Los Angeles since 2004. She earned her bachelor of science degree in biology from the University of California, Los Angeles with the goal of working in the healthcare industry. Currently, she serves as a language and cultural specialist II and is a CHI certified healthcare interpreter. She has 15 years of rewarding healthcare experience ranging from direct to indirect patient care, where the last 10 years has been in the capacity of a hospital interpreter. To work side by side with healthcare professionals including health educators and in different education modalities over the course of the years has sparked an overall interest in health education and the key importance of patient and family education in a hospital setting.

Victor M. Collazo, NIC-Master, AZ Legal-A

ASL Operations Manager
CyraCom Language Solutions

Victor Collazo is a nationally certified, professional American Sign Language (ASL) interpreter. He holds a master-level national interpreter certification, and has more than 10 years' experience interpreting for the Deaf and Hard of Hearing. Collazo has held the position of ASL operations manager for CyraCom, a national interpreter company specializing in over-the-phone and video remote interpretation, for the past 3 years. His primary responsibilities include overall management of the ASL interpreters and overseeing CyraCom's ASL-interpretation line of business. Collazo holds a bachelor's degree from Rutgers University in science and earned a degree from Camden County College in ASL interpretation. He is fluent in three languages—English, Spanish, and ASL—and is currently studying German. He hosts annual community forums for the Deaf and Hard of Hearing community, where he discusses relevant issues pertaining to video remote interpretation.

Christina L. Cordero, PhD, MPH

Associate Project Director
The Joint Commission

Christina Cordero is an associate project director in the Department of Standards and Survey Methods, Division of Healthcare Quality Evaluation at The Joint Commission. Cordero is currently focused on standards development projects for the hospital and laboratory accreditation programs. She developed the patient-centered communication standards and The Joint Commission monograph *Advancing Effective Communication, Cultural Competence, and Patient- and Family-Centered Care: A Roadmap for Hospitals*. Cordero has also provided research and technical support to The Joint Commission's *Hospitals, Language, and Culture: A Snapshot of the Nation* study. Prior to joining The Joint Commission, she conducted basic science and public health research at Northwestern University's Feinberg School of Medicine. Cordero earned both her doctor of philosophy in immunology and microbial pathogenesis and her master of public health degrees from Northwestern University.

Immacolata Dall'Oglio, RN, MSN

Manager–Professional Development, Continuing Education, and Nursing Research
Bambino Gesù Children's Hospital IRCCS, Italy
Professor on Pediatric Nursing Sciences at Master in Nursing Sciences of the University of Rome, Tor Vergata

Immacolata Dall'Oglio, MSN, is a manager at the Professional Development, Continuing Education, and Nursing Research Unit at Bambino Gesù Children's Hospital IRCCS.

She is an expert on the support of breastfeeding in high-risk infants (IBCLC) and promoted a specific program to improve breastfeeding in such settings. She is the author of a national booklet for parents about breastfeeding of the child in the hospital. She is an expert regarding family-centered care and developed this issue at an Italian level. Moreover, she has developed a research line regarding the issue of child- and family-centered care, considering the parental role in the risk prevention, too. She is a PhD student and the subject of her research is the evaluation of family-centered care in the NICU by the parent's satisfaction and experience.

David J. Davis, RN, MN

Vice President and Chief Quality Officer
Children's Hospital Los Angeles

David Davis is vice president and chief quality officer at Children's Hospital Los Angeles. He has 26 years of experience as a pediatric nurse and more than 18 years of administrative experience serving inpatient, ambulatory, home care, and hospice patients across the continuum. Davis has been at CHLA for a total of 22 years and served in a variety of roles including director of Ambulatory Clinical and Support Services, director of Clinical Informatics and, most recently, director of Patient Care Services for medical and surgical services. In these roles, Davis led implementation of the children's care continuum care delivery model, operational reorganizations, initial phases of KIDS clinical system design and implementation, and the launch of the patient care services collaborative governance model and structure. He is a member of the Executive Leadership Team and serves on multiple committees.

Crystal Xiang Ding, RN, MSN

Senior Nurse in Pediatrics
Hunan Children's Hospital China

Crystal Xiang Ding has worked at Hunan Children's Hospital since 2003 serving in different wards including Orthopedics, Rehabilitation Center, Emergency Department, and International Exchange and Cooperation Department. During her 12-year nursing journey, she has been trained in Alexandra Hospital in Singapore for 2 years and Children's Hospital Los Angeles in the United States for 2 months. She is a senior pediatric nurse who has extensive experience in Critical and Emergency Nursing, Family Center Care, and Parents' Education. She wrote three nursing articles that focus on family center care and international cooperation in medicine and nursing with developing countries. She also participated in writing two nursing books, *Clinical Pathway* and *Pediatric Nursing Routine.*

Karen N. Drenkard, PhD, RN, NEA-BC, FAAN

SVP/Chief Clinical Officer/Chief Nurse
The O'Neil Center at GetWellNetwork, Inc.

Karen Drenkard is the SVP/chief clinical officer and chief nurse of the O'Neil Center at GetWellNetwork, Inc. in Bethesda, Maryland. She is responsible for the clinical direction and brings the voice of nursing to patient engagement and the innovation of technology for nursing practice. Drenkard is the immediate past executive director at the American Nurses Credentialing Center and the Magnet Recognition Program®. Prior to that, Drenkard served for 10 years as the SVP of nursing/chief nurse executive of Inova Health System. She is currently the chair of the Advocacy Committee of the Friends of the National Institute for Nursing Research (FNINR) and is an editorial advisor to *Journal of Nursing Administration (JONA)* and *Nursing Administration Quarterly (NAQ).* She is a member of the Board of Visitors for the University of Pittsburgh School of Nursing, GWU School of Nursing Advisory Council, and is a board member for Inova Loudoun Hospital in Leesburg, Virginia. She is a fellow in the American Academy of Nursing and the National Academies of Practice. Drenkard received her doctorate in nursing administration from George Mason University. She is a Wharton Nurse Executive Fellow and a Robert Wood Johnson Executive Nurse Fellow.

Scott Ferguson, MSW, LCSW, ACM

Administrator, Family-Centered Care Support Services
Children's Hospital Los Angeles

Scott Ferguson oversees the departments of Clinical Social Work, Child Life, and Expressive Arts and Therapies at Children's Hospital Los Angeles. He has also served as a lecturer on the topic of medical social work practice at the Luskin School of Public Affairs at the University of California, Los Angeles. Ferguson is an active member of the Society for Social Work Leadership in Healthcare, serving as a board member and president.

Cathrine Fowler, RN, RM, BEd (Adult), MEd (Adult), PhD

Professor Tresillian Chair in Child and Family Health
Faculty of Health, University of Technology, Sydney

Cathrine Fowler holds the Tresillian Chair in Child and Family Health and is a member of the Centre for Midwifery, Child and Family Health at the University of Technology, Sydney. Fowler is a child and family health nurse who has extensive experience in the provision of professional, parent, and community education. Her research and clinical experience has involved working with families with complex and multiple vulnerabilities and parental learning.

Linda Frommer, MPH

Veteran & Family Centered Care Coordinator and VHA Clinical Champion, VA Palo Alto
Healthcare System, VHA Office of Patient Centered Care & Cultural Transformation

Linda Frommer, the veteran and family centered care coordinator for the VA Palo Alto Healthcare System, has been advancing patient- and family-centered care practices since 2009. She oversees the Veteran & Family Advisory Program and works to create systems change to positively impact veteran and family experience and clinical care for the more than 85,000 veterans served in the Bay Area. Additionally, she conducts workshops for staff working in VA hospitals throughout the United States on establishing and sustaining effective patient and family advisory councils. Frommer received her MPH from UC Berkeley in 1986. Prior to working at the VA, she managed the health education program at Kaiser Permanente in the New York area.

Troy Garland, RN, BA, MBA

Senior Director Outcomes and Clinical Innovation
GetWellNetwork, Inc.

Troy Garland is a registered nurse who has dedicated his professional life to improving the care delivery process within the profession. Focused on transformational leadership, Garland challenges the status quo and promotes innovative solutions in the industry to advance care delivery. He currently serves as senior director of clinical transformation and outcomes at GetWellNetwork. In this role, he consults with hospital administrators and staff to develop interactive patient care (IPC) strategies that leverage technology to engage patients for improved outcomes. In the relatively young field of patient engagement through IPC, Garland is one of the top leaders in clinical process alignment and organizational change management. He has been a registered nurse for 20 years and has a broad range of clinical and leadership experience in the healthcare industry. Prior to joining GetWellNetwork, Garland served Dignity Health at Chandler Regional Medical Center as the executive director of nursing. He holds a bachelor's degree in nursing from Gustavus Adolfus College and an MBA in health-care management from the University of Phoenix.

Orsola Gawronski, RN, MSN

Special Projects–Professional Development, Continuing Education, and Nursing Research
Bambino Gesù Children's Hospital IRCCS, Italy

Professor on Pediatric Nursing Sciences at Master in Nursing Sciences of the University of Rome,
Tor Vergata

Orsola Gawronski is a nurse currently working for the Professional Development, Continuing Education, and Nursing Research Unit at Bambino Gesù Children's Hospital (BGCH) IRCCS. She is a PhD student at the University of Rome Tor Vergata, researching the Bedside Pediatric Early Warning System (BedsidePEWS) and escalation of care in the ward setting. She received her nursing degree in 1996 and her master's in nursing science in 2007. She's been teaching research methods at the Catholic University of Rome at the master's of nursing science degree for the last 3 years. She has worked extensively for BedsidePEWS implementation as a nurse educator, as BGCH was randomized to intervention for the "Evaluating processes of care & the outcomes of children in hospital (EPOCH): A cluster randomized trial of the Bedside Pediatric Early Warning System." In the past she has worked in pediatric and neonatal critical care and emergency services. She is also a BA graduate from the University of Steubenville, Ohio.

Jacqueline E. Gilberto, MPH

Health Education Services Coordinator
Children's Hospital Los Angeles, Children's Center for Cancer and Blood Diseases

Jacqueline Gilberto obtained a bachelor of science degree from Cal State Polytechnic University, Pomona, in nutrition, and a master's of public health in biostatistics/epidemiology from the University of Southern California. Gilberto has served in several public health settings, including federal and community programs. As a health educator at Children's Hospital Los Angeles, Gilberto works collaboratively with inpatient and outpatient staff, as well as with representatives from community agencies to provide health education and related activities to patients and families coping with childhood cancer and blood diseases. Gilberto is an active member of the hospital's Patient Family Education Committee and has contributed to various research projects focused on family-centered care, health literacy, and quality of life.

Shannon K. Goff, MPH, RD, CNSC, CSP

Lead Dietitian
Children's Hospital Los Angeles

Shannon Goff has been a practicing registered dietitian since 2001 and CHLA dietitian since 2004. She collaborates on nutrition interventions with her interprofessional team in the Pediatric Intensive Care Unit on a daily basis. In addition to having a bachelor's degree from California Polytechnic University, San Luis Obispo, and a master's degree in public health from the University of California, Los Angeles, Goff is a certified nutrition support clinician and a certified specialist in pediatrics. She has been a strong advocate for nutrition within the collaborative governance structure at CHLA and an active leader within her professional organizations. She balances her work-life by playing with her two young sons, running with her dog, and relaxing with her husband, even if it is for just a few moments.

Susan K. Gorry, MA, CCLS

Child Life Specialist Lead
Children's Hospital Los Angeles

Susan Gorry is a child life specialist lead at Children's Hospital Los Angeles working in the Pediatric Intensive Care Unit to support developmentally appropriate education and experience for patients and family members. She supervises a group of nine child life specialists who work on subspecialty inpatient units and intensive care units. As a member of the Child Life Department at CHLA since 2004, she has focused on providing child life services to adolescents and young adults including in the Teen Lounge. Previously, Gorry was the adolescent/young adult life specialist at University of Texas M.D. Anderson Cancer Center in Houston, Texas. Prior to becoming a child life specialist, she was an elementary school teacher. She has an MA in child development/child life from Mills College, and a BS in elementary education from Boston University. Gorry has been a certified child life specialist for over 14 years.

Yvonne R. Gutierrez, MD, FAAP

Medical Director, AltaMed General Pediatrics Clinic
Attending Physician, Division of General Pediatrics
Assistant Clinical Professor of Pediatrics, Keck School of Medicine at USC

Gutierrez joined the faculty at Keck School of Medicine in 1996. Originally from Texas, Gutierrez obtained her BA at Stanford University and then her MD at the University of California, San Francisco. She completed her internship, residency, and ambulatory fellowship in pediatrics at Children's Hospital Los Angeles. She received board certification in pediatrics in 1995. She is medical director of the AltaMed General Pediatrics Clinic and co-chair of Patient and Family Education at Children's Hospital Los Angeles. She has been a physician champion for the GetWellNetwork since July of 2011.

Elsie Jalian, PharmD

Clinical Pediatric Pharmacist
Children's Hospital Los Angeles

Elsie Jalian received her bachelor of science in psychobiology from the University of California, Los Angeles. She then pursued her doctorate of pharmacy from the University of California, San Francisco. After completing her internship at Children's Hospital Los Angeles, she was hired on as a pharmacist. She has since been working as a lead pharmacist for the medical and surgical floors. Jalian has participated in numerous hospital-wide initiatives and committees involving patient education and safety. She was also elected co-chair of the hospital's collaborative governance overseeing body. In that position, she helped to mold and promote the use of collaborative governance within the hospital.

Outside of her clinical work, Jalian is involved in many teaching endeavors. She is the main preceptor and rotation coordinator for University of Southern California (USC) pharmacy students who come to Children's Hospital Los Angeles for a pediatric rotation. She also lectures in pediatric pharmacotherapy at the USC schools of pharmacy and physician assistant.

Tere Jones, RN, CPN

Nurse Care Manager, Complex Care Service
Children's Hospital Los Angeles

Tere Jones began her nursing career at Children's Hospital Los Angeles in 1983 as staff and relief charge nurse on a post-surgical care unit. This is where her passion for patient and family education started. In addition to working with CHLA over the past 31 years, she worked in the home health arena teaching new mothers how to care for new infants, working with a population of mainly teenage mothers. In 2001, Jones worked for B. Braun Medical Inc. as a nurse educator for the Western U.S. She was responsible for educating nursing staff on newly acquired state-of-the-art equipment and conducting equipment trials prior to pur-chase. In 2006, she returned to full time work at CHLA and joined the Patient and Family Education Committee, also chairing a subcommittee of the larger group. It was here that she put her writing and editing skills to use, helping to develop and implement education materi-als and class content for the PFE and later the Family Resource Center at CHLA. She has also been involved in training the trainers for the GT education class. During her years at CHLA, she has played a key role in several house-wide education projects and continues to educate staff, patients, and families in her current role as nurse care manager with the Complex Care Service.

Michelle Kelly, RN, MN, BSc, PhD

Senior Lecturer; Director–Simulation and Technologies
Faculty of Health, University of Technology, Sydney

Kelly is leading the integration of simulation and technologies across Faculty of Health curricula and collaborating with science, pharmacy, and medical disciplines to introduce simulation into other programs. Involvement with emerging and professional simulation groups, including project work, extends beyond Australia to North America, Europe, the Middle East Gulf countries and emirates, and Asia Pacific regions. Research areas include simulation and clinical judgement as preparation for practice; incorporating information and communication technologies (ICT) within curricula; exploring the pedagogy of healthcare simulation; and evaluating best practice guidelines for OSCEs. Current projects include in-novative learning activities within mental health and midwifery practice and simulation role plays to rehearse conversations around organ and tissue donation. Kelly contributes in an advisory capacity to a number of national and international healthcare simulation projects and groups, and is the immediate past chair for the Australian Society for Simulation in Healthcare (ASSH).

Mae-Fay Koenig, MPH

Administrative Director, Center for Global Health
Children's Hospital Los Angeles

Mae-Fay Koenig has been administrative director for the Center of Global Health since 2012. Previously she was the director of strategic business innovation since 2010. She is responsible for international business development and strategic planning activities, as well as overseeing the operations for International Patient Services for CHLA. Koenig started at Children's Hospital Los Angeles in 2003 as the administrative manager for the Children's Center for Cancer and Blood Diseases and in 2006 became a project manager in Strategic Planning and Business Development. Prior to CHLA, she worked in Strategic Planning and Business Development at Health Net of California and also in Community Medical Services (external contracting) at Kaiser Permanente. Koenig obtained her master's in public health from the University of California, Los Angeles and her bachelor of science in biology and sociology from the University of California, Riverside.

Regina Little, BA, IS

Language Access Analyst
CyraCom, Inc.

Regina Little is an analyst for the Language Access department at CyraCom, an international interpreter company that specializes in phone and video interpretation. For the past 3 years, she has been a member of CyraCom's Language Access department, which consistently produces materials on the importance of language services for patient safety in healthcare. Little interfaces with clients daily, compiling hospital best practices and data for case studies, articles, and research papers. She graduated from the University of Arizona with a bachelor's degree in international studies, East Asia focus, and a creative writing minor. She spent 2 years in Japan as an exchange student and attended Nanryo High School and Chiba University.

Kimberly A. Loffredo, OTR/L

Occupational Therapist III
Children's Hospital Los Angeles

Over the past 15 years, Kim Loffredo has practiced occupational therapy in a variety of inpatient and outpatient settings. After graduating from Quinnipiac University in Hamden, Connecticut, in 1999, she began a career focused in neuro-rehabilitation and gerontology at Rancho Los Amigos National Rehabilitation Center in Downey, California, where she began her training in assistive technology with mentoring from experts at CART, Center for Applied Rehabilitation Technology. She is currently a pediatric OT at Children's Hospital Los Angeles, where she continues to use electronic aides of daily living and augmentative technologies to serve a culturally diverse inpatient and outpatient population.

Samar Mroue, RN, BSN

Patient Family Educator; Clinical Nurse
Children's Hospital Los Angeles

Mroue has been a registered nurse at Children's Hospital Los Angeles since 2010 in a medical surgical unit. Prior to that, she began her career in 2001 as a pediatric nurse in a major hospital in Lebanon, and later worked briefly in 2008 to 2009 as a nurse in the outpatient clinics in adult Rheumatology & Nephrology. Mroue has been a member of the CHLA's Patient Family Education committee since 2012. She also is a teacher in the hospital's Family Resource Center, where she helped develop the PICC line class for families, which later became an all-inclusive CVC line care class. She has also been involved in training the trainers for the class. During her time at CHLA, Mroue has also been involved in other house-wide councils and projects.

Marifel Pagkalinawan, RN, BSN, CPHON

Patient Family Educator, Clinical Nurse
Children's Hospital Los Angeles

Marifel Pagkalinawan discovered her passion for teaching very early on in her career. She became a director for staff development at a skilled nursing facility not too long after graduation. As a staff nurse and charge nurse at Children's Hospital Los Angeles responsible for assuring that caregivers and patients acquire certain skills prior to discharge, she has amassed, over the last 23 years, a cache of techniques to impart knowledge. For over 15 years, she has been a well-regarded instructor for a chemotherapy and biotherapy provider course; a skills lab instructor for both the RN residency program and Camp CHLA, where adolescents explore careers in the healthcare field; and a preceptor for new graduates and newly hired registered nurses. She has been a member of the committee involved in teaching the staff when CHLA transitioned to the electronic medical record. As a CPR instructor, Pagkalinawan also finds fulfillment in teaching life-saving skills to caregivers at the Family Resource Center and at her local church. Her enthusiasm for family-friendly education has spilled over to the development of curriculum content for central line care. Her ultimate goal is to empower learners by assisting them in finding meaning in their task and gaining confidence in their skills.

Katy Peck, MA, CCC-SLP, CBIS, CLE, BCS-S

Speech-Language Pathologist
Children's Hospital Los Angeles

Katy Peck is a pediatric speech-language pathologist (SLP) recognized as a board certified specialist in swallowing, certified brain injury specialist, and lactation educator with 15 years of experience working with high-risk populations. She is a lead speech pathologist responsible for training staff in swallowing, instrumental assessment, and assessment/intervention for multiple high-risk patient populations. She was a guest presenter for multiple internationally broadcasted webinars. Peck presented a lecture on Pediatric Tracheostomy and Swallowing at the American-Speech-Language-Hearing Association Annual Convention in 2010, 2012, 2014, and multiple state conferences. She has presented short courses across North America (ranging from half- to full-day lectures) on tracheotomy and impacts on speech and swallow function. Peck was nominated to serve on the ASHA Program Planning Committee in 2014. She was nominated to mentor clinicians in the United States and Canada seeking BCS-S certification. She has been an adjunct professor on faculty at Chapman University since July 2014.

Nancy A. Ramirez, CHI

Language & Cultural Specialist II, CHI Certified Healthcare Interpreter
Children's Hospital Los Angeles

Nancy Ramirez has worked at Children's Hospital Los Angeles since 2002, serving in a variety of roles. She has over 10 years of experience in healthcare. The last 4 years she has dedicated to serving LEP families in the Cardiothoracic Intensive Care Unit, CV Acute Unit, and supporting outpatient areas in her role as a language and culture specialist II. Due to her passion for sharing knowledge, she has served as chair of the Education committee for Diversity Services since 2013. In this role she has been able to help support the creation of continuing education hours approved by CCHI to maintain certification.

Helen Rowan, RN, MSN, DipMgt

Manager, Family Services and Volunteers
The Royal Children's Hospital Melbourne

Helen Rowan trained in nursing midwifery and maternal and child health nursing before moving on to education as a clinical nurse educator in the area of adult education.

Rowan has worked with the Royal Children's Hospital, Melbourne for the past 35 years. Initially she worked in health promotion, in particular safety promotion and injury prevention.

Rowan completed post-graduate courses in leadership and management before leading the Royal Children's Hospital Family Services and Volunteers Department as manager for the past 10 years. She has always been passionate about family-centered care. She leads her department with a strong vision to not only support the hospital's vision to be a great children's hospital, leading the way, but also to make a positive difference in the hospital experience for patients, families, caregivers, and friends through the application of family-centered care principles.

Allison Noyes Soeller, PhD, MA

Outcomes Specialist; Researcher and Instructor
Children's Hospital Los Angeles and the Annenberg School for Communication and Journalism at the University of Southern California

Allison Soeller earned a PhD and MA in communication from the USC Annenberg School for Communication and Journalism. Before graduate school, she worked for the National Archives and Records Administration as an outreach specialist. From this experience, she developed an interest in how organizations function and communicate, which became the focus of her work in graduate school. She has gained experience working with a variety of different kinds of organizations, including the U.S. Navy, the World Bank, media companies, and healthcare organizations. In her research, Soeller is primarily interested in organizational collaboration, change processes, and strategic communication. Most recently, her work has focused on healthcare collaboration and the role that communication plays in developing collaborative capacity at the team and organizational levels in a hospital. She's currently working with a group at Children's Hospital Los Angeles on research and interventions aimed at improving patient and family education.

Ellen Swartwout, PhD, RN, NEA-BC

Vice President, Research & Analytics
O'Neil Center at GetWellNetwork

Ellen Swartwout is the vice president for Research & Analytics at the O'Neil Center/
GetWellNetwork. She is currently responsible for building the research agenda in the
field of patient engagement. Prior to this role, she led programs at the American Nurses
Credentialing Center (ANCC) as senior director of Certification and Measurement Services
and the director of the Pathway to Excellence program. Prior to ANCC, she was responsible for strategic planning, performance improvement, and program development at Inova
healthcare system. Swartwout has also served as a nurse consultant for QSEN, conducting
program evaluation analysis. She was a recipient of the 2013 AONE research seed grant
and STTI Epsilon Zeta Chapter research grant for her dissertation study and received the
Nursing Research Dissertation Award from George Mason University (GMU). She received
her doctorate and master's degree from GMU and her BSN from the College of New Jersey.
Swartwout is board certified as nurse executive, advanced and served as adjunct faculty for
biostatistics at GMU.

Emanuela Tiozzo, RN, MSN

Director–Professional Development, Continuing Education, and Nursing Research
Bambino Gesù Children's Hospital IRCCS, Italy
Professor on Pediatric Nursing Sciences at Master in Nursing Sciences of the University of Rome,
Tor Vergata

Emanuela Tiozzo has been the head of the Professional Development, Continuing Education,
and Nursing Research Unit at Bambino Gesù Children's Hospital (BGCH), Rome, Italy,
since 2007. She has worked as the nursing director of the BGCH site in Palidoro for 10
years. Before, she practiced as a registered nurse and ward sister in the pediatric setting. She
has been responsible for numerous national and international training events and research
projects realized at BGCH, some in collaboration with the National Board. She graduated
in pediatric nursing in 1984. She obtained the diploma in nursing management in 1989, the
diploma of nursing director in 1992, and her master's degree in nursing science in 2006. She
leads and promotes nursing research at BGCH. She leads the clinical audit program and is
a member of several hospital committees. She teaches pediatric nursing at the University of
Rome Tor Vergata.

Alberto Tozzi, MD

Pediatrician/Epidemiologist
Gesu Bambino Children's Hospital, Rome

Tozzi is a pediatrician and an epidemiologist with experience in vaccine trials and in surveillance of infectious diseases. He has worked as a researcher with the Italian National Health Institute for more than 15 years. In 2004, Tozzi moved to the Bambino Gesù Children's Hospital, a large clinical and research center where he joined the epidemiology unit. He has also been a consultant for WHO for activities on polio eradication and for the investigation on a cluster of severe adverse events to vaccines in India. He is also a component of the Expert Vaccine Group of the European Center for Diseases Control, Stockholm, Sweden. Tozzi is responsible for the research area of Multifactorial Diseases and Complex Phenotypes at the Bambino Gesù Children's Hospital. His group is conducting research concerning the preparation of apps for smartphones for delivering immunization indications, maintaining a clinical diary, and finding health resources in the field for families of chronic patients; the acceptability of personal health records in families with children with genetic diseases supported by smart TVs; the development of assisted support systems for patients with asthma and cardiac arrhythmias; and the remote monitoring of surgical patients at home. In 2013, Tozzi was made responsible for the Telemedicine Unit. Nearly 400 children with cardiac arrhythmias, 500 with diabetes type 1, and 50 with cystic fibrosis are included in hospital telemonitoring programs.

Karla Velasquez, CHI

Language & Cultural Specialist II, CHI Certified Healthcare Interpreter™
Children's Hospital Los Angeles

Karla Velasquez started working in Children's Hospital Los Angeles in 2003 as an admitting patient representative and joined its department of Diversity Services in 2004. She is passionate about her role as language and culture specialist II, as it allows her to help her non-English speaking community. She has been a part of the Patient Family Education committee at CHLA, and is very much involved in helping to interpret for support groups held by different specialty divisions in CHLA such as the rheumatology division, the Hemostasis and Thrombosis Center, Neurofibromatosis/Neurology, and for the nonprofit agency Lupus Los Angeles.

Gloria Verret, RN, BSN, CPN

Patient Family Educator, Clinical Nurse
Children's Hospital Los Angeles

Gloria Verret has been a pediatric nurse for 19 years. At Children's Hospital Los Angeles for the past decade, she is a charge and clinical nurse on a solid organ transplant/surgical/ EMU unit and serves on the unit leadership council. She is a DAISY Nurse, a blogger for RN Remedies, a member of CHLA Champion Committee for Magnet® Re-designation, and a CPN Champion. She has placed several years in the hospital Nurse Week Essay contests, with one essay published. She has presented nationally on projects such as the unit-based Journal Club she initiated, and in 2014, her research study, an innovative mentorship program for new graduate nurses. She has taught in the CPN Review Course for 9 years, helping to re-write the curriculum in 2014. She teaches in the Family Resource Center, co-wrote the PICC/ CVC curriculum, and has been invited to speak at Nurse Week Education Day on how to teach families. She has a degree in history as well as a BSN.

Jennifer R. Ward, RN, BSN

Registered Nurse, Clinician 2
Student with the University of Cincinnati-MSN-AGNP program

Jennifer Ward has a bachelor of science degree in nutrition science from Indiana University in Bloomington, Indiana, and she has a bachelor of science degree in nursing from the University of Virginia in Charlottesville, Virginia. Ward has worked in long-term care, on- cology, and in the medical-surgical sector. Her focuses of practice have dealt extensively with nursing informatics, shared governance, pain management, and wound care. She plans to further obtain her certification as a wound and ostomy care nurse. Moreover, she holds a sincere appreciation for nursing policy development and nursing within the political sector. And, she has devoted vast attention to mentoring new graduates, and to leading teams within the acute care arena. She appreciates the theoretical contributions of Patricia E. Benner, RN, PhD, FAAN, FRCN. As she progresses in her education, Ward plans to further research ini- tiatives and make contributions to nursing in both the long-term and the acute care arenas.

David W. Wright, MPH

Senior Vice President/Chief Strategy Officer
GetWellNetwork, Inc.

David Wright serves as GetWellNetwork's chief strategy officer. In this role, he advises health system leaders on the development of strategy for patient engagement across the care continuum. For more than a decade, he has worked closely with clients to integrate IPC as a care delivery model and to plan, measure, and validate its impact on quality, safety, service, and financial performance. Wright has been recognized as an outstanding preceptor and adjunct faculty member, and he has received numerous healthcare awards in marketing, strategy, and physician integration. Most recently, he served on the board of directors of the American Nurses Credentialing Center (ANCC) and the Institute for Interactive Patient Care, which he founded to conduct and validate third party research on the impact of IPC. Wright has a BS degree from Virginia Polytechnic Institute and State University and a master's degree in public health from the University of California, Los Angeles.

Julie Lihui Zhu, RN, MSN

Vice-president; Professor of Nursing
Hunan Children's Hospital China and Hunan University of Chinese Medicine China

Lihui Zhu was designated as the candidates of "225" High-level Talents Project, and Experts of "121" Talents Project in Hunan Province. Currently, she is the chairman of the Health Education Committee of Nursing Association in Hunan Province, associate chairman of the Nursing Management Committee, member of the Editorial Board of *International Nursing Journal,* and so on. She published professional nursing articles and reviews for more than 50 journals. There are five professional books under her general editorship, and she participated in another five books. She has more than nine nursing research projects, and one of them won the Provincial Medicine Science and Technology Award.

Table of Contents

Part I: Building Foundations for Promoting Self-Care Management 1

1 Patient-Family Education: A Health System Approach 3
Lori C. Marshall, PhD, MSN, RN; and Allison Noyes Soeller, PhD, MA

2 Nurses as Educators Within Health Systems 25
Lori C. Marshall, PhD, MSN, RN; Immacolata Dall'Oglio, RN, MSN;
David Davis, RN, MN; Gloria Verret, RN, BSN, CPN; and Tere Jones, RN, CPN

3 The Nurse's Role in the Era of Accountable Care: A Catalyst for Change 57
Linda Alexander, BSN, MBA, RN, CCM; Lori C. Marshall, PhD, MSN, RN;
Tere Jones, RN, CPN; Scott Ferguson, MSW, LCSW, ACM; and Linda Frommer, MPH

4 Interprofessional Education Strategies 81

Shannon Goff, MPH, RD, CNSC, CSP; Katy Peck, MA, CCC-SLP, CBIS, CLE, BCS-S;
and Susan Gorry, MA, CCLS

5 Advancing Patient and Family Education Through
Interprofessional Shared Governance 105

Lori C. Marshall, PhD, MSN, RN; Marifel Pagkalinawan, RN, BSN, CPHON;
Elsie Jalian, PharmD; Yvonne R. Gutierrez, MD, FAAP; and Jennifer Ward, RN, BSN

Part II: Maximizing Knowledge-Transfer:
Tools and Technology........................ 123

6 Use of Simulation for Patient and Caregiver Education 125

Michelle Kelly, RN, MN, BSc, PhD; Lori C. Marshall, PhD, MSN, RN; and
Cathrine Fowler, RN, RM, BEd, MEd, PhD

Foreword

When Lori Marshall asked me to write the foreword for this book, I was quickly reminded that sometimes we choose our path in life, and other times it chooses us.

In 1999, I had recently gotten engaged and was about to graduate from Georgetown University with business and law degrees. I was, as they say, going places. Two days before my 28th birthday, I was diagnosed with non-Hodgkin's lymphoma. Overnight, the place I was going was decided by three words you never want to believe your doctor will reveal… *you have cancer.*

I was fortunate to go to a hospital with some of the best doctors and nurses in the world. I spent 10 days as an inpatient after surgery to remove a tumor from my stomach, and then I went through four cycles of CHOP chemotherapy. I am incredibly grateful to have had such an exceptional medical outcome, but my healthcare experience was really challenging.

It felt like I was on the outside looking in on my own care. They gave me a few old cancer pamphlets to read. The 12 channels on the TV in my room worked some of the time. Smartphones and tablets weren't around back then, and I wasn't allowed to bring my laptop. Wearing a floral hospital gown 24/7 was at the bottom of my list of concerns, so clearly I was not in a great frame of mind. The main thing about chemotherapy—apart from being confusing, terrifying, and painful—is that it can be quite boring. I sat for 6 hours at a time while a mysterious cocktail of medications that I still cannot pronounce today slowly filtered into my bloodstream.

Luckily, I had a nurse named Jane Diaz during my treatment. Of course, she cared for me as all nurses do—took my blood, gave me my medications, wheeled me around, and helped me to the bathroom. The difference with Jane, though, was that she also cared *about* me. She asked me lots of questions and answered mine. She asked me about my goals and what I wanted to do after graduating. She got to know how close I was to my family, how over-the-top in love I was with my fiancée, and the guilt I felt for getting sick during what was supposed to be the happiest time in her life. She shared things about herself and about her husband, who was fighting brain cancer at the same time I was battling. We cried together as she described his treatments and how afraid he was about dying. She made the effort to connect, and that made all the difference.

With her knowledge, Jane helped prepare me and my family to live through, and after, my treatment. With her compassion and interest, she helped restore my confidence to take control of my future. I finished chemotherapy ready to live my life fully and attack my goals with even more resolve and enthusiasm than I had before cancer. Only I channeled it in a different direction, as my cancer journey shaped my life. Jane helped me realize *what I wanted my health for* … and I was on a mission.

My care experience—the good and the bad—led me to realize something that, on the face of it, is kind of intuitive: An engaged patient is a better patient with better outcomes. When people have something important they are reaching for, and when you give them the information and resources to participate actively in their care, they will attack it with attention to detail and commitment. And that, together with their family, friends, and care team, lays a foundation for them to succeed.

Today, I am blessed to take part in the transformation of healthcare to a person-centered model. And, I am honored to call Dr. Marshall a colleague and friend in this important work. In this book, you'll read about a number of strategies from healthcare experts who are much smarter and more experienced than I am. Even though these experts all have different backgrounds, you'll probably notice a trend among them. They don't just care for people; they care about them.

Ultimately, the most important people in the care process are the patient and the family. To put them in a position to succeed, we have to help educate and activate them in a way that works best for them. But first, we have to take the opportunity to try and know them. And to know them we just have to ask.

To the healthcare facilities and caregivers who do all of these things every day, I simply say thank you on behalf of all patients and families. Dr. Marshall assembled a group of incredible global healthcare leaders to provide chapters for her book. I am honored to help get you started on what will be a great read.

–Michael O'Neil, Founder & CEO, GetWellNetwork, Inc.
Twitter: @GetWellCEO

Introduction

This book draws from practicing experts who represent many healthcare disciplines. Interprofessional collaboration is paramount to improving people's health and wellbeing. Our hope is that you as the reader will take initiative to improve the way you engage patients and families in the learning exchange. We also hope that you will encourage others to do the same, leading to a more seamless exchange of patient and family education across and between health systems. This book is about creating a new paradigm that moves patient education to the central part of a health system. The paradigm shift requires nurses to think beyond their current teaching encounters and needs toward the future, to consider the next setting and life-continuum needs. Such a paradigm shift requires a new approach.

Nurses must gain a health systems view that goes beyond their moment in time to develop patients and families as self-regulated learners. The nurse must also see value in the planned care handoffs—whether it is to bedside nurses, clinical staff, or a new care setting—with part of the handoff to include the patient, family, and caregiver.

Second, an organization must allocate the right tools and resources for patient and family education programs so they are embedded into the health system. Classes are needed that support population health management, including decision-making and appropriate access and utilization of services and care, as part of a coordinated effort between the patient and families and the health system. (Nielsen-Bohlman, Panzer, & Kindig, 2004; Maher & Lutz, 1997; Scheck McAlearney, 2003).

It is recognized that care needs are different across the life span. Adherence to treatment plans happens with engaged patients and families and is a critical component of building the platform for successful self-care management. Self-care management is best achieved through a multicultural and linguistic lens, drawing from metacognition/information processing concepts and social learning theory. Patients who understand their predispositions, genetic road map, current conditions, and treatment options and plans are more likely to take an active role in decisions regarding their care (Drenkard & Wright, 2014).

Third, a health system's population health management strategy should align with self-care management education processes and outcomes. Patient and family education is focused on helping learners apply sets of complex knowledge and skills to participate in care, make decisions, navigate the health system, and communicate and interact with providers and healthcare staff (Nielsen-Bohlman, Panzer, & Kindig, 2004).

Thus the book is divided into three parts:

> **PART I:** Building Foundations for Promoting Self-Care Management

> **PART II:** Maximizing Knowledge-Transfer: Tools and Technology

> **PART III:** Establishing a Health System Approach for Patient and Family Education

Each chapter builds on the previous one and serves to advance your knowledge, which then enables you to apply the content to organizational and role-relevant changes.

On behalf of all the book contributors, please join us in leading one of the most important components that significantly impacts health and wellbeing at the individual and community levels: patient and family education. Ultimately, the book is meant to be a practical resource providing a general model and framework that can be applied around the world.

References

Drenkard, K., & Wright, D. (2014). Patient engagement and activation. In J. Barnsteiner, J. Disch, & M. K. Walton (Eds.), *Person and family centered care* (pp. 95–111). Indianapolis, IN: Sigma Theta Tau International.

Maher, K., & Lutz, J. (1997). Identifying opportunities to improve the management of care: A population-based diagnostic methodology. *Journal of Ambulatory Care Management, 20*(2), 18–36.

Nielsen-Bohlman, L., Panzer, A. M., & Kindig, D. A. (Eds.). (2004). *Health literacy: A prescription to end confusion.*

Scheck McAlearney, A. (2003). *Population health management: Strategies to improve outcomes.* Chicago, IL: Health Administration Press.

Building Foundations for Promoting Self-Care Management

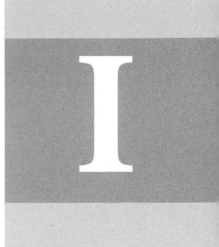

I

"People know themselves much better than you do. That's why it's important to stop expecting them to be something other than who they are."
–Maya Angelou, 2011

Patient-Family Education: A Health System Approach

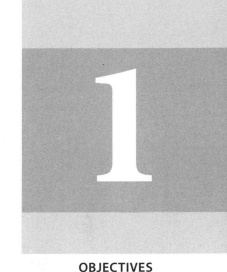

Lori C. Marshall, PhD, MSN, RN
Allison Noyes Soeller, PhD, MA

Introduction

This chapter explains the need for an evidence-based patient and family education model rooted in a health systems perspective. It reviews the key findings from the literature and best practices and introduces the Marshall Personalized Patient-Family Education Model (PPFEM). Additionally, the chapter builds a case for the important role of a well-designed, nurse-led patient-education system to address population health, complex care, and self-care management needs.

Why Patient-Family Education Is Becoming Increasingly Important

You don't have to look too far to find practical and concrete evidence showing how important patient-family education is becoming in a patient's care, especially as it relates to readmission rates or emergency department visits:

- Effective patient and family education can reduce readmissions, shorten lengths of stay, and reduce or optimize service use (Boutwell, Griffin, Hwu, & Shannon,

OBJECTIVES

- Discuss the key components of the Marshall Personalized Patient-Family Education Model (PPFEM).
- Discuss the importance of using a nurse-led patient and family education (PFE) model across the care continuum.
- Apply the PPFEM to your practice setting as a way to approach patient and family education.

2009; Hernandez et al., 2010; Jones et al., 2011; Nielsen-Bohlman, Panzer, & Kindig, 2004).

- Patients are 30% less likely to return to the emergency department or be re-admitted when they understand their after-hospital care instructions, how to take their medication, and when to make follow-up appointments (Agency for Healthcare Research and Quality [AHRQ], 2009).

- Patient and family education affects children and adults by reducing readmissions and enabling the management of complex care needs. Readmission rates were highest for children aged 13 to 18, with 6.5% of all children hospitalized being readmitted in 30 days and 61.6% of the readmissions occurring within 14 days after discharge (Berry et al., 2013).

- Readmission rates increase according to the number of chronic conditions present, with 82% of adults 65 and older having at least one chronic disease that requires ongoing care and management. Hypertension, arthritis, heart disease, cancer, and diabetes are the top five most common conditions requiring regular care (Committee on the Future Health Care Workforce for Older Americans, Board on Health Care Services, & Institute of Medicine, 2008).

- Readmissions also increase for patients with public insurance, such as Medicaid and Medicare, as compared to the uninsured or other payer types (AHRQ, 2010; Berry et al., 2013). For children, 10 admission diagnoses account for 27.7% of all readmissions, with anemia or neutropenia, ventricular shunt procedures, sickle cell anemia crisis, cystic fibrosis, and asthma being the top five conditions (AHRQ, 2013). Healthcare expenditures increase with three or more conditions and are even higher when five or more conditions are present (AHRQ, 2013).

Changing Demographics Call for New Approaches

One key factor affecting the development of an effective patient and family education program is the changing demographic profile of patients and families. By 2030, close to one in five Americans (19%) will be 65 or older (Committee on the Future Health Care Workforce for Older Americans et al., 2008). People 65 and older make nearly twice as many physician office visits per year as adults 45 to 65 (Krupa, 2012). The average annual healthcare costs among Medicare enrollees age 65 and over are higher among non-Hispanic African Americans. By 2030, 30% of the country will be comprised of minorities, and by 2050, minorities will encompass 54% of the population. Minorities will become 50% of the youth population by 2023 (Shrestha & Heisler, 2011). Children and youth have unique needs as compared to the elderly, and young adults require a different focus as compared to adults in general. Patient and family education is a moving target; like life, each day becomes a new page in the learning chapter. Therefore, it is crucial to have a flexible methodology to support PFE that takes into account culture, language, age, and other personal patient and family factors and encourages the development of self-regulated learners who can communicate and navigate the networks and complex decisions around health and wellbeing.

In addition to changing demographics, there is significant variation in how education programs are set up to support health systems (Boutwell et al., 2009). That's where the Marshall Personalized Patient-Family Education Model-Health System Approach comes in.

Understanding the Marshall Personalized Patient-Family Education Model

The Marshall Personalized Patient-Family Education Model-Health System Approach (PPFEM-HSA) was developed to address the several issues found in patient and family education efforts, including the need to have a standardized approach across health systems that serves as a shared mental model and a connected proactive framework best led by the nursing roles (see Figure 1.1).

Why use a shared mental model for PFE? It's important for nurses to develop a shared mental model between patients/families and care teams, as this mental model is critical to the success of patient and family education across and between health systems.

Creating a shared mental model involves networking, organizing, and arranging information into a mental image or representing the concepts and actions coupled with a preliminary plan or schematic to process information regarding team goals and objectives (Langan-Fox, Code, & Langfield-Smith, 2000; Paris, Salas, & Cannon-Bowers, 2000). As such, shared mental models help nurses and other healthcare providers coordinate their patient education roles and responsibilities, manage relationships and interactions, and coordinate decision-making (Paris et al., 2000) to match the healthcare team's objectives with the patient and family central to that team.

"When patients, families, nurses, other healthcare providers, and ancillary care staff have a similar way of perceiving, encoding, retrieving, and storing information, it enables teamwork (Langan-Fox et al., 2000) and successful collaborative care."

Why is the PPFEM-HSA an effective framework to help nurses address the problems? The PPFEM-HSA helps nurses and other healthcare professionals visualize the connections between the PFE concepts and required actions and outcomes. The model is an interprofessional framework that leverages the nurses, who comprise the largest group in the healthcare workforce (U.S. Bureau of Labor Statistics [USBLS], 2014). Because of this, nurses are in a central position to ensure that patient education is truly personalized and successfully supported across the life and healthcare continuum. Additionally, they have a vital role in patient safety and quality of care (AHRQ, 2015) and are central to building a system in which clinical effectiveness, including research, is a more natural byproduct of the care process (Olsen & McGinnis, 2010).

The PPFEM-HSA explicitly aligns and connects the nurse's role in educating the patient with these core nursing functions:

- Negotiating and planning care means that medical errors and "failure of a planned action to be completed as intended or the use of a wrong plan to achieve an aim" (Kohn, Corrigan, & Donaldson, 1999) are both greatly reduced.
- Nurses serve a fundamental role in assessing and monitoring the patient's progress toward the outcomes of care. This is particularly important when patients and families are negotiating and navigating the healthcare journey.
- The management and maintenance of a person's health is more likely to be achieved by nurses, who can coordinate care and facilitate the integration of services from multiple providers (American Nurses Association [ANA], 2012).

Care coordination, self-management, and health literacy are essential to transform healthcare quality, and nurses by scope of practice are at the core of this work (Adams & Corrigan, 2003).

The Marshall Personalized Patient-Family Education Model: A Health System Approach

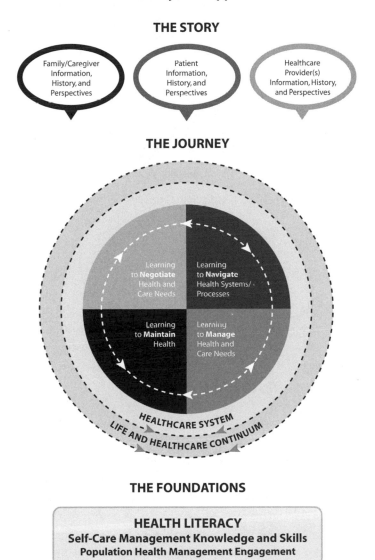

THE STORY

Family/Caregiver Information, History, and Perspectives

Patient Information, History, and Perspectives

Healthcare Provider(s) Information, History, and Perspectives

THE JOURNEY

Learning to **Negotiate** Health and Care Needs

Learning to **Navigate** Health Systems/Processes

Learning to **Maintain** Health

Learning to **Manage** Health and Care Needs

HEALTHCARE SYSTEM

LIFE AND HEALTHCARE CONTINUUM

THE FOUNDATIONS

HEALTH LITERACY
Self-Care Management Knowledge and Skills
Population Health Management Engagement

Figure 1.1   The Marshall Personalized Patient-Family Education Model-Health System Approach (PPFEM-HSA). Copyright © 2015 Lori C. Marshall.

The PPFEM-HSA makes some assumptions about healthcare:

- Healthcare is a journey, not a linear process. Patients and families progress forward through each core learning need toward health maintenance, but given time and changes in health, they can also return to a previous point in this dynamic process.

- The role of a nurse is to facilitate interprofessional collaboration for patient and family education that supports knowledge-transfer across the continuum and between health systems.

- A patient's and family's degree of self-regulated learning is based on the life and healthcare continuum.

The PPFEM-HSA has three main components, described in the following sections:

- The story
- The journey
- The foundations

Definition 1.1*: Patient-Family Education (PFE). Anything that provides patients and families with information that enables them to make informed choices about their care, health, and wellbeing and that helps them gain knowledge and skills to participate in care or healthy living processes. Healthcare workers can provide this education through a verbal, written, or multimedia approach as part of independent or instructor-led learning activities. Examples of patient and family education include but are not limited to: learning about admissions and the surgical process, new diagnoses, medication, and insurance; paying for healthcare services; understanding the roles of healthcare providers; learning how to access care and talk with providers; and mastering complex care skills such as central-line and total-parenteral nutrition. Other patient education examples are geared toward health prevention and promotion and address topics such as home safety, healthy eating, and strategies to maximize the patient's or family's coping skills.*

The Patient's Story Initiates the Education Experience

When patients and families/caregivers recount their health stories to their care provider(s), this initiates the personalized patient education experience (see Figure 1.2). Along the healthcare journey, healthcare providers contribute their own perspectives to the narrative. Personalization (the patient's story) helps determine which core learning components are needed and *when* they are needed. Personalization shapes the approach to these learning encounters and ensures that the educational approach you take is aligned with the patient's age/development, culture, and language.

THE STORY

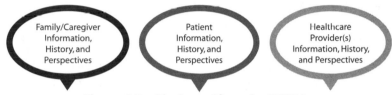

Figure 1.2   The "story" from the PPFEM.

The goals of understanding the patient's story are to:

- Personalize the healthcare experience
- Identify health risk factors
- Establish good communication
- Build the nurse-patient relationship
- Meet the expectations patients and families have regarding the healthcare experience
- Create self-awareness in patients regarding coping skills

The narrative/story approach personalizes care by recognizing that people "are as much valuing as they are reasoning animals" (Fisher, 1978, p. 376). People do not reason about health decisions and actions objectively; their thoughts are filtered through personal, familial, cultural, and professional value systems. In order for the story to make sense to patients and families as well as to healthcare providers, it has to be jointly created so that it takes into account multiple different value systems.

This story draws from:

- Patient information, history, and perspectives
- Family/caregiver information, history, and perspectives
- Healthcare provider(s) information, history, and perspectives

Information About the Patient

Information is multifaceted. It encompasses a discrete set of behaviors, actions, and capabilities in a moment in time. Patient information includes age, language, race/ethnicity, religion, spiritual beliefs, and education level. It includes use of senses such as hearing, vision, touch, and smell. It includes mobility and cognition/metacognition. Information also includes the patient's current state of health and wellbeing, which is the absence or presence of a specific illness, condition, or disease (whether genetic or through injury/trauma). Other components of patient information include disabilities, functional losses, factors contributing to disease burden (environmental—like air pollution, poor water quality, or infectious diseases), personal habits (such as smoking or overeating), and factors imposed by a caregiver (second-hand smoke or preparing/serving high-fat foods). Information also includes a degree of self-regulated learning and engagement in self-care management.

History of the Patient

A *history* is the sum of a person's interaction with life and includes people, places, and events. It pulls all the information from birth to the current date and serves as a foundation to predict, prevent, or mitigate changes in health and wellbeing that affect one's healthcare journey.

Perspectives of the Patient

Perspectives are the beliefs that people hold about what constitutes, influences, and contributes to health, wellness, illness, disease, and injury. Perspectives manifest via internal or external behaviors such as the attitudes, actions, and reactions toward people, places, and events in one's life. Perspectives include self-efficacy, locus of control, goal orientation, and degree of forward/future thinking and proactivity. It is important to consider the patient's or caregiver's mental-health status and functioning, which shape their perspectives.

Connecting the Patient's Story to Effective Communication

The patient's story influences his or her interactions and communication with healthcare providers, and these stories collectively contribute to her experiences across the health system. These interactions are tied to motivational processes via the relationship between provider and patient/families. A relationship with positive communication promotes self-regulated learning and encourages the use of the PPFEM foundations (health literacy, knowledge, and skills and engagement in health activities) to achieve healthcare goals. The healthcare provider (HCP)—such as the nurse—plays an important role in supporting this connection and fostering the relationship. The HCP either strengthens or weakens the connection through his or her own "story" and directly influences the patient's and family's:

- Healthcare journey
- Experience within the health system
- Use of their "personal foundations"

The Patient's and Family's Healthcare Journey

A patient's and family's healthcare journey is made up of a series of interactions within a health system or across systems and across the life and healthcare continuum (see Figure 1.3). A health system provides population health management prevention, promotion, and progression tools and resources with changes in health across the continuum of care and throughout the life span. The health system includes a communication network bound by information systems, technology, policies, and processes. Health systems can work in partnership or independently when it comes to meeting the goals that support health and wellbeing. Intersecting health systems form a network of essential resources that might not originate from within the same system. Health systems have their own inherent complexities and uniqueness, which make for an unpredictable experience from system to system—especially when there is an intersection between multiple systems. As healthcare professionals who also have close contact with patients, nurses play an important role in facilitating interprofessional collaboration within and between health systems. They are the main line of offense in providing consistent and quality patient and family education.

Definition 1.2: *Health system. A collection of resources, healthcare professionals, healthcare workers, paraprofessionals, community volunteers, places, processes, and organizations that help people with their health and wellbeing. There are several types of health systems, including hospital health systems, community health systems, and home health systems.*

THE JOURNEY

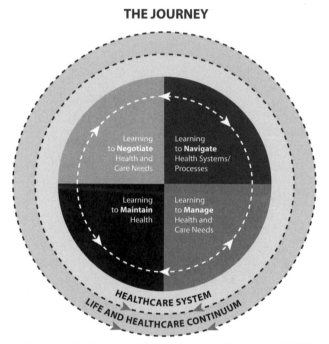

Figure 1.3 The "healthcare journey" from the PPFEM.

Central to the journey is a set of core patient and family learning needs. When these are completed in a sequence, they help the patient maintain health. The progression, however, is not linear. Core learning needs are dynamic. They change throughout life and across the healthcare continuum. Patients and families must learn to:

- Negotiate their healthcare needs
- Navigate the health systems and its many processes
- Manage their healthcare needs
- Maintain their health

Negotiating Healthcare Needs

In this model, the patient begins negotiating his or her healthcare needs by gaining an accurate self-reflection of his current state of health and wellbeing. This includes assigning value to a higher state of health and wellbeing. The patient does this through self-talk, discussion, and consultation with family, friends, and healthcare providers. The concept of self-determination plays out at this level, and a person's choices may or may not resonate with family, caregivers, or providers.

It's important that you consider the patient's story in order to understand how they make choices and what influences them, as this will help when you're attempting to mediate conflicting ideas regarding care between a patient and his or her caregivers. Two common areas that come to mind are autonomous decision-making and locus of control. For example, a patient and family coming from a collectivist culture may place less emphasis on autonomy and self-determination. Another example is that in some cultures, a condition or illness may be attributed to an extrinsic power or cause, something that is outside of the person's control (Betancourt, Green, Carrillo, & Ananeh-Firempong, 2003).

The goals at this stage are:

- Adhering to the treatment plan
- Creating a patient/family/caregiver/healthcare provider partnership
- Establishing effective interprofessional collaboration

A nurse's efforts should focus on helping the patients and caregivers reach these goals.

Navigating Health Systems and Processes

In order to navigate the health system and its many processes, patients must have or gain a general understanding of how healthcare is organized, provided, and coordinated in their area. In order to navigate the health system, patients must have a basic understanding of their health issues. You must help them find their way through the health system by helping them to understand the basic organizational procedures and the communication networks.

The goals at this stage are:

- Learning the health system
- Establishing a support plan and resources
- Learning how to obtain information
- Establishing a peer mentor and support network

A nurse's efforts at this stage should focus on helping the patients and caregivers reach these goals.

Managing Healthcare Needs

This stage focuses on helping the patient acquire self-care management knowledge and skills. It's vital that the patient or caregiver have a solid understanding of the condition or illness. You must be able to recognize any gaps in knowledge and predict how these affect care routines and treatment plans.

The goals at this stage are:

- Establishing self-care management
- Preparing for transition of care
- Promoting care coordination
- Modifying/strengthening coping strategies
- Determining long-term goals

A nurse's efforts at this stage should focus on helping the patients and caregivers reach these goals.

Maintaining Health and Wellbeing

This is the patient's terminal learning goal of a healthcare journey. Health and wellbeing are uniquely defined by each person and are based on his or her story. It is not necessarily the absence of disease or lack of issues.

The goals at this stage are:

- Maintaining functional status
- Preventing disease progression
- Promoting health and wellness

A nurse's efforts should focus on helping the patients and caregivers reach these goals.

Personal Foundations Support Knowledge-Transfer

To achieve these learning needs, a patient and family must build a foundation individually and collectively. This foundation can help all parties involved negotiate and manage the patient's healthcare needs, navigate confusing systems and processes, and maintain the patient's health. These foundations directly impact the degree of self-directed learning the patient will do. The PPFEM foundations are health literacy, self-care knowledge and skills, and engagement in population health management activities (see Figure 1.4).

> **Definition 1.3:** *Population health. "The design, delivery, coordination, and payment of high-quality health care services.... to improve the health of patient populations, improve patients' experience of healthcare, and reduce per capita costs of healthcare for a population using the best resources we have available to us within the health care system." (Institute for Healthcare Improvement [IHI] 2015a, para. 8)*

> **Definition 1.4:** *Population health management activities. Offered by a health system as a portfolio of interdependent tools and resources to support the healthcare journey. These include employee wellness programs, just-in-time/on-demand learning resources, genetic counseling, lifestyle and behavior change classes, disease-based medical care follow-up programs, health promotion/prevention programs, and coping/support resources. These offerings range from a focus on a select population to a region or community. Activities can be provided exclusively by the health system, in partnership with community/regional agencies or as part of state/national health initiatives. Academic, public health, faith-based, community, and regional partnerships are beneficial when there is a need to address social and environmental conditions, such as*

quality or water and air, toxins, pollution, and urban planning. These partnerships are also leveraged to address the social factors such as educational systems, unemployment, income level, and support that impact the health of a population. Adapted from McAlearney, 2003; IHI 2015b; Kindig & Stoddart, 2003.

THE FOUNDATIONS

HEALTH LITERACY
Self-Care Management Knowledge and Skills
Population Health Management Engagement

Figure 1.4   The PPFEM "foundations" that impact the healthcare journey.

Health literacy is the patient's ability to understand and process health-related information in order to make good decisions and apply health-related information to care-giving situations, include the delivery of care. "Health literacy skills are needed for dialogue and discussion, reading health information, interpreting charts, making decisions about participating in research studies, using medical tools for personal or familial health care" (Nielsen-Bohlman, Panzer, & Kindig, 2004, p. 31). It is viewed as the initiating and essential foundation in the PPFEM and is required to achieve health maintenance.

Self-care management knowledge and skills refers to learning about health needs, conditions, health systems of processes, support systems, coping strategies, and care-giving skills. The healthcare provider helps by coaching, mentoring, and transferring or handing off knowledge and skills effectively to patients and caregivers.

Population health management engagement refers to a patient's, family's, or caregiver's level of activation or participation in a health system's population health management activities.

Engagement and activation are essential components of healthy living and are positively related to patient outcomes. They influence the degree of self-regulation and motivation for maintaining health and wellbeing. As such, highly self-directed, active, and engaged patients:

- Have a primary care provider and regularly see them to negotiate and establish goals for health and wellbeing

- Set goals with a focus on changing habits that reduce disease burden, such as healthy eating, making lifestyle changes, and adopting healthy behaviors

- Monitor progress of goals and regulate factors as needed to continue meeting goals

- Attend self-care-management education sessions and engage in their health system's health management programs and services

- Have access to and use health information technology resources such as a patient portal for monitoring and tracking health information

- Have access to and use interactive patient-care systems and/or resource centers to further their knowledge and skills

- Use tools for planning and organizing their healthcare needs, which include being connected to a centralized resource for coordinating and planning care

- Use multiple communication methods to communicate with specialty and support providers when complex care issues exist

- Update contact information routinely and keep appointments

Developing Self-Regulated Learners

It is important to have a solid understanding about *self-regulation* in learning, which is the use of special strategies intended to facilitate a learner's acquisition of skills or knowledge established as part of a learning goal (Zimmerman, 1989). Zimmerman describes self-regulated learners "by the degree they are metacognitively, motivationally, and behaviorally active participants in their own learning process" (1989, p. 329) such as with patient activation and engagement.

The metacognitive strategies used to support population health and self-care management include helping learners with monitoring, planning, regulating (Driscoll, 1994), and integrating technology and tools (McKnight, 2012). Self-regulated learning builds on principles from social-cognitive theory, including self-efficacy or agency, effort, and goal-setting. There are varying degrees of self-regulation from person to person and situation to situation (Zimmerman, 1989). As a learner's self-efficacy increases, so does his use of self-regulation strategies such as metacognitive strategies, which helps him remain motivated about learning (Bandura, 1991; Schunk, 1994, 1996; Zimmerman, 1989). These concepts are discussed in greater detail in Chapter 2.

Efficacy beliefs are linked with a person's "motivational" processes; they influence goal choice, level of effort invested, persistence, and resiliency in the event of disappointment or failure (Bandura, 1995, 1997). People improve their efficacy by working through goals with focused, persistent effort (Bandura, 1995, 1997).

Thus the more capable, or efficacious, a person judges herself to be:

- More likely to choose challenging learning goals (Dweck, 1990; Zimmerman, 1989).
- Invest more effort to achieve a goal (Bandura, 1991; Clark, 1997; Marshall et al., 2003; Marshall et al., 2004).
- Persist longer to achieve a goal (Schunk, 1994, 1996; Zimmerman, 1989).
- More successfully and frequently use self-regulatory learning strategies (Dweck, 1990; Meece, 1994).

NOTE

In learning, *attributions* are a learner's beliefs as to the cause of a learning outcome (positive or negative) (Weiner, 1985). This is important to explore and understand in order to support knowledge-transfer. Attributions are also a component of the patient story related to cause of disease or illness which may be influenced by cultural beliefs. It is always best to ask the learners what they believe is the cause for their learning outcomes, either positive or negative, in order to personalize their approach to learning.

Improving Patient-Provider Communication

Communication is a process woven throughout the PPFEM and through which patient-family education occurs. Early transmission models of communication assumed a uni-directional flow of information from sender to receiver (Shannon & Weaver, 1949). A common metaphor used to explain these models is that of a hypodermic needle full of information that the sender injects into the receiver (Bineham, 1988). If these models were accurate, patient and family education would be quite simple, but research and theory have shifted to advocate more interactive models, which are also more complex. These models suggest that "communication involves the creation and exchange of meaning between the parties in a communication activity" (Hallahan, Holtzhausen, van Ruler,

Vercic, & Sriramesh, 2007). This perspective assumes a bi-directional flow of information through which meaning is created jointly via dialogue.

This interactive approach has implications for nurses who want to provide high-quality patient-family education. The assumption that staff and care providers can simply "inject" information into a patient or family member and that this information will mean exactly what they intended is based on an outdated model of communication. Instead, education is a process of dialogue between staff/care providers and patients/families in which shared meaning is jointly created.

Empowering Patients and Sharing in the Decision-Making

The interactive model for patient and family education represents an ideal, but in practice it can be difficult to implement. Dialogue requires all those involved in an interaction be engaged and empowered to participate. However, when the people involved in an interaction are patients/families with little to no formal expertise in healthcare and staff/providers with extensive expertise, the latter group often becomes the primary communicator and the interaction can become unidirectional. Although this may seem appropriate given the formal expertise of staff and providers, research suggests that when you empower patients and families to be more involved and engaged in the care process, you get improved self-efficacy (Anderson et al., 1995).

Patient empowerment is a key component of *shared decision-making (SDM),* defined as "a two-way exchange of information between the parties concerned with the medical decision either from the professional or from a patient's point of view" (Kasper, Légaré, Scheibler, & Geiger, 2012, p. 4). This perspective on communication and information exchange can also be applied to the education process. If information is the dynamic product of creating joint meaning, the exchange process is critical. Focusing on the exchange process requires attention not only to the process itself but also to the interpersonal relationship between patients/families and the staff/care providers (Kasper et al., 2012).

Creating Reliable Communication Networks

At the interpersonal level, patient and family education is a process of creating meaning through dialogue among individuals. At the systems level, education remains a communicative process of creating meaning, but it extends across unit, disciplinary, and even organizational boundaries. The complexity of modern healthcare often means you have to involve multiple staff and providers in the education process. These groups and individuals form a communication network. As a nurse and an educator, one of your roles is to facilitate communication among the different groups and individuals across this network. Because you typically interact with the patient and family most often, you are in an ideal position to recognize whether shared meaning is truly being created across the different groups and individuals in a network.

If there are disconnects, you must work to bridge these by facilitating communication among groups. You need to think of yourself as a *connector* within your organization and among organizations within a health system. You also need to develop the knowledge and skills that will enable you to play this role, including:

- Interpersonal and leadership skills
- A mental map of your organization
- An understanding of different patient care roles
- Knowledge of other organizations often involved in the care process for your patients (e.g., community organizations)

Conclusion and Key Points

It is essential to adopt a shared mental model such as the PPFEM as a way to organize and structure patient and family education systems and processes:

- It promotes teamwork and successful collaborative care because the patients, families, nurses, other healthcare providers, and ancillary care staff have a similar image of the PFE concepts and actions.
- It helps nurses and other healthcare providers coordinate their patient education roles and responsibilities.
- It makes the information less confusing by managing communication, relationships, and interactions, and coordinates decision-making to match the patient and family objectives with the healthcare team's goals.

As you read this book, you are asked to consider your role in advancing the developing health system approach to PFE at this crucial time. Adopt a greater willingness, if you haven't already, to hand off knowledge and skills to your patients and families. It is also important to reflect upon your role in facilitating interprofessional collaboration to ensure that critical knowledge is transferred between providers and patients and families.

When communicating with your patients and families, remember these key points, which will lead to greater success with your interactions:

- Communication during patient and family education should be a process of dialogue through which you create joint meaning between staff/providers and the patient/family.

- If communication becomes a simple process of information transfer in which staff/providers "inject" information into the patient/family, it is unlikely that shared meaning will be created, and this will result in unsuccessful communication.

- Enabling dialogue might require interventions aimed at empowering the patient/family to participate and engage in the care process.

- The process of communication as dialogue has to work at the systems level as well as the interpersonal level for patient and family education to be truly successful.

- Nurses play a critical role in facilitating communication across a patient care network because of their role in facilitating interprofessional collaboration and care coordination.

As a nursing professional, it is paramount that you ensure that patient and family education remain a core component of your nursing practice. Consider this your call to action. Consider this your opportunity to elevate the professional power of the nursing profession in shaping the health and wellbeing of your patients and their families.

References

Adams, K., & Corrigan, J. (2003). *Priority areas for national action: Transforming health care quality.* Washington, DC: Institute of Medicine of the National Academies. Retrieved from www.nap.edu/openbook.php?record_id=10593

Agency for Healthcare Research and Quality (AHRQ). (2009, February 2). *Educating patients before they leave the hospital reduces readmissions, emergency department visits and saves money* [Press Release]. Retrieved from http://archive.ahrq.gov/news/press/pr2009/redpr.htm

Agency for Healthcare Research and Quality (AHRQ). (2010). *30-Day readmission rates to U.S. hospitals* (Infographic No. 153-4). Washington, DC: Agency for Healthcare Research and Quality. Retrieved from www.hcup-us.ahrq.gov/reports/statbriefs/statbriefs.jsp

Agency for Healthcare Research and Quality (AHRQ). (2013, July). Pediatric readmission rates vary by condition and hospital type. *AHRQ Newsletter.* Retrieved from www.ahrq.gov/news/newsletters/research-activities/13jul/0713ra31.html

Agency for Healthcare Research and Quality (AHRQ). (2015). *Nursing and patient safety.* Retrieved from www.psnet.ahrq.gov/primer.aspx?primerID=22

American Nurses Association (ANA). (2012). The value of nursing care coordination. A white paper of the American Nurses Association. Retrieved from www.nursingworld.org/carecoordinationwhitepaper

Anderson, R. M., Funnell, M. M., Butler, P. M., Arnold, M. S., Fitzgerald, J. T., & Feste, C. C. (1995). Patient empowerment: Results of a randomized controlled trial. *Diabetes Care, 18*(7), 943–949. http://doi.org/10.2337/diacare.18.7.943

Angelou, M. (Interviewee) & Winfrey, O. (Interviewer). (2011). *Lesson 13: When people show you who they are, believe them* [Video]. Retrieved from Oprah's Life Class website: www.oprah.com/oprahs-lifeclass/Lesson-13-When-People-Show-You-Who-They-Are-Believe-Them?_escaped_fragment_

Bandura, A. (1991). Self-regulation of motivation through anticipatory and self-reactive mechanisms. In *Perspectives on motivation: Nebraska symposium on motivation* (Vol. 38, pp. 69–164). Lincoln, NE: University of Nebraska Press.

Bandura, A. (1995). Exercise of personal and collective efficacy in changing societies. In *Self-efficacy in changing societies* (Vol. 15, p. 334). Cambridge, UK: Cambridge University Press.

Bandura, A. (1997). *Self-efficacy: The exercise of control.* New York, NY: Freeman.

Berry, J. G., Toomey, S. L., Zaslavsky, A. M., Jha, A. K., Nakamura, M. M., Klein, D. J., … Kaplan, W. (2013). Pediatric readmission prevalence and variability across hospitals. *JAMA, 309*(4), 372–380.

Betancourt, J. R., Green, A. R., Carrillo, J. E., & Ananeh-Firempong II, O. (2003). Defining cultural competence: a practical framework for addressing racial/ethnic disparities in health and healthcare. *Public Health Reports, 118*(4), 293.

Bineham, J. L. (1988). A historical account of the hypodermic model in mass communication. *Communication Monographs, 55*(3), 230–246. http://doi.org/10.1080/03637758809376169

Boutwell, A., Griffin, F., Hwu, S., & Shannon, D. (2009). *Effective interventions to reduce rehospitalizations: A compendium of 15 promising interventions.* Cambridge, MA: Institute for Healthcare Improvement.

Clark, R. E. (1997, November). *The CANE model of motivation to learn and to work: A two-stage process of goal commitment and effort.* Paper presented at the University of Leuven, Belgium.

Committee on the Future Health Care Workforce for Older Americans, Board on Health Care Services, & Institute of Medicine. (2008). *Retooling for an aging America: Building the health care workforce.* Washington, DC: National Academies Press. Retrieved from http://www.nap.edu/openbook.php?record_id=12089&page=40

Driscoll, M. (1994). *Psychology of learning for instruction.* Boston, MA: Allyn and Bacon, Inc.

Dweck, C. S. (1990). Motivation. In R. Glaser & A. Lesgold (Eds.), *Foundations for a cognitive psychology of education* (pp. 87–136). Hillsdale, NJ: Erlbaum.

Fisher, W. R. (1978). Toward a logic of good reasons. *Quarterly Journal of Speech, 64*(4), 376–384.

Hallahan, K., Holtzhausen, D., van Ruler, B., Vercic, D., & Sriramesh, K. (2007). Defining strategic communication. *International Journal of Strategic Communication, 1*(1), 3–35.

Hernandez, A. F., Greiner, M. A., Fonarow, G. C., Hammill, B. G., Heidenreich, P. A., Yancy, C. W., … Curtis, L. H. (2010). Relationship between early physician follow-up and 30-day readmission among Medicare beneficiaries hospitalized for heart failure. *JAMA, 303*(17), 1716–1722.

Institute for Healthcare improvement (IHI). (2015a). The IHI Triple Aim. Retrieved from http://www.ihi.org/engage/initiatives/TripleAim/Pages/default.aspx

Institute for Healthcare improvement (IHI). (2015b). http://www.ihi.org/communities/blogs/_layouts/ihi/community/blog/itemview.aspx?List=81ca4a47-4ccd-4c9c-89d9-14d88ec59e8d&ID=50

Jones, S., Alnaib, M., Kokkinakis, M., Wilkinson, M., Gibson, A. S. C., & Kader, D. (2011). Pre-operative patient education reduces length of stay after knee joint arthroplasty. *Annals of the Royal College of Surgeons of England, 93*(1), 71.

Kasper, J., Légaré, F., Scheibler, F., & Geiger, F. (2012). Turning signals into meaning—"Shared decision making" meets communication theory. *Health Expectations, 15*(1), 3–11.

Kindig, D., & Stoddart, G. (2003). What is population health? *American Journal of Public Health, 93*(3), 380–383.

Kohn, L. T., Corrigan, J. M., & Donaldson, M. S. (1999). *To err is human: Building a safer health system.* Washington, DC: Committee on Quality of Health Care in America, Institute of Medicine.

Krupa, C. (2012, October 29). Gerontologists outline how doctors can bridge communication gap with older patients. *amednews.com.* Retrieved from http://www.amednews.com/article/20121029/health/310299947/4/

Langan-Fox, J., Code, S, & Langfield-Smith, K. (2000). Team mental models: Techniques, methods, and analytic approaches. *Human Factors, 42*(2), 242–271. doi: 10.1518/001872000779656534

Marshall, L. C., O'Neil, H. F., Abedi, J., Johnston, L., Visocnik, F., & Kainey, G. (2003, April). *Reliability and validity of the Healthcare Teams Questionnaire (HTQ).* Paper discussion session presented at the 2003 annual meeting of the American Educational Research Association, Chicago, IL.

Marshall, L. C., Wunch, K., Haydon, K., Visocnik, F., Thomas, P., Rosenfeld, C., & Abbas, L. (2004, October). *Efficacy, effort and teamwork skills in an interdisciplinary rehabilitation team.* Paper discussion session presented at the 2004 annual conference of the American Rehabilitation Nurses Association, Atlanta, GA.

McAlearney, A. S. (2003). *Population health management: Strategies to improve outcomes.* Health Administration Press. Chicago, IL.

McKnight, S. (2012). Telehealth: Applications for complex care. *Online Journal of Nursing Informatics (OJNI), 16(3).* Retrieved from http://ojni.org/issues/?p=2034

Meece, J. (1994). The role of motivation in self-regulated learning. In D. H. Schunk & B. J. Zimmerman (Eds.), *Self-regulation of learning and performance: Issues and educational applications* (pp. 25–44). Hillsdale, NJ: Lawrence Erlbaum Associates, Inc.

Nielsen-Bohlman, L., Panzer, A. M., & Kindig, D. A. (Eds.). (2004). *Health literacy: A prescription to end confusion.* Washington, DC: National Academies Press.

Olsen, L., & McGinnis, M. (2010). *Redesigning the clinical effectiveness research paradigm: Innovation and practice-based approaches (workshop summary)*. Washington, DC: Institute of Medicine National Research Council of the National Academies. Retrieved from http://iom.edu/Reports/2010/Redesigning-the-Clinical-Effectiveness-Research-Paradigm.aspx

Paris, C., Salas. E., & Cannon-Bowers, J. (2000). Teamwork in multi-person systems: A review and analysis. *Ergonomics*, *43*(8), 1052–1075.

Schunk, D. H. (1994). *Self-regulation of self-efficacy and attributions in academic settings.* Retrieved from http://psycnet.apa.org/psycinfo/1994-97658-003

Schunk, D. H. (1996, April). *Self-efficacy for learning and performance.* Paper presented at the annual meeting of the American Educational Research Association, New York, NY.

Shannon, C., & Weaver, W. (1949). *The Mathematical Theory of Communication*. Urbana, IL: The University of Illinois.

Shrestha, L. B., & Heisler, E. J. (2011). *Changing demographic profile of the United States*. Washington, DC: Congressional Research Service. Retrieved from http://fas.org/sgp/crs/misc/RL32701.pdf

U.S. Bureau of Labor Statistics. (2014, January 8). *Registered Nurses: Occupational outlook handbook* [Handbook]. Retrieved from http://www.bls.gov/ooh/healthcare/registered-nurses.htm

Weiner, B. (1985). An attributional theory of achievement motivation and emotion. *Psychological Review*, *92*(4), 548–573.

Zimmerman, B. J. (1989). A social cognitive view of self-regulated academic learning. *Journal of Educational Psychology*, *81*(3), 329–339.

Nurses as Educators Within Health Systems

Lori C. Marshall, PhD, MSN, RN
Immacolata Dall'Oglio, RN, MSN
David Davis, RN, MN
Gloria Verret, RN, BSN, CPN
Tere Jones, RN, CPN

OBJECTIVES

- Explain the nurse's role in leading patient and family education.

- Discuss the core components of the Marshall Personalized Patient-Family Education Model-Health System Approach (PPFEM-HSA) and highlight the specific actions that nurses need to take to achieve the learning goals.

- Recognize the different self-regulated learning strategies used by patients and caregivers.

Introduction

This chapter focuses on the nurse's unique and important role as a leader in patient and family education. It emphasizes a paradigm shift toward forward thinking and includes systems thinking when it comes to planning and coordinating patient and family education. Age/developmentally appropriate population-health management and self-care management strategies are presented here, with a focus on patients from vulnerable populations, including pediatrics, patients with cognitive processing issues including traumatic brain injury, and gerontology.

Toward a New, Not-So-New, Paradigm

Why is it important for nurses to embrace a *new* paradigm in which they view patient and family education as a primary role function? Nurses have the power to shape their care environment (Ponte et al., 2007). In particular, bedside nurses are with the patient more than any other discipline, and out of all the healthcare providers, play the most critical role to observe, detect, advocate, and "ensure patients receive high-quality care" (Agency for Healthcare Research and Quality [AHRQ], 2015, para. 1).

> *"Nurses, in concert with other health professionals, need to adopt roles as care coordinators, health coaches and system innovators." (The Institute of Medicine, 2011, p. 66)*

One of the nurse's core roles is coordination of care, with patient and family education being one of the most important elements, to ensure there is continuity of care across the continuum for all care settings (American Nurses Association [ANA], 2015). It's fundamental for the nurse to know the difference among self-care, complex care, and population health management for patients. Understanding the principles and tools you might use as a coordinator of care for each of these, as well as how they might be applied in different settings across the continuum, is also key. Each of these is fundamentally different within the care-coordinator role.

One of the focuses of self-care is to ensure competency of the patient and/or family to carry out aspects of basic care of themselves, developing their knowledge of care tasks such as activities of daily living (ADLs), medication administration, and care of supplies or equipment necessary to meet their health needs. Engaging the patient is essential for the patient to demonstrate competency. How do you achieve this? The nurse must listen to the patient's point of view, explore how the patient feels, and determine how confident the patient is to care for the problem.

The nurse must assess these issues about the patient and caregivers:

- What is their knowledge about the problem? (*What do they know?*)
- What are they already doing to address the issue/problem? What have they tried? (*What do they know to do?*)
- What is their feeling about the problem? (*What do they feel?*)
- What do they think could be done differently? (*What do they think to change?*)
- What matters to them?

You must ask these questions from both a short-term and long-term perspective, because the answers may be different.

Coordinating complex care involves being a health coach and helping patients navigate within and across the systems they must directly interact with to meet their health needs. Population health management is a higher level of aggregate coordination, and it involves assessing the needs of a specific patient population, analyzing population outcomes, and making adjustments in care. These changes will ultimately affect the population as a whole, but also the individual patient within the population.

In today's dynamic healthcare environment, with its constant changes and new initiatives, healthcare team members, and specifically nurses, can often get lost in the shuffle of competing elements. Among all their other duties, nurses must remember their primary role as an educator. Common barriers that keep nurses from adopting this paradigm include the perception of lack of time, knowledge of how to teach, and a commitment and investing effort into patient education (Boswell, Pichert, Lorenz, & Schlundt, 1990; Carpenter & Bell, 2002).

Adopting a *new* paradigm involves thinking differently, as well as adopting and integrating behaviors for leading patient and family education within health systems into your practice as a nurse.

Self-Reflecting on and Assessing Your Competencies

How ready are you for change? The nurse's role is a facilitator and clinical leader for patient and family education. According to the ANA *Scope and Standards of Nursing Practice,* Standard 5B, Health Teaching and Health Promotion, states, in part, "that the registered nurse employs strategies to promote health and a safe environment" (ANA, 2010, p. 10). The registered nurse:

- "Provides health teaching that addresses such topics as healthy lifestyles, risk-reducing behaviors, developmental needs, activities of daily living, and preventive self-care" (ANA, 2010, p. 41).
- "Uses health promotion and health teaching methods appropriate to the situation and the healthcare consumer's values, beliefs, health practices, developmental level, learning needs, readiness and ability to learn, language preference, spirituality, culture, and socioeconomic status" (ANA, 2010, p. 41).

By your licensure as a professional nurse, you are obligated to these standards, which expect all nurses to play a significant role in patient and family education.

Do you take charge of your own career? Assuming accountability and taking responsibility for developing one's competencies are critical and basic to being a professional. While it's valid to say that some nursing professionals have a passion or propensity for patient and family education, every nurse must maintain a basic competency for educating patients and families. Nurses have a professional obligation and responsibility to perform the core functions of nursing. Regardless of the degree to which an individual nurse participates in each function, all of the functions come into play throughout our practice, including patient-family education.

The core competencies you must embody as a nurse are related to the following core functions:

- Understanding the patient and family educational process
- Coordinating care
- Reinforcing patient and family partnerships and engaging them

The healthcare team begins and ends with the patient (and family) as the core team member. *Engaging* patients in their own care and constructing the patient-clinician partnership determines in part how successfully the patient moves from illness to wellness (or in maintaining wellness).

Are you a good communicator? A nurse who educates others must learn to be a good communicator. Open and transparent communication is vital. It is a partnership of educating that involves give and take. You learn from the family and patient, and they learn from you the things they still need to know to provide the best care moving forward. Be conscious that the patient, parents, family, and friends are all invaluable resources. Everyone represents a resource at their own level.

Do you facilitate self-efficacy? Another core element of the nurse's role is to facilitate the development of self-care or independence through teaching and education. This is key to the professional and therapeutic role of the nurse. Many clinicians develop close relationships with patients, especially those with chronic conditions, because they provide clinical care over extended periods of time. To facilitate independence, nurses must pay special attention to cultivating self-care as opposed to enabling dependence on clinicians and on the system.

When you deliver on these competencies, you'll see various benefits to clinical care outcomes. The Institute of Healthcare Improvement (IHI) Triple Aim focuses on improving the patient experience of care (e.g., US CAHPS, patient experience/satisfaction), improving the health of populations (e.g., health functional status, morbidity and mortality), and reducing the per capita costs of healthcare (e.g., total costs per member per month, hospital and ED utilization rate) (IHI, 2015). Patient and family education not only directly contributes to each of these outcomes but is a necessity to enable them to occur.

The Nurse's Role in Educating Patients and Families

As stated previously in this chapter, educating patients and families is fundamentally *the* most important role of the nurse. To achieve better learning outcomes, we'll walk you through the core model components and highlight the specific actions that nurses need to achieve the PPFEM-HSA learning goals.

Using a Patient's and Family's Story

Starting with the patient's and family's story, Table 2.1, you are reminded to modify your instructional approach in a linguistically appropriate manner and to consider relevant age and developmental aspects, as needed. Also take into account the patient's and family's culture, because "concepts of illness, health, and wellness are part of the total cultural belief system. Culture is one of the organizing concepts upon which nursing is based and defined" (ANA, 1991, Para 3).

Thus, you must use the patient's story to support knowledge-transfer by customizing the approach you take to each patient. This way, you:

- Build prerequisite/foundational knowledge.
- Structure content and simplify concepts (low to high level of abstraction).
- Select the right approach, e.g., text vs. visual (handouts, hands on, or pictures/graphics).

- Organize care routines with calendars (week/month), symbols (sun/moon), color codes, and daily events (breakfast, lunch, and dinner or when you first get up/right before you go to sleep).
- Plan for more time as needed to provide the instruction in small doses, yet more frequently.

Table 2.1 The Goals of the Marshall PPFEM, "Story" Component

Goals	Nurses Achieve Goals Through Collaboration
Personalize the healthcare experience	Understanding factors influencing health and care needs
Identify health risk factors	
Establish communication	Understanding country/regional perceptions of disease, conditions, or disability
Build relationship	
Define expectations	Understanding expectations
Create self-awareness of coping	Determining risk factors and degree of risk
	Determining health and care needs

Once you determine the approach you'll be taking, you need to partner with the patient and family to map out a plan.

Assessing a Patient's Motivation and Desire for Wellness

You map out a plan by determining the learning goals, understanding exit coping strategies, and developing forward thinking, as shown in Table 2.2. Imagine the patient has the Aladdin lamp: Ask the patient or family, "regarding your situation, what would be your three desires?" This approach could be useful to share and understand the self-awareness of the patient and his expectations. It clarifies what you can do for and with him. This is also useful for understanding expectations that might be difficult to meet given the circumstances.

Show the general outline of a process. Create a plan and adjust it based on readiness. While they know it is important, most staff go in without a plan. If you are conscious about the process, you can understand your role because you are one part of a larger plan. And it is important to know when another person—be it a nurse or other specially trained educator—is needed or coming back at another time to continue the learning process.

For this negotiation to be successful and to successfully support self-regulation of learning, there are two important concepts that you need to consider:

- **Self-reflection:** First, learning to negotiate is influenced by the learner's ability to accurately reflect and evaluate, which is essential to self-regulated learning. Self-reflection includes emotional reactions (such as stress or mood) and physiological indicators (such as heart rate or being tired) to make efficacy judgments (Bandura, 1986, 1997). For patients, self-reflection is the process of determining if they have the capacity to do what they are being asked to do. It also includes determining whether they feel like doing what they are asked to do. As a nurse, your role is to coach, mentor, and support opportunities for this process. This is where the value of interprofessional collaboration comes in, as other disciplines might need to support this aspect more directly in certain situations.

- **Motivation:** Secondly, learning to negotiate is influenced by the learner's motivation. Motivational processes play out in the following ways. If the learner chooses a learning goal, how hard is that goal, and how hard will they work at it or how much "effort" will they invest in reaching the goal? Thus, learning to negotiate is pivotal because it happens at the beginning stage of goal setting, which lays the foundation for adherence to treatment plans. It is also why patients and families must be part of the process when choosing a treatment plan, because the goals linked to that plan are tied to a motivational process.

Clark's (1997) Choice and Necessary Effort (CANE) model (see Figure 2.1) provides an easy way to connect three components—personal agency, emotion, and value. All three components must be in place for a learner to choose a goal. If a learner does not "feel like" working on a goal, they will not choose it unless they are able to create the value around it. Each of us sometimes face situations in which we don't feel like doing something, but through self-talk and connecting to a greater purpose, we move forward with a goal.

PERSONAL AGENCY X	**EMOTION** X	**VALUES** =	**GOAL CHOICE**
Efficacy (Can I do it)	Do I feel like it	Utility (Value later)	**COMMITMENT=**
Context Barriers		Interest (Am I curious)	Continued choice to
		Importance (Is this me)	act or not (persistence)

Figure 2.1   Clark's Choice and Necessary Effort (CANE) model. Used with permission. Richard Clark © 1997.

It is worth mentioning that a learner may over- or underestimate their efficacy levels. Figure 2.2 shows the relationship among the amount of effort a learner will invest, based on his level of confidence in completing a goal or learning a task. *Effort* is defined as the amount of new knowledge, in the form of cognitive strategies, that must be generated to achieve a goal (Clark, 1997). The information gathered from the story helps you know what the patient and family have previously done so you can appropriately guide the learner to a goal that will be enough of a stretch without seeming impossible. Hence the recommendation to set both short-term and long-term health goals.

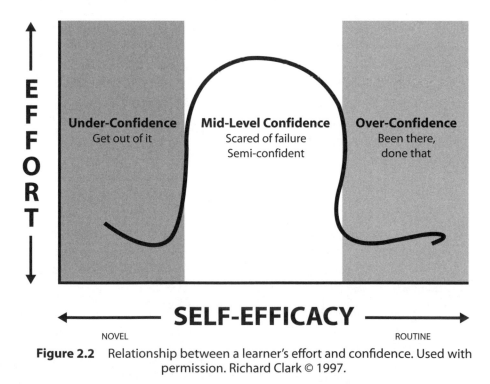

Figure 2.2   Relationship between a learner's effort and confidence. Used with permission. Richard Clark © 1997.

Giving Patients Confidence in Their Own Abilities

In order to navigate learning needs, patients and families have to feel confident that they can take on healthcare providers and the health systems. They also have to feel confident that they can manage their health needs and actions to maintain health. Having confidence or higher efficacy is critical to navigate the healthcare journey. In Chapter 1 it was mentioned that efficacy is related to goal choice and effort. The higher one's efficacy, the harder a goal will be selected and the more effort one will invest in achieving that goal. In looking at Table 2.2, these learning goals help with the structure and process needed to take charge of one's health journey.

Table 2.2 Using the PPFEM to Achieve Learning Goals		
Model Component	*Goals*	*Nurses Achieve Goals Through Collaboration*
Learning to negotiate healthcare learning needs	Adhere to treatment plan Create a patient/family/caregiver-provider partnership Establish interprofessional collaboration	Determining immediate goals Establishing forward thinking (hope and believing there is a future) Identifying early coping mechanisms Brokering interprofessional partnerships
Learning to navigate the health system and processes	Learn health system Establish support plan and resources Learn how to obtain information Establish peer mentor and support network	Identifying locations and settings Brokering support (peer level or groups) Identifying resource needs including transportation and access to care Helping to use the Internet and interactive patient-care technology for learning support Learning how to evaluate the resources

continues

Table 2.2 Using the PPFEM to Achieve Learning Goals (continued)		
Model Component	**Goals**	**Nurses Achieve Goals Through Collaboration**
Learning to manage healthcare needs	Establish self-care management Prepare for transition of care Promote care coordination Modify/strengthen coping strategies Determine long-term goals	Identifying learning and self-care management needs Preparing patient for self-care management Facilitating knowledge-transfer Supporting transition of care across life continuum Teaching new coping skills
Learning to maintain health	Maintain functional status Prevent disease progression Promote health and wellness	Reinforcing self-care management skills Helping patients control the environment they live in Ensuring access to care Providing opportunities for positive coping strategies to be reinforced Providing support across continuum of care Assessing functional health status Presenting transfer of care option Providing education and development (schooling, training, etc.)

Whereas negotiation serves as an essential component for setting goals, successful navigation helps build efficacy, which is a critical foundation for applying knowledge and skills in managing care.

If you find that a patient has underestimated his efficacy, he may have adequate knowledge but does not realize that he knows how to do it. The patient might see himself as unable and/or see his environment as preventing success. You would see him avoid a task, get easily distracted, or try to find an honorable way out. This patient values the task at hand but does not invest enough effort.

Clark (1997) provides tips on what a nurse can do to help an under-confident patient engage. Start by reducing the challenge by focusing on the task, and point to prior knowledge if available. Nurses should:

- Provide daily goals
- Structure the task
- Provide procedural advice
- Attribute mistakes to effort (rather than ability)
- Show coping models
- Model positive mood
- Monitor and give feedback

If a patient overestimates her skill level, she may have adequate knowledge but treat novel tasks as routine and use the wrong approach to solving problems; if she fails or performs poorly, she then blames others (Clark, 1997). This might be due to her incorrectly perceiving a task or goal as familiar when it is in fact novel and requires much thought and effort to handle. This patient values the task but underestimates the effort needed to perform it.

Using the CANE concepts (Clark, 1997), you can help these kinds of patients by adjusting their belief about the goal or task. In these cases, nurses should:

- Show novelty and difficulty
- Prove that the current approach might lead to failure
- Attribute failure to effort
- Show peer performance
- Request a new approach
- Monitor progress closely
- Give feedback

Providing Access to Support Groups and Systems

Support groups and systems are critical to a patient's success. Nurses can help support higher efficacy beliefs via support groups in two ways. First, through the use of "social persuasion" by telling patients or caregivers they're capable of performing a goal or can meet a goal; this provides temporary or situational efficacy (Bandura, 1986, 1997). Unless social persuasion is followed by a positive experience, the influence is not long lasting (Bandura, 1986, 1997).

The second is to influence learners "vicariously" by brokering peer models and support through social models. This is a comparative element of self-reaction and is aided when models are perceived as similar to the learner (i.e., when the patient perceives the model group to be true peers) (Bandura, 1986, 1997). Patients increase their efficacy by observing and interacting with a "social model." In this regard, always be thinking about the resources you can use for these types of experiences. The nurse is not the only resource of the educational process; the nurse is a facilitator and a supporter.

Using a patient's peers as a resource and as part of the process is important. You should begin brokering these relationships early in the learning process. Peers provide different motivational benefits, including learning new coping skills.

Helping Patients and Families Find Information

Searching online for healthcare information shows initiative and active involvement in healthcare by the family or patient. Not all sources, however, are valid. Some are advertisements by corporations or special interests, so it is important to teach the family to search for reputable sources. It may be valuable to offer a list of some valid sources and to discuss what the family has found online. The discussion should be open and accepting of the initiative shown by the family, but also a careful examination of the sources, their relevance to the patient, and their scientific/medical value.

Maximizing Knowledge-Transfer Through Collaboration

At this point, you must focus on identifying and preparing for the learning need. This section addresses how you can maximize learning. You can structure a learning event to maximize knowledge-transfer. You have probably done this yourself when you hear the patient or family member has learning needs: You grab a handout or two and go in to start teaching. When you arrive at the room, you realize that what you brought with you, or thought you would do, won't work. A key problem for nurses when it comes to patient and family education is not having a plan. As Carpenter and Bell say, "Patient education is approached best in an organized manner in which each education encounter, regardless of the length of time, is more likely to produce a quality session, thereby influencing patients to make positive changes in behavior" (2002, p. 157).

A learner's efficacy is highly influenced by achieving mastery, which is tied to managing care needs. *Mastery* is defined as experiencing the actual completion of a goal/task (Bandura, 1986, 1997) and is considered the most effective form of influence on self-efficacy. It is important to note that failure can undermine efficacy unless a person has had the chance to build up enough resiliency through multiple successes. Mastery is also connected to motivated behavior and completion of goals.

You help patients achieve mastery through thoughtful planning in the way you design and organize the educational experience. We will cover foundational concepts about instructional design and information processing that serve as powerful tools that support self-directed learning. This is the pinnacle of knowledge-transfer, where you hand off what you know to the patients and families.

Although multiple learning theories and models exist, the goal of this chapter is to keep your attention focused on what matters most, which is having a plan.

Structuring the Learning

A simple way to remember how to organize and structure an educational experience draws from the evidence on cognition (how people process information). Figure 2.3 highlights the instructional design process. This is flexible enough to apply to both formal and informal education needs. For informal use, the bedside nurse would write notes to organize her approach or run through this mentally in preparation for education. That is the operative phrase… prepare in advance.

Start with an introduction by stating the learning goals, explain why they are important, and give a brief overview of what you will cover. Motivationally, this is a critical step, because the reason for needing to learn a particular task or skill may not be one the learner has "bought into." As such, it is at this stage the nurse would also seek to understand the learner's side of it and leverage that. Refer back to the CANE model to review the value component (utility, interest, and importance). It is also at this introductory phase that the nurse would propose a way for the patient to have a shared mental model of the concepts to be learned. For example, healthcare providers will start teaching about asthma medications, specifically relievers and controllers. The patient or caregiver leaves that encounter and heads home. Upon a return visit to the clinic, it is discovered that only one medication, the reliever, is being frequently used. Upon further exploration, the patient thought the nurse demonstrated the same thing. If the previous education started by using a shared mental model, the learner could then connect the condition (asthma) to the different types of medications needed to help bronchospasms (reliever) and reduce inflammation (controller). The simplest model to use is the lungs and how they work. Without this knowledge of what is "normal," that learner cannot easily connect what happens with asthma.

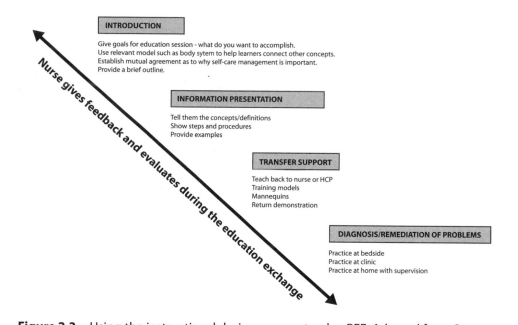

Figure 2.3   Using the instructional design process to plan PFE. Adapted from Gagne, Wagner, Golas, & Keller (2004).

Next, present or tell the learners the information starting with foundational concepts and then build to steps, procedures, and examples. Knowledge-transfer is supported by using tools and showing the learner how to do it. For mastery, the learner must have the opportunity to demonstrate or show you the steps. Employ the use of good communication and feedback to ensure they are confident. Highlight the aspects of the learning task they do well and show them the areas that need to be changed to the right step. This is part of practice and feedback, where your role is to evaluate their knowledge and skills for self-care management.

Connecting Structure to How People Process Information

The next concept that is important to understand is how learners process information. When you have a good understanding of this process, you'll be able to work better with a variety of learners. Figure 2.4 provides an overview of how information is processed based on the work of Driscoll (1994).

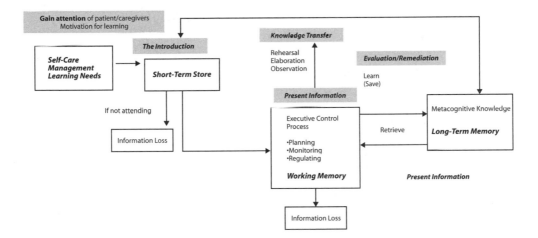

Figure 2.4   The basic information-processing model connected to the instructional design components. Adapted from Driscoll (1994).

The introduction component of your education is key to gaining the learners' attention. They need this to help retain the information so it can become part of their future self-care management knowledge and skills toolkit. If not, the information is lost, because short-term memory is a temporary holding zone. To make information part of the long-term memory, the learner must use metacognition or higher-level "executive processing" to control learning. Executive processing includes planning, monitoring, and regulating. *Planning* is choosing the right strategies, approaches, and resources to meet one's health goals. *Monitoring* is checking on the progress or status of a health goal. *Regulating* is one's ability to adjust or organize the self-care environment.

A learner then uses other strategies to hang onto the information so it is accurate and available later. Learners rehearse, reorganize, or elaborate on the information to make the knowledge theirs. This is why the process of learners explaining back what they learned is valuable. It is also why nurses must afford every opportunity to have patients and families practice skills and share their knowledge during their healthcare journey. Keep in mind that many conditions and injuries greatly affect information processing and require a focused approach. A few strategies will be presented later in the chapter.

Helping Patients Maintain Their Health and Wellbeing

Setting and choosing goals is a small part of maintaining health and wellbeing. The greatest challenge lies in the long term. This is when choices are tested, when held up against time. This is where you as the nurse must be aware of and know how to address the concept of commitment. Commitment differs from choosing a goal in that people can choose many goals, but the actions leading to sustainably acting on that goal day after day, year after year, are unique to commitment. Commitment is the ability to keep working on a goal regardless of the distractions (Clark, 1997).

How do you determine if your patient and family are self-regulated learners? Maintaining health and wellbeing requires a daily recommitment to one's goals. Table 2.3 provides examples of the words, actions, and language your patients, their family, and/ or caregiver will use that give you an indication as to their degree of self-regulation. The nurse's role is to help patients and caregivers develop strategies to increase self-regulatory processes, which lead to consistently performing self-care management behaviors.

This supports the use of metacognitive learning strategies (planning, monitoring, and organizing) that have been discussed in Chapter 1 and in a previous section in this chapter. The goal is that patients can connect their actions in the educational process with greater intent. In order to do this, they must gain greater awareness of their own actions and understand the intentions behind them.

> **TIP**
>
> Make one of your goals to commit to developing patients and families as future self-regulated learners. As such, it is important to recognize opportunities to coach, encourage, and mentor patients and families to use these strategies.

Table 2.3   Examples of Self-Regulated Learning Strategies for Patients and Caregivers

Strategy	Definition	Example
Self-evaluation	Statements indicating learner-initiated self-reflection and evaluations of their progress in meeting a goal or evaluating health status	"I checked over my weight loss chart to make sure I was on track." "I used my child's asthma action plan to check David's number from this morning, with the number the doctor wrote. Since it was lower, I gave him more medicine and called the doctor."
Organizing and transforming	Statements indicating learner-initiated overt or covert re-arrangement of information they need to learn to improve learning	"Before I met with my doctor, I made an outline using the handout about what I needed to learn."
Goal setting and planning	Statements indicating learner's setting of health goals or sub-goals and planning for sequencing, timing, and completing activities related to those goals	"I started eating lower-fat foods 2 weeks before my surgery, and now I pace myself to eat a little butter each week."
Seeking information	Statements indicating learner-initiated efforts to secure further task information from non-social sources when undertaking an assignment	"Before beginning the new chemotherapy, I went to the Cancer Society website to get as much information as possible concerning the topic."
Keeping records and monitoring	Statements indicating learner-initiated efforts to record events or results	"I wrote down my peak flow numbers." "I keep a list of the questions I want to ask my doctor."

continues

Table 2.3   Examples of Self-Regulated Learning Strategies for Patients and Caregivers   (continued)

Strategy	Definition	Example
Environmental structuring	Statements indicating learner-initiated efforts to select or arrange the physical setting to make meeting the learning goal easier	"To help with my asthma, I vacuum and keep the house dusted a few times a week." "I had a ramp built so I can get in and out of the house on my own."
Self-consequating	Statements indicating a learner's arrangement of rewards or punishments for success or failure	"If I keep my HbgA1c below 6.0, I will treat myself to a new outfit or movie."
Rehearsing and memorizing	Statements indicating learner-initiated efforts to memorize material by overt or covert practice Types of rehearsal: **Maintenance rehearsal** is the direct cycling of information in order to keep it active in short-term memory. **Elaborative rehearsal** is relating the information to be remembered to other information to promote deeper processing.	"In preparing to take my father (or child) home from the hospital, I have to learn how to give IV medicines. I keep writing the order of what I'm supposed to do until I remember it." "After my nurse told me about the medicine, I explained what it was for and why I was taking it. I was able to tell her the difference between the two inhalers."
Seeking social assistance	Statements indicating learner-initiated efforts to solicit help from (a) peers, (b) parent/family, and/or (c) healthcare providers	"If I have problems, I ask my mother [or friend] for help."
Reviewing records	Statements indicating learner-initiated efforts to re-read (a) notes, (b) websites, and/or (c) documents from healthcare visits to prepare for interactions with healthcare providers	"When getting ready to see my doctor, I review my _____."

Adapted from Zimmerman (1989).

In contrast to the examples of self-regulated learning strategies in Table 2.3, a patient lacking self-directed behavior makes statements indicating learning behavior that is initiated or driven by others, such as parents, friends, or healthcare providers. These statements (such as "I just do what the nurse or doctor tells me to do") indicate that the learner has not internalized or bought into the goal.

Developing Population-Specific Strategies

Patient-education strategies for three vulnerable and at-risk populations are explored next, using the Marshall PPFEM as a framework (see Figure 2.5).

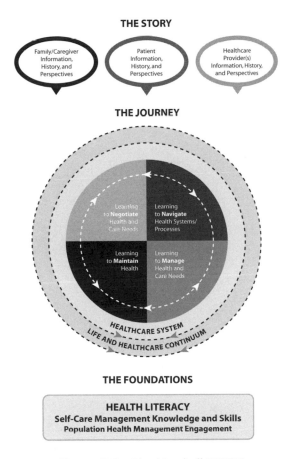

Figure 2.5   The Marshall PPFEM.

Patient-Family Education Applied to Pediatrics

Pediatrics is a challenging patient population due to the wide range of approaches you have to take. Although the patient is the focus of the healthcare experience, the family/caregivers become equally important in the journey.

Consider the "story" from the pediatrics perspective:

- Pediatric patients must be treated according to age and developmental needs, which are very different from infant to school-age to adolescent.
- Pediatric patients are not little adults; dosing of medication is different and approaches to healthcare teaching must be different than with adults.
- Pediatric care extends to 26 years of age.
- Young adulthood is an extremely vulnerable time. Young adults are still developing and must be approached in a way that considers that adult thinking may not be fully developed. They are at great risk for falling into coverage gaps, and this is critical for those with complex care needs.

Next, consider the "journey" from the pediatrics perspective. Recall that the journey includes negotiating health and care, navigating health systems and processes, managing health and care, and maintaining health.

In negotiating health and care from the pediatrics perspective:

- Engage the child at the appropriate developmental level.
- Address and engage the child as well as the parent.
- Toddlers often need a "broken record" response, with the consistent message repeated.
- Offer realistic choices such as "you can choose which medication to take first."
- Keep instructions simple.
- Use playful songs, nursery rhymes, current movies, and other play to engage the child and build trust.
- Be truthful when talking about painful procedures or the taste of medications.
- Use eye contact and real words, even for infants, and pause to let the child respond.

- Watch for signs of overstimulation or stress, through body language with the infant or small child, who may turn away, close eyes, and sneeze. Watch for acting out in school-age or older children. You may see withdrawal in teens.

In navigating health systems and processes from the pediatrics perspective:

- The goal is to achieve developmental milestones, which may have to be modified due to illness/disabilities.
- Prolonged hospital stays can impact normal growth and development, so care must be given to optimize growth and development through special therapies.
- Younger children rely on parental support and guidance, whereas peer support is important to adolescents.

In managing healthcare from the pediatrics perspective:

- Education on proper nutrition, adequate sleep, and adequate time to play and exercise is important. Teenagers in particular need adequate sleep.
- Do not ask the child to "be brave," but state that you understand if the child is in pain and do something to ease the pain.
- In the hospital setting, seek out Child Life professionals, who help children cope with procedures and let them be kids.
- Educating parents about medications or other care is necessary.
- Different disease processes require dietary adjustments, so enlist dietitian support.

In maintaining health from the pediatrics perspective:

- Medication adherence is problematic for adolescents with chronic diseases. They may rebel against the restrictions of the disease process, so using text messaging, social media support groups, or other peer support may help.
- Children do not realize their limitations, so safety is key. Keep medications out of reach, anchor tubing to keep it from being entangled, and cover any wounds or intravenous access sites.

The foundations of pediatrics-based education involve:

- **Supporting the pediatric population with health literacy as well as mastery of knowledge and skills.** For small children, or those with delays, the first transition in care is from healthcare provider to family. However, the children should always be included in teaching whenever possible. For younger children, use play to engage the child and let the child explore. For example, let the child hold an empty syringe or examine a tube, or have a doll with devices such as tubes or casts if the child has any devices. The child should be at the center of this activity, although the family needs special attention and education to become autonomous in caring for their child.

- **Advancing the education as the child ages.** Education should advance with the child's development to maximize the child's independent self-care, and the child should receive specialized, individualized teaching. When possible, encourage self-care to transition the pediatric patient to independent self-care. Encourage parents to embrace maximum independent self-care by the child so the family can optimize whatever growth and development is possible for this child. The goal is to achieve maximum functioning for the child. The parents may need special attention to allow this separation due to fears and feelings of protectiveness for the sick or impaired child.

Note that adolescence is a particular challenge, because this stage is naturally expressed in some opposition to control, desire to fit in with peers, and resentment against strict medical regimens such as medications or restrictions in diet or activity. Enlisting peer support can help, such as online support groups or camp activities.

Patient-Family Education Applied to Children and Adults with Cognitive Processing Issues

Cognitive processing issues present a challenge to patient educators. This is an issue found across the life span. In children, it may be due to congenital issues or events surrounding birth or due to accidents, brain traumas, or neurological diseases. In adulthood, it is often due to degenerative changes, including Alzheimer's disease, which alters memory and cognition, or traumatic injury. While this section covers cognitive processing issues, PFE for traumatic brain injury will also be covered, because some of the same approaches are leveraged to facilitate knowledge-transfer.

Consider the "story" from the perspective of treating someone with a traumatic brain injury or other cognitive processing issue. The concept of "learning about previous health and care experiences current knowledge and skills" is essential (Lash, 2000). What makes traumatic brain injury unique regardless of age, for example, is the drastic change in the patient's story in one moment's time.

Next, consider the "journey" from the perspective of treating someone with a traumatic brain injury. Recall that the journey includes negotiating health and care, navigating health systems and processes, managing health and care, and maintaining health.

In negotiating health and care from the traumatic brain injury perspective:

- Developmental age will be different after the injury, depending on its severity.
- Patient's developmental age may be less than the age in years.
- Capacities and cognition may change on a daily basis.
- Patient may be forgetful; short-term memory loss is not uncommon, so be patient, repeat with kindness, and avoid showing frustration.
- Patients may grieve loss of function and isolation, especially teenage patients, so optimize any visitors, texting, and online groups with supervision.
- Encourage others to interact with the patient when appropriate, when patient is not too tired, hungry, or upset.
- Family members will likewise grieve the loss of function, potentially the loss of personality and future hopes and dreams.

In navigating health systems and processes from the traumatic brain injury perspective:

- Sensorimotor capacities will be impacted.
- Patient may no longer be independent in any or all of activities of daily living.
- Patient may not be able to eat, swallow, urinate, or have bowel movements spontaneously or under their control.
- Goal is to maximize function for the individual with appropriate gradient expectations.

In managing health and care from the traumatic brain injury perspective:

- Therapists will teach you how to work with the patient to avoid inducing helplessness or atrophy from disuse, and, on the other hand, how to avoid frustrating the patient with unrealistic expectations.
- Many patients will need assistive/adaptive devices for mobility such as braces, casts, crutches, walkers, reachers, visual or hearing aids, or communication devices.
- Safety is key, because mobility deficits may make patient unable to sit/stand/walk as they could in their pre-injury status.
- Use simple words according to developmental age, not age in years.
- You may need to reword directions or communications to achieve understanding.
- Keep directions simple and to the point.
- Talk to the patient gently and clearly, maintaining eye contact.
- Patient may need constant monitoring to avoid injury.
- Patient may be agitated and combative, so safe handling is needed.
- Keep stimulation to a minimum, with a quiet environment and soft lighting.

In maintaining health from the traumatic brain injury perspective:

- TBI patients need rest and sleep.
- TBI patients need good nutrition and may have eating difficulties.
- Skin care is important if the patient is not continent.
- Bladder and bowel functions may not be normal; careful assessment and monitoring of intake and output is vital; patient may require bowel training, catheterization.
- Move toward normalizing life, accepting the new baseline for the patient, and optimizing all function.

The foundations of PFE for traumatic brain injury patients are as follows.

Health Literacy

Health literacy by its very definition can be a significant issue in the brain-injured patient. To have health literacy, one must, to some degree, have the capacity to obtain, process, and understand health information. One also must be able, on some level, to make health decisions based on the information one has and understands. A brain-injured patient can have varying degrees of memory loss, confusion, agitation, and issues with judgment, among other behavioral changes. A family and caregiver assessment is a big part of any complete learning assessment, but here it becomes a crucial part in the planning of education and goal setting.

The gradient approach to competent literacy—with intermittent and consistent assessments of the positive steps in the learning process—is very important here, because the learning process can be slow in this population, resulting in discouragement and setbacks along the way. Focusing repeatedly on the gains made in any education can go a long way, but especially here, to promote functional literacy.

Self-Care Knowledge and Skills

In patients with cognitive dysfunction, self-care skills must not only be thoroughly assessed, but the overall goal must be allowing and promoting as much *safe* independence as possible. Along with the patient assessment, assess patient support both in the home and in the community. A person with a brain injury can sometimes remember parts of their pre-injury life and abilities, and frustration is common. Again, it is vital to engage the family for support and promote positive feedback; repetitive instruction and reinforcement of gains is key. This will help to preserve motivation and safe independence.

A multidisciplinary team approach that leverages many areas of expertise is absolutely necessary to put in the overall plan and implementation. It is important to address all areas of deficit and provide an appropriately planned gradient education program that can engage the patient, family, and caregivers to meet their maximum function and potential.

Population Health Engagement

There are support groups for all kinds of issues, but not all are accessible when and where they are needed. The coordinating professionals on the multidisciplinary team are responsible for finding and sharing the appropriate resources so that those groups can be utilized.

Community outreach projects can assure public education on the pertinent issues and connect people needing services and support with those delivering it. This can make a difference in the progression toward changing the paradigm to a forward-thinking plan across the entire continuum of care and responsibility.

Resources for Cognitive Processing Issues/TBI

Brain injuries in children: http://www.biausa.org/brain-injury-children.htm

Office of Head Start, Early Childhood Learning and Knowledge Center (US HHS), information about traumatic brain injury: http://eclkc.ohs.acf.hhs.gov/hslc/tta-system/teaching/Disabilities/Services%20to%20Children%20with%20Disabilities/Disabilities/disabl_fts_00019rev_081806.html

Alzheimer's information: http://alzheimers.gov/

Patient-Family Education Applied to the Elderly (Gerontology)

An elder's story is rich with life experiences and history. Reflection on a lifetime of experiences, career, and travels shapes who they are. Keep in mind elders' variation in health status, because the term "elder" does not equate to unhealthy or inactive. However, the body does experience changes as we age, and common issues for the elderly population include vision, hearing, and mobility (see Figure 2.6).

Next, consider steps in the "journey" from the perspective of gerontology.

In negotiating health and care from the perspective of gerontology:

- Be sure to account for patients' outlook on life and living, including the importance of family and friends.
- Set realistic goals and be sure to include family members in the process.

In navigating health systems and processes from the perspective of gerontology:

- Modify activity such as driving, socialization, and engagement determined by baseline function.

In managing healthcare from the perspective of gerontology:

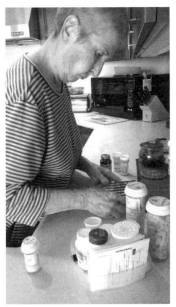

Figure 2.6   Elder organizing weekly medications.

- Encourage patient to be as engaged as possible.
- Although the patient is an important focus for patient and family education, this is where the transition back to family and caregivers becomes important. As in the pediatric population, the child begins to learn routines as part of care transition, so does the transition of care need to be brought back to the family of the elderly.
- Educate caregivers on where/how to support their loved ones.
- Educate caregivers on how to maintain self-care.
- Teach new coping skills. In part, this is derived from the level of forward thinking in play. Self-determination is a critical component.

In maintaining health from the perspective of gerontology:

- Ensure there are transportation services to keep appointments.
- Set up communication processes, including technology, to remain connected to providers and health system.
- Maintain solid community and family support and network.

The foundations of PFE for gerontology patients are as follows:

Health Literacy

In gerontology, it is important to dispel the myth that behaviors are set and cannot be changed. It is very possible when the educational process is well paced and individualized to change the way things are done (Best, 2001). Tools are needed for planning and organizing things like the daily routine and medication regimens (Shen et al., 2006).

Technology tools can be used here, because many elderly people are now engaged with some form of technological device. You must be cognizant that changes can be both upsetting and even dangerous if not monitored until the new regimen is solidly in place. As with TBI patients, you may encounter impaired decision-making and judgment with elderly patients (Centeno, 2011). The difference here is that they are more likely to worsen over time, requiring reassessment and new goal setting.

Self-Care Knowledge and Skills

Here, maintenance of independence is the goal. A threat to self-care can be upsetting to your patient, because it creates the feeling of a loss of independence. It is important to assess for safety factors and encourage support for the areas deemed the most unsafe if performed solely by the patient, but it is also important to find and maintain areas where self-care can be performed safely.

Focus should also be on *safe* independence, as in the TBI patient, because falls can be common here and lessen independence by causing setbacks in function. It is important to recognize that muscle weakness and loss of muscle tone is not necessarily a function of aging, but more a function of inactivity. It is a vicious cycle, because inactivity breeds weakness and that in kind produces more inactivity. A well-paced and consistent exercise program is key to preserve tone and strength and prevent injury due to falls. According to the CDC website, "strengthening exercises, when done properly and through the full range of motion, increase a person's flexibility and balance, which decrease the likelihood and severity of falls. One study in New Zealand in women 80 years of age and older showed a 40% reduction in falls with simple strength and balance training" (CDC, 2011, paragraph 5).

Patient communication skills are also important to assess, because the patient may be able to communicate to other caregivers some basic cares that are needed when they are unable to perform them safely on their own. This piece can be crucial to foster the idea of independence, because the patient, from his own level of knowledge, may be able to direct the action of those things that he cannot do by himself. The key here being engagement of the patient with his care and with his caregivers based upon his level of cognition and ability.

Population Health Engagement

Connecting to one's health system and preventing isolation is an important part of health and wellbeing. This can be accomplished via community groups and through the use of social media. Facebook can be a wonderful way to keep family connected from around the world. Skype and other Internet-based tools are good to support emotional health. The responsibility of the professionals on the care team is educating, coordinating, and facilitating the connection between the aging patient and the world around them. Connection is vital to maintaining the feeling of self-worth.

Elder Resources

Administration on Aging (AoA): http://www.aoa.gov/

Medicare.gov, information on coordinating care: http://www.medicare.gov/manage-your-health/coordinating-your-care/coordinating-your-care.html

Conclusion and Key Points

One of the most important nursing roles is in educating the patient and family. This component is directly responsible for influencing health outcomes. Yet, when it comes down to it, medication administration and other task-related aspects of a nursing professional's job often overshadow these priorities. How do you shift your paradigm as a nursing professional so you can simultaneously serve the needs of the moment and of the future?

First, you must become an active and accountable exchange agent in educational activities and in the knowledge-transfer process. This means being willing to "let go of" and "hand off your knowledge" to the patient and family. To make it easy to remember the educational priorities, we leave you with the Five Rights of Patient-Family Education.

> *"The Five Rights of Patient-Family Education: The Right Approach (the Story) aimed at the Right Context (Continuum of Care) with the Right Content (Health Literacy) using the Right Methods (Self-Care Management Knowledge and Skills) followed by the Right Support (Population Health Engagement)."*

Second, you need to adopt a broader framework for patient and family education that accounts for the current setting but within a global context. This includes ensuring that the treatment plans reflect the setting where the patients and families will continue their care after your involvement. For example, you plan a rehabilitation program for a child from a low-income country.

Finally, consider your role in shaping your own healthcare system and take into account that this perspective could change greatly and thus could influence the social, political, and cultural approach. This impacts the sustainability of the educational tools and resources available for patients and families. This may be one of the most important messages, that while focusing on improving health and wellbeing of people, nurses turn the PPFEM toward creating a health system that actually supports patients and families. In some cases, this focus should be a priority over the personal perspective (family, patient, and provider) that the HCP interprets as a professional.

References

Agency for Healthcare Research and Quality, U.S. Department of Health & Human Services (AHRQ). (2015). *Nursing and patient safety.* Retrieved from psnet.ahrq.gov/primer.aspx?primerID=22

American Nurses Association. (1991). *New position statement: Cultural diversity in nursing practice.* Accessed March 1, 2015 at http://nursingworld.org/MainMenuCategories/Policy-Advocacy/Positions-and-Resolutions/ANAPositionStatements/Archives/prtetcldv14444.html

American Nurses Association. (2010). *Nursing: Scope and standards of practice.* (2nd ed.). Silver Spring, MD: American Nurses Association.

Bandura, A. (1986). *The social foundations of thought and action.* Englewood Cliff, NJ: Prentice Hall.

Bandura, A. (1997). *Self-efficacy: The exercise of control.* New York, NY: Freeman.

Best, J. T. (2001). Effective teaching for the elderly: Back to basics. *Orthopedic Nurse, 20*(3), 46–52.

Boswell, E. J., Pichert, J. W., Lorenz, A. L., & Schlundt, D. G. (1990). Training health care professionals to enhance their patient teaching skills. *Journal of Nursing Staff Development, 6*(5), 223–239.

Carpenter, J., & Bell, S. (2002). What do nurses know about teaching patients? *Journal for Nurses in Staff Development, 18*(3), 157–161.

Centeno, J. (2011). Methods of teaching and learning of the elderly: Care in rehabilitation. *CJNI: Canadian Journal of Nursing Informatics, 6*(1), Article Two. Retrieved from http://cjni.net/journal/?p=1147

Centers for Disease Control and Prevention (CDC). (2011). *Why strength training?* Retrieved from http://www.cdc.gov/physicalactivity/growingstronger/why/index.html

Clark, R. E. (1997, November). *The CANE model of motivation to learn and to work: A two-stage process of goal commitment and effort.* Paper presented at the University of Leuven, Belgium.

Driscoll, M. (1994). *Psychology of learning for instruction.* Boston, MA: Allyn and Bacon, Inc.

Gagne, R., Wager, W., Golas, K., & Keller, J. (2004). *Principles of instructional design.* Boston, MA: Cengage Learning.

Institute for Healthcare Improvement (IHI). (2015). The IHI Triple Aim. Retrieved from http://www.ihi.org/engage/initiatives/TripleAim/Pages/default.aspx

Institute of Medicine. (2011). *The Future of nursing: Leading change, advancing health.* Washington, DC: The National Academies Press, 2011.

Lash, M. (2000). Teaching strategies for students with brain injuries. *TBI Challenge!, 4*(2). Retrieved from www.biausa.org/LiteratureRetrieve.aspx?ID=48657

Ponte, P. R., Glazer, G., Dann, E., McCollum, K., Gross, A., Tyrrell, R., … Washington, D. (2007). The power of professional nursing practice—An essential element of patient and family centered care. *OJIN: The Online Journal of Issues in Nursing, 12*(1), Manuscript 3.

Shen, Q., Karr, M., Ko, A., Chan, D. K., Khan, R., & Duvall, D. (2006). Evaluation of a medication education program for elderly hospital in-patients. *Geriatric Nurse, 27*(3),184–92. Retrieved from http://hospitalmedicine.ucsf.edu/improve/literature/discharge_committee_literature/med_reconciliation/evaluation_of_medication_education_program_for_elderly_hospital_inpatients_shen_geriatr_nurs.pdf

Zimmerman, B. (1989). A social cognitive view of self-regulated academic learning. *Journal of Educational Psychology, 81,* 329–339.

The Nurse's Role in the Era of Accountable Care: A Catalyst for Change

Linda Alexander, BSN, MBA, RN, CCM
Lori C. Marshall, PhD, MSN, RN
Tere Jones, RN, CPN
Scott Ferguson, MSW, LCSW, ACM
Linda Frommer, MPH

OBJECTIVES

- Describe the shifting paradigm of healthcare in the United States due to the Patient Protection and Affordable Care Act of 2010.

- Explain the changing role of nursing in the transition to globally accountable care.

- Understand the critical need to view patient and family education/interventions across the continuum.

- Understand the interdependence of multiple systems of care.

Introduction

This chapter focuses on systems thinking when it comes to planning and coordinating patient and family education and care management. It will address the connection among accountable care organizations (ACOs), case management, home health, and community/public health.

This chapter shares ideas on how to align education and interventions to support population health with emphasis on self-care management, and on how to support complex care across the continuum. Information about transition and transfer of care includes comprehensive handoffs (exchange of clinical and nonclinical information). This chapter imparts insights on common issues, barriers, and challenges affecting care coordination and cross-continuum partnerships.

Finally, this chapter helps the reader (whether nurse, nursing student, or nurse leader) understand the importance of having a dual mindset now and in the future, as leaders guiding patient and family education across multiple systems of care. Direct-care staff tend to focus on their shift and not about what's next or next month. This is the impetus to change.

Overview of U.S. Healthcare Reimbursement Models

Nurses play a pivotal role in shaping care outcomes for patients. As the care team member who interfaces with the patient on a more frequent and consistent basis, nurses have the ability to promote disease self-management and wellness promotion through education, person-centered interventions, and integration of supportive services. Leveraging this access to patients and their caregivers is paramount as we navigate this era of accountable care. To do this, nurses need an understanding of how their health system works, the interdependence of multiple systems of care, and the critical need to view patient and family education and engagement across the continuum.

This section is intended to provide a brief overview of major reimbursement models in the United States and their impact on access to healthcare. Compared to other countries, the United States spends more money per capita on healthcare. Other healthcare systems are far more efficient with better outcomes, especially in the management of complex care needs (World Health Organization [WHO], 2000).

Historically in the United States (prior to 1965), access to healthcare services was limited to those who had the resources to pay. Those less fortunate relied on natural remedies, in-kind services, or traditions to treat ailments that had been passed down through the generations. Primary care physicians generally provided medical care in the community, and reimbursement was mostly cash-based, with a fee schedule for defined services (fee-for-service or FFS). Before Medicare, it is estimated that 60% of those over 65 had health-insurance coverage, with coverage often unavailable or unaffordable to the rest because older adults paid more than three times as much for health insurance as the younger population (Berenson & Rich, 2010). Let's fast-forward to the advent of Medicare and Medicaid.

The Advent of Medicare and Medicaid

In 1965 (yes, only 50 years ago!), Medicare and Medicaid programs were added to Title XVIII and Title XIX, respectively, of the Social Security Act, extending healthcare coverage to seniors age 65 and over, as well as to low-income, vulnerable populations (such as orphaned children and disabled adults and children) (Centers for Medicare & Medicaid Services [CMS], 2005–2006). Medicare was implemented in 1966, providing coverage to more than 19 million seniors during this time. In the same year, state funding was made available to implement Medicaid programs. Over the years, modifications to the Medicare and Medicaid programs designed the mature program that we experience today (CMS, 2005–2006).

A collateral effect of the implementation of Medicare and Medicaid was the expansion of hospital-based care. This new payment model spurred a care-delivery shift from primary/community-based care to hospital-centric care. With this shift came rising healthcare costs due to the operational costs associated with hospital care. A benefit to hospital care was the ability to improve access to healthcare services and treat more complicated illnesses. However, the rising costs became difficult to manage under the existing payment structure.

The Health Maintenance Organization ACT

The Health Maintenance Organization ACT of 1973, signed into law by President Richard Nixon, was an amendment to the Public Health Service Act that provided "assistance and encouragement for the establishment and expansion of health maintenance organizations, and for other purposes" (Library of Congress, 1973, p. 1). It was intended to reduce unnecessary healthcare costs through a variety of mechanisms, including economic incentives for physicians and patients to select less costly forms of care, programs for reviewing the medical necessity of specific services, increased beneficiary cost-sharing, controls on hospital admissions and lengths of stay, and intensive management of high-cost healthcare … hence the term "managed care" (CMS, 2015a). Managed Care Organizations (MCOs) and Health Maintenance Organizations (HMOs) were charged with creating systems or networks of care to manage the rising costs of care. Although markets with HMOs somewhat slowed rising healthcare costs (Larkin, 1999), overall they continued to rise in the United States (AHRQ, 2002). As coverage expansion continued, costs continued to rise. Access to care was no longer an issue, as it was prior to 1965. Cost became a pressing concern for lawmakers, because the Medicare and Medicaid programs would no longer be sustainable with their current cost structure. "Healthcare accounts for a large and growing share of economic activity in the United States, nearly doubling as a share of gross domestic product (GDP) in the period between 1980 and 2011, from 9.2% to 17.9%" (The Medicare Payment Advisory Commission [MedPAC], 2013, p. 3).

The Patient Protection and Affordable Care Act

On March 23, 2010, President Barack Obama enacted the Patient Protection and Affordable Care Act (PPACA) (U.S. Department of Health and Human Services [USDHHS], 2015b). Specific provisions of the PPACA are to be phased in through January 1, 2018. The law is the principal healthcare reform legislative action of the 111th U.S. Congress. Unlike the Social Security Act, which houses the Medicare and Medicaid programs, the PPACA reforms certain aspects of the private health-insurance industry and public health-insurance programs. These reforms include increasing insurance coverage for pre-existing conditions, expanding access to insurance to over 30 million Americans, an increased enrollment in federal healthcare programs, and additional policy changes to reduce the long-term costs of healthcare (USDHHS, 2015a).

The PPACA has three key components relevant to this chapter: accountable care organizations, value-based reimbursement, and care integration.

Accountable Care Organizations (ACOs)

Accountable care organizations, or *ACOs,* refer to entities that manage care for an assigned membership to improve health outcomes and reduce costs of care. ACOs create alignment with the hospital and physician communities to achieve common objectives based on the Institute for Healthcare Improvement (IHI) Triple Aim philosophy: improve the health of patient populations, improve patients' experience of healthcare, and reduce per capita costs of healthcare (IHI, 2015). "The components of the Triple Aim are not independent. Changes pursuing any one goal can affect the other two sometimes negatively, sometimes positively" (Berwick, Nolan, & Whittington, 2008, p. 760). Elements of an ACO may involve primary care (wellness promotion and disease prevention); quality outcomes; community/stakeholder collaboration; data sharing and integration; capitated payments (a monthly payment per member instead of FFS); and a shared savings model (sharing of savings with practitioners and the ACO).

Value-Based Reimbursement

Value-based reimbursement involves innovations in payments for healthcare services to include quality measures or outcomes instead of payment for the volume of services rendered. An example of this payment change is Medicare readmission penalties to hospitals. The advent of a penalty for hospital readmission rates above a specified threshold produced readmission reduction strategies at hospitals across the United States. Despite receiving reimbursement for Medicare admissions and readmissions, hospitals could face millions of dollars in penalties if this quality measure is not managed.

Another element of value-based reimbursement is transparency. This relates to information sharing via health-information exchanges and transparency of costs/charges to providers and patients, as well as quality performance. Disclosure of financial relationships of providers and physicians with manufacturers, distributors, and their subsidiaries is also pertinent to the notion of value-based reimbursement. It is believed that undisclosed, these relationships can undermine care decisions and lead to increased costs, thereby reducing value (Weintraub, 2010).

The Medicare Payment Advisory Commission is "a non-partisan policy and technical advice to the Congress on issues" such as "payments to private health plans participating in Medicare and providers in Medicare's traditional fee-for-service program that" affect the Medicare program (2015a). MedPAC helps analyze other issues that impact Medicare such as care access and quality of care. In 2010, MedPAC published data revealing that 37% of hospitalized Medicare beneficiaries used one or more post-acute settings with an average payment of $30,000 per beneficiary for post-acute care. The report further depicted that utilization of post-acute services was tied to hospital readmission rates (see Table 3.1).

Table 3.1	Post-Acute Settings by Readmission to Hospital and Discharge to Secondary PAC Setting		
Post-Acute Care (PAC) Setting	*Percent Discharged from Hospital to PAC*	*Percent Readmitted After PAC Setting*	*Percent Discharged to Second PAC Setting*
Skilled Nursing Facility	17.3	22.0	29.3
Home Healthcare	15.0	18.1	2.3
Acute Rehabilitation Facility	3.2	9.4	56.8
Hospice	2.1	4.5	2.4
Long-Term Acute Care Hospital	1.0	10.0	53.4
Psychiatric Care	0.5	8.7	25.4
Total Patients	40.0	18.0	19.8

Adapted from MedPAC, 2010.

Care Integration

Care integration refers to deconstructing the silos that have evolved in the healthcare delivery system over the years and creating a care delivery plan that crosses all settings of care and is shared among all care team members, including family and caregiver support. As one would imagine, this can occur in varying degrees. There has been an insurgence of entities to facilitate this transition with multiple naming conventions, but all focused on integrating care: Integrated Delivery Network (IDN), Clinically Integrated Network (CIN), Continuing Care Network (CCN), and even ACOs meet this qualifier. An integration network is simply "a network of organizations that provides or arranges to provide a coordinated continuum of services to a defined population and is willing to be held clinically and fiscally accountable for the outcomes and health status of the population served" (Shortell, Gillies, & Anderson, 1996, p. 7).

A clinically integrated network is the solution to what is called the *silo effect*. The silo effect refers to the lack of communication and support often found in acute-care episodes. Providers focus primarily on their own goals, often ignoring the needs of others along the care delivery system. Technology adoption has simplified the ability to integrate care; however, this task remains in its infancy across the U.S. healthcare market.

> *"The larger healthcare market poses additional barriers to investment in IT. Payment systems that tie reimbursement to the volume of services delivered, for example, may penalize providers who improve quality in ways that result in fewer units of service. To the extent that IT investments lead to reduced volume, many who make the investment will not reap all of the benefits. Systems that integrate care across settings tend to be more advanced users of IT because they are able to capture some of these efficiencies. In addition to barriers posed by payment systems, a fragmented delivery system leads to redundant investments by multiple providers who lose the benefit of economies of scale. Although this aspect of our delivery system is a barrier to adoption, widespread use of IT could help providers coordinate care across settings, overcoming some of the problems of fragmentation."*
> *(MedPAC, 2004, p. 158)*

Another strategy proposed in the PPACA (USDHHS, 2015b) that supports care integration is episodic care, as opposed to encounter- or visit-based care. *Episodic care*—the re-engineering of the acute episodes derived from acuity-based expectations of patient care requirements, devoid of provider preference, and driven by the least restrictive/costly care environment—encourages involved care providers to work collaboratively to optimize patient outcomes and utilization of resources. The episodic reimbursement approach rewards providers based on patient outcomes or units of service over a period of time, rather than based on volume.

In 2009, Jencks, Williams, and Coleman explored adult hospital readmission rates and found of the readmissions in 30 days, over 77% were related to medical conditions and 22% were from surgical conditions. In both conditions, heart failure and pneumonia accounted for the most frequent reason for readmission. This paved the way to recognition that hospitals need to become more involved in preventing readmission. It also heightened awareness that the 30-day post-acute care episode is a critical time. According to Krumholz (2013), it is best to focus on the first 30 days after discharge, when the patient is temporarily more vulnerable. Patients are at greater risk due to stress of being hospitalized and the effects of the illness that lingers. They are also at greatest risk for adverse events connected to recovering from the illness and hospitalization. The premise behind this suggestion is related to the need for acute and post-acute providers to address non-clinical contributors to hospital readmissions post-discharge.

In December 2014, MedPAC made the recommendation to Congress to institute "site-neutral" payments for post-acute services for specified Medicare patients with medical rehabilitation needs (MedPAC, 2015b). This recommendation is based on the premise that certain medical rehabilitative services are consistent and should not cost more, based on the clinical setting. In today's reimbursement structure, similar medical rehabilitation services in an acute rehabilitation hospital would cost more than in a skilled nursing facility. A site-neutral payment would nullify the discrepancy due to the care setting.

Connecting ACOs and Bundled Payments

Hospitals and physicians view ACOs as a key strategy to adapting to changes under healthcare reform. Many healthcare executives and thought leaders view ACOs and value-based payments as a precursor to bundled payments for episodic care (National Conference of State Legislators [NCSL], 2010). In 1999, post-acute Medicare payments grew 25% to 35% a year (Assistant Secretary for Planning and Evaluation [ASPE], 1999) and continue to grow 5% yearly (Rau, 2013a). If variation in Medicare spending for post-acute services, such as home health, long-term care, and skilled nursing were addressed, it would account for a 73% decrease in variation (Rau, 2013b).

Thus, post-acute entities must be prepared to deliver a "value-based" service that aligns with referring source priorities, as part of the episode of care.

$$ACO + VBP = SBP$$

Single bundled payment (SBP) is defined as a "single negotiated episode payment of a predetermined amount for all services (physician, hospital, and other provider services) furnished during an episode of care. This could be paid prospectively or retrospectively" (CMS, 2011, p. 39).

Value based purchasing (VBP) is defined as "linking provider payments to improved performance by health care providers. This form of payment holds health care providers accountable for both the cost and quality of care they provide. It attempts to reduce inappropriate care and to identify and reward the best-performing providers" (healthcare.gov, 2015).

Now that you have the connection, it is important to understand why post-acute care is crucial. The other important factor to success is connecting people and care across the continuum.

Due to siloed care-delivery systems, many healthcare leaders have segmented experiences. Each segment of the continuum has unique challenges, payment systems, and so on. You need to spell out the settings of care along the continuum. That includes ambulatory care, acute care (hospital and rehab), long-term acute care, skilled nursing care, extended/long-term care, home care, palliative care, and hospice care. Community, mental, and public health services may also be described here. This is a great opportunity to depict the interdependence of the different settings and the need to break down silos.

Managing Populations Instead of Managing Encounters

Population health management (PHM) has become the hallmark to an accountable care strategy. As a person-centered approach to care management over a period of time, PHM seeks to look at a continuum of care (not an encounter); integrates acute, post-acute, and community-based care; and considers root causes to implications that affect the health of a population. Episodic care is essential to PHM. To shift from encounter-based care to person-centered episodic care, caregivers and clinical teams must consider the whole person when developing care plans.

Key "accountable care concepts" consist of:

- Nursing assessments that include community needs post-discharge
- Monitoring care for an extended period of time (i.e., 30 days)
- Following care protocols based on clinical indicators vs. volume
- Accountability and care coordination with downstream partners

- Including quality as a key factor for selection of partners
- Considering risk-based models to drive change (shared savings)
- Including behavioral health (assessment and action plans)

CASE EXAMPLE

Hospital That Shifted from an Encounter-Based Approach to Care to an Episodic, Person-Centered Approach

Hospital X identified that it discharged patients to more than 100 non-affiliated skilled nursing facilities (SNF) each month. Upon evaluation of readmission rates, 80% of patients readmitted within 30 days were from SNFs. Hospital X decided to implement a "population health" strategy for its patients discharged to SNFs. An overview of the strategy follows:

- Integrated care protocols were developed for the top discharge and readmission diagnoses.
- Select SNFs were selected as preferred providers, based on quality outcomes, including readmission rates.
- SNF staff and Hospital X discharge planning/nursing staff were trained on the use of developed care protocols.
- Nurse-to-nurse handoffs were instituted for all SNF transfers from Hospital X.
- A community integration assessment was conducted by Hospital X prior to transfer to SNF, to identify barriers to patient self-management.
- Hospital X established a care coordination committee to evaluate adherence to care protocols and identify solutions to barriers.

Hospital X experienced a reduction in its overall readmission rate by 50% in year one!

The hospital focused on the following changes:

- Bundled payment pilot program
- Looked at acute and post-acute treatment for a 30-day episode
- Coordinated with downstream/community partners
- Shifted culture from "encounter" to "episode"
- Realigned the physicians

In addition to reducing readmission, the hospital realized other outcomes, including:

- Increased patient/caregiver engagement
- A savings of $600,000 during the pre-pilot phase

Embracing Downstream Accountability

As discussed, the silo effect refers to the lack of communication and support often found in acute care episodes where providers focus primarily on their own goals, often ignoring the needs of others. Changing this focus comes by embracing a downstream accountability beyond your role, setting, and moment. In the United States, nearly 63% of all nurses work in a hospital, as shown in Figure 3.1, yet it is estimated that 70% to 90% of medical care is performed in the home setting (WHO, 2000).

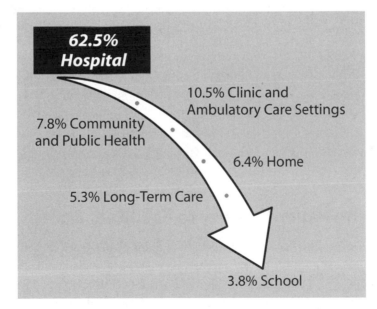

Figure 3.1   The downstream impact of a nurse role by percent of nurses working in a setting in the United States (Institute of Medicine [IOM], 2010).

As you move through the rest of the chapter, please consider the significance of your role in what happens to your patients and families after your involvement with them. The role of the nurse who shares this accountability is to:

- Look at continuum, not merely hospital stay
- Use a holistic assessment and care-management approach
- Integrate hospital and community care providers
- Evaluate outcomes for chronic-disease management
- Consider other factors (psychosocial, community) affecting population health

Downstream accountability is critical to the success of a health system approach to patient and family education regardless of region or county. No matter where you are working, it is imperative to develop a perspective and understanding forward from where you are in the health system. Your patients and their care providers will be continuing on with the goals and plans that were developed in your setting. It is vital to be accountable to formulate a feasible plan and then take the responsibility to ensure that this plan is forwarded to the providers in the next step of the care continuum, beyond the walls of your unit or facility.

Referring back to the Marshall PPFEM introduced in Chapter 1, the following tables expand on the model components and goals to provide respective health-systems strategies to achieve them. While a particular setting may have unique attributes relevant to care delivery, a common set of strategies can mitigate a majority of care coordination issues and enhance efficiency, as well as increase patient satisfaction with the care experience.

Sharing the Patient's Story to Facilitate Care

Leveraging shared knowledge about the patient and family increases consistency of care and enhances communication among and between settings. Efficient and effective care coordination and case management are keys to providing consistency and organization for this process (Adam & Corrigan, 2003). The level of oversight and foresight necessary in these roles can be very helpful to augment the patient's and family's story. As the nurse helping to form this story and share this knowledge, look to use the patient (and their family) as one of your key resources. The new health system PFE-focused paradigm encourages you to keep the next handoff in mind to ensure that your knowledge is moving with the patient on his journey through the health system.

This is a level of mindfulness that promotes the value of shared knowledge in the best interest of the patient and family. This paradigm recognizes that care delivery in your current setting can be improved when armed with important information about your patient that comes from another setting (see Table 3.2).

Table 3.2 PPFEM Health Systems Strategies to Achieve Goals of the Story	
Goals	*Health System Strategies to Achieve Goals*
Personalize healthcare experience	Assessments/screening tools
Identify health risk factors	Strong collaboration between nursing and other interdisciplinary team members
Establish communication	
Build relationship	
Meet expectations	Embedded mechanisms to ensure that patient story is accurately heard and understood
Create self-awareness of coping	

As mentioned previously in this chapter, the common thread for accountable care delivery is via partnerships using patient-centric processes, which maximizes the patient-family education experience across health systems

Connecting the Experiences on the Journey

One of the most important benefits when using a health system approach to PFE is the provision of a consistent learning experience that is coordinated among and between the various settings and systems. This is accomplished by supporting partner handoffs and by proactive planning, coordination, and communication. Health systems can successfully achieve this by realigning structure and processes within one's health system to support external handoffs (see Table 3.3).

Additionally, sharing tools used by healthcare providers not only supports consistency between settings but also creates standardized messaging and language throughout the journey. As discussed in Chapter 2, a shared mental model helps to clarify roles and responsibilities and leads to enhanced functioning of the healthcare team inclusive of the patient, family, and caregivers.

Table 3.3	**PPFEM Health System Strategies Required to Achieve a Healthcare Journey Component**	
Model Component	*Goals*	*Health System Strategies Used to Achieve Goals*
Learning to negotiate healthcare learning needs	Adhere to treatment plan Patient/family/caregiver-provider partnership Establish interprofessional collaboration	Create treatment plan Create provider care management and coordination plan Assign peer coach or mentor Assign nurse care manager
Learning to navigate the health system and processes	Learn health system Establish support plan and resources	Assign family-centered care education coach or peer mentor Assign nurse navigator Create a support plan
Learning to manage healthcare needs	Establish self-care management Prepare for transition of care Promote care coordination Modify/strengthen coping strategies Determine long-term goals	Provide classes Support groups Engage in mentoring sessions Use technology-based interaction Assign nurse care manager Perform home environmental assessment

Learning to maintain health	Maintain functional status	Assist in environmental re-design
	Prevent disease progression	Provide medical home visit program
	Promote health and wellness	Enroll in support groups
		Use nurse-lead health screening
		Engage in community partnerships
		Leverage technology-based interactions
		Assign nurse care manager

For example, Table 3.3 shows that a goal for negotiating health and care needs includes establishing a partnership among the patient, family, and/or caregivers and the healthcare providers. This is accomplished by using information from the story and by engaging everyone to develop a care management plan in which roles and responsibilities are clarified. The inclusion of the patient/family ensures a transparent communication, which leads to better working relationships, especially if expectations are clear and the story is understood.

In a health system approach, this plan is patient-centric and can be shared across the continuum. For complex care purposes, planning tools should be either shared on patient portals or become part of a health information exchange. They can also be organized for the patient and family in a binder and brought to any healthcare setting for ease of information sharing. Binder organization is a helpful tool in creating independence for the patient and caregivers. It essentially puts them in the more responsible position of ensuring that their information moves forward to the next step.

Connecting the Health System Components

Outside of hospital and clinics, the most common cross-continuum settings include home health, skilled nursing/extended care facilities, and the use of community-based and/or public health services.

Home Care

There is a range of services that comprise delivering care in the home, also known as "home care." A set of factors determines the home care portfolio (see Table 3.4). For example, home health staff augment the patient's and family's resources for a specified part of the day or day of the week (respite care) or deliver a majority of the care.

Table 3.4 Factors Impacting the Home Care Portfolio	
Patient	*Family/Caregivers*
Access and use of technology	Access and use of technology
Age/developmental level	Age/developmental level
Backup caregivers	Backup caregivers
Complexity of care	Caregiving to others
Coping skills	Coping skills
Diseases, conditions	Diseases, conditions
Employment status and job flexibility	Employment status and job flexibility
Financial resources	Financial resources
Frequency of care	Home setting
Home setting	Level of physical ability
Insurance type	Life stressors
Level of disability	Location to the patient
Mobility	Mobility
Number of medications	Rapport with patient
Social support system	Social support system
Transportation	Transportation

A home care portfolio includes one or more of the following:

- Nutrition support feeding through a tube
- Medications TPN, lipids, and antibiotics
- Therapies (OT, PT, speech)
- Nursing care (injections and changing catheters and wound dressings)
- Assistance with activities of daily living, such as a home health aide
- Medical supplies: dressing changes/wound care, feeding tubes, and ostomies
- Social or emotional support (social work)
- Pain and comfort care
- End of life/palliative care

It is important to keep in mind that opening up one's home as the setting for the delivery of care changes dynamics among the patient, family/caregiver, and healthcare providers, and more intimate partnerships form with healthcare providers. Although the home is a more cost-effective setting, it comes at a price to the caregivers and family who lose privacy and have to share caring for a loved one in exchange for support with the physical delivery of care. The decision-making authority and knowledge about the patient are not, however, lost in this partnership. Within the delicate dynamics of a home-care setting, remember to focus the patient and family involvement in care to support self-determination and move away from dependence.

With this in mind, the following should be considered when establishing a partnership with a home-health agency (HHA). Since seamless transitions of care are important, you must ensure an HHA partner:

- Has a physician who sees the patient in the setting.
- Starts care within 24 hours or less from a patient being sent home from the hospital.
- Has easy outpatient access to services and care.
- Develops processes for when things go wrong between hospital and home and at home.

The HHA must support the partnership by having information and reporting systems to:

- Identify system/process for communication and coordination.
- Integrate data for sharing of clinical information.
- Measure outcomes and reporting, including transparency of quality and safety data.

As the upstream partner, you must also address knowledge and competencies by:

- Clearly defining clinical vulnerabilities and helping to strengthen them.
- Sharing the responsibility to educate/develop your partner home-health agency.

Hospice Care

Hospice care is care provided to those with life-limiting illness. This care is usually given toward the expected end of life. It is care with a philosophy that focuses on medical care, pain management, and spiritual and emotional support. The plan of care is based on the individual's needs and desires regarding their quality of life. Hospice care also involves providing support to the patient's family members and loved ones.

An important nursing role across the life span is honoring end-of-life decisions. There is no single approach to decision-making or end-of-life practices around the world or experienced by humankind. Although it is ideal to get preferences in writing, it is not common. If someone has a written document, its focus tends to be on life quality. Younger people, those who are white, and those who come from lower socioeconomic backgrounds are not likely to have a document. Thus, is it through discussions that these preferences are uncovered. You must "ask the patient—that is, have 'the conversation'— and do so as often as necessary" (Institute of Medicine [IOM], 2015, p. 11).

Skilled Nursing Facility (SNF)/Extended Care

Skilled nursing care may be temporary or the primary setting where a person lives their life. Each situation has unique effects on the patient and the family. When an SNF or extended care setting is a continuation of a hospital stay as a transition to home, the patient (and family) sees their life, home, and belongings within their reach. Although not easy, coping with this temporary situation is manageable with the right types of support.

When the placement into an SNF or extended care is a permanent transition, early planning and preparation of patient and family are key. Remember to always return to the patient's story in order to incorporate a new healthcare experience.

For home care, the critical health-system strategy is to establish goals of care prior to transferring from one setting to the next. This also illustrates the dynamic learning state across the healthcare continuum. For example, establishing goals prior to care expectations requires the patient's and family's story to be updated. New expectations are set, new perspectives are gained. This kicks off a new learning cycle on the healthcare journey as needs are negotiated, a new setting must be navigated, and new processes learned. Once the healthcare goals are established, it may require learning new care routines or skills.

Ensure that discharge orders are clear and complete to avoid unnecessary and/or unplanned utilization of emergency department and hospital services.

Nurse-to-nurse report is critical. This is where the story and knowledge are shared for the creation of safe and effective care and plans moving forward. For patients who live in extended care or alternate care facilities, it is imperative to understand fully how a family member is involved and not make assumptions about the presence or absence of family. In addition, staff working in the hospital setting may hesitate to complete the admissions or learning needs assessments if parents or family members are not involved. This can result in an incomplete story to share and carry forward.

Like the home health setting, it is important to know the capabilities of your SNF partners, including the frequency of physician visits, types of providers delivering care, and the competency level of staff:

- An SNF and extended care setting must have physician oversight. This is a medical director who reviews orders.
- Process to monitor goal-attainment and when to transition to home or community LOS is based on clinical indicators, not on reimbursement.

Connecting Community and Public Health with the Home Health System

Community-based health settings form an important link in a "home health system." It is important to think of the home as a health system, because the patient and family draw off of a variety of resources for health and wellness needs and broker them accordingly. Community and public health connections serve as some of the most important educational resources aimed at maintaining health and wellbeing. Increasing awareness of vital resources and ways to access services strengthens the home health system (Alper, 2014).

As part of the dynamic process, early learning needs related to navigating health systems should support patient's self-determination. In other words, build the education and resources around what they have chosen for their life path. This fact presents another opportunity for nursing to draw upon strong partnerships with professionals from other disciplines, such as social work, case management, and chaplaincy, to name a few. Assessments and treatment plans from a varied group of professionals will potentially lead to the most effective post-discharge care plans, in that the broad spectrum of patient goals will form the basis of planning.

A robust, interdisciplinary treatment team that enjoys efficient and patient-centered communication will lead to the greatest success in identifying and deploying resources such as the following:

- Assistance with basic life needs, such as food, shelter, and transportation
- Intensive case management serving the patient's specific community or population
- Mental health services and support groups
- Spiritual support
- Access to financial assistance programs
- Psychosocial wraparound services
- Area agencies on aging
- Community agencies (e.g., exercise and wellness)
- Faith-based organizations

- Support groups
- Chronic disease self-management
- Telehealth resources (including tele–mental health)
- Creative arts/therapies
- Health coaching

This list of resources highlights the importance of ensuring that patients' basic life needs are met, because it is only then that patients and families will be able to fully engage in the educational process. It is possible that nurses may find themselves working in an environment that does not include access to an interdisciplinary team. In such situations, patients would benefit from nurses' efforts to identify key community partner agencies that can be deployed for assessment while the patient is still hospitalized. Such collaborations are invaluable and frequently have no associated cost to the patient or healthcare institution. An excellent first step in the process of forming partnerships is to contact the local department of social services and request consultation with a community expert on available resources.

The home learning context is enhanced when connected to other health systems, including:

- Primary care coordination
- Behavioral health assessment and treatment
- Maximized hospital-based resources (e.g., navigators, peer mentors, case managers, or health coaching)
- Integrative health modalities
- Psychosocial rehabilitation

Conclusion and Key Points

Healthcare reform is driven by rising costs and continuing care quality and safety issues. It is here to stay. Learning to manage and maintain health, for many, occurs predominately outside of the hospital or care institution. It is essential to consider the home environment and surrounding resources if you want to truly impact health and wellbeing. You must also understand that post-acute care and community integration are key for hospitals to manage populations, including behavioral health services. In addition, integrated care networks are one way that hospitals can begin the shift from volume- to value-based systems. This includes leveraging risk as a way to create alignment with physicians and downstream providers. Ultimately, the home health system may be the most important to understand, support, and strengthen.

What You Can Do to Lead Patient Education Between Health Systems

This is a time for you to reflect and recommit to upholding your professional nursing responsibility for patient and family education with a lens that transcends your immediate practice environment.

Make it a priority to:

- Review and understand your organization's processes for cross-continuum handoffs.
- Recognize the need for change and become involved in facilitating that change.
- Become involved.
- Work with your organization to develop a health system structure and process for the patient and family education. This includes establishing partnerships and knowledge sharing.

Other resources to explore:

- Prepare yourself as an effective facilitator of collaborative interprofessional relationships. The ANA has a wonderful resource on the principles of collaborative relationships: http://www.nursingworld.org/MainMenuCategories/ThePracticeofProfessionalNursing/NursingStandards/ANAPrinciples/Principles-of-Collaborative-Relationships.pdf.
- Consider advancing your practice as a Clinical Nurse Leader and explore master's degree programs that develop you as a CNL. The American Association of Colleges of Nursing (AANC) has a listing of programs: http://www.aacn.nche.edu/cnl/about/cnl-programs.
- Become a certified Clinical Nurse Leader through AANC's certification process. Check out the AANC site: http://www.aacn.nche.edu/cnl/frequently-asked-questions.

References

Adams, K., & Corrigan, J. (2003). *Priority areas for national action: Transforming health care quality.* Washington, DC: Institute of Medicine of the National Academies. Retrieved from http://www.nap.edu/openbook.php?record_id=10593

Agency for Healthcare Research and Quality (AHRQ) (September 2002). Reducing costs in the health care system: Learning from what has been done. Retrieved from http://archive.ahrq.gov/research/findings/factsheets/costs/costria/costsria.pdf

Alper, A. (2014). Roundtable on *Population Health Improvement*; Board on Population Health and Public Health Practice; Institute of Medicine. *Population health implications of the Affordable Care Act: Workshop summary.* Washington, DC: The National Academies Press. Retrieved from http://www.nap.edu/catalog.php?record_id=18546

Angelou, Maya (1998). "One isn't necessarily born with courage, but one is born with potential. Without courage, we cannot practice any other virtue with consistency. We can't be kind, true, merciful, generous, or honest." Interview in *USA TODAY* (March 5, 1988).

Assistant Secretary for Planning and Evaluation (ASPE), United States Health and Human Services. (1999). *Medicare's post-acute care benefit: Background, trends, and issues to be faced.* Retrieved from http://aspe.hhs.gov/daltcp/reports/1999/mpacb.pdf

Berenson, R., & Rich, E. (2010). U.S. approaches to physician payment: The deconstruction of primary care. *Journal of General Internal Medicine, 25*(6), 613–618.

Berwick, D., Nolan, T., & Whittington, J. (2008). The Triple Aim: Care, health, and cost. *Health Affairs, 27*(3), 759–769. doi: 10.1377/hlthaff.27.3.759

Bundled Payments for Care Improvement (BPCI) Initiative: General information. Retrieved from http://innovation.cms.gov/initiatives/bundled-payments/index.html

Centers for Medicare & Medicaid Services (CMS). (2005–2006) Key milestones in Medicare and Medicaid history, selected years: 1965–2003. *Health Care Financing Review, 27*(2). Retrieved from http://www.cms.gov/Research-Statistics-Data-and-Systems/Research/HealthCareFinancingReview/downloads/05-06Winpg1.pdf

Centers for Medicare & Medicaid Services (CMS). (2011) Bundled Payments for Care Improvement Initiative Request for Application. Retrieved from http://innovation.cms.gov/Files/x/Bundled-Payments-for-Care-Improvement-Request-for-Applications.pdf

Centers for Medicare & Medicaid Services (CMS). (2015a)

Centers for Medicare & Medicaid Services (CMS). (2015b)

Centers for Medicare & Medicaid Services (CMS). (2015c) Retrieved from http://www.cms.gov/About-CMS/Agency-Information/History/downloads/CMSProgramKeyMilestones.pdf

Healthcare.gov (2015). Accessed at https://www.healthcare.gov/glossary/value-based-purchasing-VBP

Institute for Healthcare Improvement (IHI). (2015). *The IHI Triple Aim.* Retrieved from http://www.ihi.org/engage/initiatives/TripleAim/Pages/default.aspx

Institute of Medicine (IOM). (2010). *Infographic—The future of nursing.* Retrieved from http://www.iom.edu/Reports/2010/The-Future-of-Nursing-Leading-Change-Advancing-Health/Infographic.aspx

Institute of Medicine (IOM). (2015). *Dying in America: Improving quality and honoring individual preferences near the end of life.* Committee on Approaching Death: Addressing key end of life issues; Washington, DC: National Academies Press. Retrieved from http://www.nap.edu/catalog.php?record_id=18748

Jencks, S., Williams, M., & Coleman, E. (2009). Rehospitalizations among patients in the Medicare fee-for-service program. *New England Journal of Medicine, 360,* 1418–1428 doi: 10.1056/NEJMsa0803563

Krumholz, H. (2013). Post-hospital syndrome—An acquired, transient condition of generalized risk. *New England Journal of Medicine, 368*(2), 100–102. doi: 10.1056/NEJMp1212324

Larkin, G. (1999). Ethical issues of managed care. *Emergency Medicine Clinics of North America, 17*(2), pages 397–415.

Library of Congress (1973). The Medicare Payment Advisory Commission (MedPAC). (2004). *Report to the Congress: New approaches in Medicare* (June 2004 Report). Retrieved from http://www.medpac.gov/documents/reports/chapter-7-information-technology-in-health-care-(june-2004-report).pdf

The Medicare Payment Advisory Commission (MedPAC) (2010). *Report to the Congress: Aligning incentives in Medicare* (June 2010 Report). Retrieved from http://www.medpac.gov/-documents-/reports

The Medicare Payment Advisory Commission (MedPAC) (2013). *Report to the Congress: Aligning incentives in Medicare* (March 2013 Report). Retrieved from http://medpac.gov/documents/reports/mar13_ch01.pdf?sfvrsn=0

The Medicare Payment Advisory Commission (MedPAC) (2015a). Website accessed May 31, 2015. Retrieved from http://medpac.gov/

The Medicare Payment Advisory Commission (MedPAC) (2015b). *Report to the Congress: Aligning incentives in Medicare* (March 2015 Report). Retrieved from http://medpac.gov/documents/reports/mar2015_entirereport_revised.pdf?sfvrsn=0

National Conference of State Legislators (NCSL) (May 2010). Episode-of-Care Payments. Accessed at http://www.ncsl.org/portals/1/documents/health/EPISODE_of_CARE-2010.pdf

Rau, J. (2013a, December 2). CMS targets post-acute care spending. *Healthcare Finance News.* Retrieved from http://www.healthcarefinancenews.com/news/cms-targets-post-acute-care-spending

Rau, J. (2013b, July 24). IOM finds differences in regional health spending are linked to post-hospital care and provider prices. *Kaiser Health News.* Retrieved from http://kaiserhealthnews.org/news/iom-report-on-geographic-variations-in-health-care-spending/

Shortell, S., Gillies, R., & Anderson, D. (1996). *Remaking health care in America: Building organized delivery systems.* San Francisco, CA: Jossey-Bass Inc.

United States Department of Health and Human Services (USDHHS). (2015a). *Affordable Care Act of 2010.* Retrieved from http://www.hhs.gov/healthcare/rights/index.html

United States Department of Health and Human Services (USDHHS). (2015b). *Patient Protection and Affordable Care Act (PPACA).* Retrieved from http://www.hhs.gov/healthcare/rights/law/index.html

Weintraub, A. (2010, April 6). New health law will require industry to disclose payments to physicians. *Kaiser Health News.* Retrieved from http://kaiserhealthnews.org/news/physician-payment-disclosures

Weisfeld, V., & Lustig, T. (2015). *The future of home health care: Workshop summary.* Washington, DC: National Academies Press. Retrieved from http://www.nap.edu/catalog.php?record_id=21662

World Health Organization (WHO). (2000). *The World Health Report 2000—Health systems: Improving performance.* Retrieved from http://www.who.int/whr/2000/en/

"Alone we can do so little, together we can do so much."
–Helen Keller

Interprofessional Education Strategies

Shannon Goff, MPH, RD, CNSC, CSP
Katy Peck, MA, CCC-SLP, CBIS, CLE, BCS-S
Susan Gorry, MA, CCLS

OBJECTIVES

- Discuss the key steps of developing an interprofessional curriculum.

- Explain the considerations when rolling out your program, including solutions for potential challenges.

- In collaboration with others at your healthcare setting, create one interprofessional education intervention.

Introduction

Historically, the professional system of healthcare delivery occurred separately, in silos. Perhaps this was simply because healthcare practitioners were trained in this isolating system where physicians taught physicians and nurses taught nurses. Each professional practitioner provided clinical care, insight, and education individually. Specialization of healthcare exacerbated the situation by consequently compartmentalizing communication. In a double-blind, peer-reviewed analysis, Matziou et al. summarized that errors and omissions in patients' care are at greater risk of emerging without interprofessional collaboration (2014, p. 526). Other evidence corroborates unnecessarily high error rates and poor patient outcomes due to poor health professional communication (Rice et al., 2010, p. 351). Fortunately, the healthcare system tenaciously advances affording the opportunity to revisit key concepts (Indiana State Nurses Association [ISNA], 2014, p. 8). This includes the way information is communicated among team members as well as how it is disseminated to patients.

Interprofessional Collaboration

Luckily, a revolution has been gradually building in the healthcare system: *interprofessional collaboration*. Interprofessional collaborative practice has been conceptualized as follows:

> *"...the continuous interaction of two or more professionals or disciplines, organized into a common effort to solve or explore common issues, with the best possible participation of the patient." (Ewashen, McInnis-Perry, & Murphy, 2013, p. 326)*

Interprofessional collaboration is promoted as a fundamental building block that will result in improved patient safety while delivering exceptional, more complex service (Rice et al., 2010, p. 350). Initially, this concept applied to improving communication among healthcare professionals and extracting health professionals from their silos. As a result, "interprofessional teams provide(d) a more clinically effective service, generate[d] better health outcomes, [and were] more patient-focused and innovative" and it was done at a cost savings (Mitchell et al., 2013, p. 2318). Interprofessional collaboration has also been linked to improved morale and job satisfaction.

Figure 4.1 illustrates how interprofessional collaboration for patient and family education has demonstrated success across several care disciplines and settings (Chung et al., 2012; Commodore-Mensah & Dennison Himmelfarb, 2012; Micklos, 2014; Willumsen, Ahgren, & Ødegard, 2012).

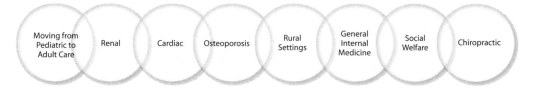

Moving from Pediatric to Adult Care • Renal • Cardiac • Osteoporosis • Rural Settings • General Internal Medicine • Social Welfare • Chiropractic

Figure 4.1   Care disciplines and settings with successful interprofessional collaboration.

Interprofessional Education

From interprofessional collaboration, *interprofessional education* was born. It has been described as follows:

> *"...when two or more professions learn with, from, and about each other to improve collaboration and the quality of care." (ISNA, 2014, p. 8)*

Traditionally, interprofessional education primarily applied to the academic setting where clinicians were jointly trained, experienced shared learning, or were taught by various disciplines and professions. One study out of England found that interprofessional education improved attitudes between medical students and their nursing colleagues (ISNA, 2014, p. 8). Within the United States, the Institute of Medicine published a report in 2003, *Health Professions Education: A Bridge to Quality,* which specifically identified that training on interdisciplinary teams should occur for all healthcare professionals (Institute of Medicine, 2003, p. 45).

A critical need exists for high-quality interprofessional communication and collaboration to help coordinate patient care in an effective manner. Collaboration is intricate and depends on all participants to actively commit to information sharing while accepting patient care responsibilities together (ISNA, 2014, p. 8). Furthermore, collaboration can be done at the grass-roots level of an organization that allows the creators of change to be the healthcare professionals (Hjalmarson, Ahgren, & Kjölsrud, 2013, p. 168). One effective, unique application of interprofessional education and collaboration redirects collaborative education from the healthcare provider as the recipient. As a result of this paradigm shift, diverse healthcare providers become the educators of a single learning need, and your patients become the recipients of interprofessional education (see Figure 4.2). Once implemented, this successful strategy will be just one of many in your toolbox. As you well know, one educational approach does not work for all, although this may work for many.

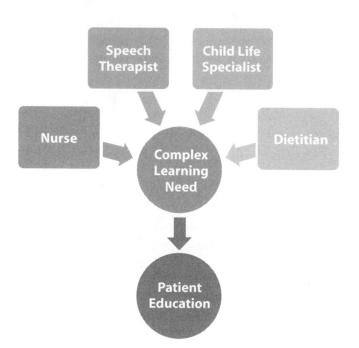

Figure 4.2 An example of the interprofessional education paradigm shift.

Interprofessional Education 2.0

This new paradigm of interprofessional education is founded on the concept that collaboration saves time, money, and confusion. This paradigm not only applies to the professionals but also to the patients and their caregivers.

> *"Integrated care gives rise to patient-centered actions including a well-planned and organized set of services or care processes, targeted at the multi-dimensional needs of an individual client or a category of patients with the same needs." (Hjalmarson et al., 2013, p. 161)*

Implementation requires an interdisciplinary team of professionals who, together, conquer a complex learning need. They work together to conduct a needs assessment, determine the best evidence-based practice, develop curriculum, integrate it into their medical system, deliver the education, and then—finally and perhaps most importantly—evaluate its effectiveness.

Implementing Interprofessional Education 2.0

This chapter guides you through creating your own interprofessional education intervention. First, you walk through building the framework and establishing the logistics of your program. Next, we lay out the approaches for curriculum development. We investigate key considerations when rolling out your program and solutions for potential challenges. Finally, we give you the tools for capturing those ever-important care outcomes.

One highly successful example of this new interprofessional education strategy will be woven throughout the chapter: gastrostomy tube (GT) class. Collaboratively conceptualized and designed, this class intended to decrease the rate of hospital readmissions related to the gastrostomy tube. The evolution of GT class is woven throughout the chapter and highlighted to help you conceptualize interprofessional education. You will learn to identify a complex learning need, recruit key players, develop curriculum, evaluate the outcome measures, and conclude for yourself the success of your intervention. The goal of this chapter is to motivate and stimulate you. It will support your efforts and direct you to improved patient safety, outcomes, and job satisfaction.

Building the Framework for Your Program

A blueprint of your plan is necessary to systematically utilize the interprofessional-education strategy. Everyday teaching efforts may transform from a process of repeating the same content across multiple daily encounters to a streamlined approach mapped for efficiency. The foundation of a collaborative approach to teaching begins with defining your topic of focus or complex learning need. Several examples of potential content areas of interprofessional education are listed in Figure 4.3. Build off of these or get your own:

- Generate ideas by contemplating content and observing areas for improvement.
- Consider the team members required to make the rooted concept for teaching take life. Ponder your audiences' needs and demographics in terms of their medical literacy, education, and receptiveness to the concepts you aim to teach. Resource availability may serve as a barrier; therefore, you must deliberately reflect on the possible hurdles early on.
- Finally, think through outreach options to extend the success of this model and meet the needs of multiple patients and families with similar education needs.

This may encompass caregivers, siblings, teachers, community healthcare workers, and peers.

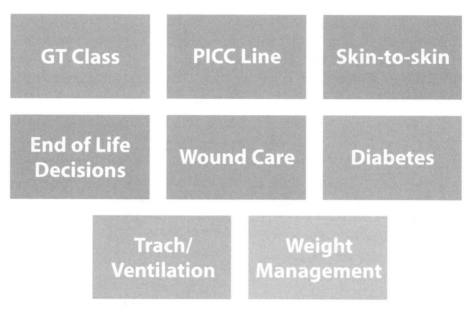

Figure 4.3   Potential content areas of interprofessional education.

Selecting a Topic

Selecting a topic area may be a challenge at first. As a healthcare professional, there is a plethora of everyday complex learning needs that could benefit from interprofessional education. Let's break down areas of need with the intent to then isolate one content area for development.

- **Family and Staff Needs:** Families and staff members may lend ideas for content areas of instruction. Questions asked repetitively during patient-family education (for clarifying purposes on behalf of the recipient) may offer a topic for immediate attention. You may witness inconsistent delivery of education between staff members, in response to high-frequency inquiries. This variability may reduce the quality of education provided between encounters. If a patient or family receives similar educational content, yet the information exchange varies between instructors, a breakdown in the education model is present.

You may ask yourself, "How can we make this less confusing for the patient or family?" And the answer may very well become your learning topic. Use these encounters during the moment of teaching as opportunities to identify recurrent educational barriers. Consider how use of an interdisciplinary education model may improve efficiency and consistency of instruction across healthcare workers.

- **Institutional Needs:** Review institution-wide statistics to prioritize specific content areas. Facility administration or your superiors may communicate the need for an interdisciplinary collaboration that lends a top-down approach to content selection and teaching. For instance, a class or instructional pathway may represent the desire to reduce return admission rates for gastronomy-tube-related concerns.

- **Streamlining Redundancy in Education:** Content identification may result from a desire to streamline education on a topic that requires input from multiple specialty divisions. For example, decision-making for tracheotomy placement is an area requiring input from multiple specialty services to offer a more comprehensive map of instruction.

Examples of common participants in content prioritization include division heads, educational leaders, caregivers, and healthcare workers in hospital-based care, outpatient facilities, specialty clinics, and skilled-nursing facilities.

Determining the Key Players

Brainstorming about your prioritized content will help to highlight associated content areas, necessary key players, and a systematic vision for rollout. For implementation to be successful, administrators must support and buy in to the program, so be sure to include them in the brainstorming process. Begin with defining the key players on your intervention team. Whether you work at a hospital, skilled nursing facility, school, or home health, you are part of a medical team. We know that working in silos as separate entities causes limitations in healthcare. This is the foundational rationale through which we strive to connect specialty ancillary services as frequently as possible to meet the multifaceted needs of the patient. Accessibility to medical team members in some settings may be a challenge, especially for home healthcare workers. Your team will need to be modified based on your work setting.

Let's explore this process through the use of a case study.

CASE EXAMPLE

PICU Nurse

Meet Kelly, a PICU nurse who experiences multiple patient encounters per month dealing with acute respiratory distress and decline due to progressive neuromuscular conditions. The acute hospitalizations force her patients and their families to decide between 'round the clock BiPAP and tracheotomy with mechanical ventilation. Kelly must guide the patient and family through a risk-benefit analysis, negotiating medical necessity, mobility, and other factors related to quality of life. During these encounters, Kelly may use visual supports to describe the changes in anatomy and physiology that her patients are experiencing. Active listening and responses to frequently asked questions take place during these exchanges between Kelly and family and physician and family.

In this example, multiple key players were not readily identified:

- Psychology
- Child-life specialist (pediatrics)
- Physical therapy
- Speech-language pathology

Consequently, this family did not receive a comprehensive insight into their options. Key players play pertinent roles as content specialists who contribute unique insight and perspective into the core curriculum development. Together, they will embody an equivalent vision and function as participants of the systematic process to improve consistency and efficiency.

Pathways: Class vs. One-on-One Teaching

Curriculum development may be a component of a larger educational pathway. As seen in the previous case example, you may want to develop content employing interprofessional education strategies to teach a class to parents and caregivers. This may be small group instruction or given to a larger audience. To offer a more standardized method of instruction based on a single content area, you may also use this model for one-on-one instruction. Regardless of whether teaching occurs in a class or one-on-one, the crucial components are standardizing the education content and training all potential educators thoroughly.

Determining Resources and Performing Cost Analysis

Now that you are aware of the tools necessary to build the foundation of an interdisciplinary education model and the benefits to both the patient and family, let's discuss factors of consideration. To make this process evolve from an idea to a systematic educational approach, take into account the current resources available. Analysis of resources and anticipated needs will help you define an efficient, cost-effective system. Essential considerations include (but are not limited to) the following items:

- Funding for staff who will be instructors
- Teaching materials
- Location
- Marketing (if class-based instruction)
- Data tracking

To justify the cost of an interprofessional gastronomy class, we simply chose to correlate the average cost of admission for a gastronomy-related readmission in 1 year to the estimated cost of the class per person (see Figure 4.4). The estimate of the gastronomy class included staff salaries, documentation time, scheduling, location, educational tools, and so on. This objective data illustrated a direct comparison between the cost of the class and the financial burden of readmissions.

As you know, there are many low-cost teaching tools used to appeal to both kinesthetic and visual learners during instruction. To promote an educational class, marketing costs can be kept low by using pre-established lines of communication such as facility-wide emails, use of communication boards, and even discussions with families. However, if the educational pathway is for one-on-one education, staff education using "super-users" may take the place of marketing efforts.

> **Definition 4.1:** *Super-Users: Staff designated to train other staff. The structure may be either unit- or organizational-specific.*

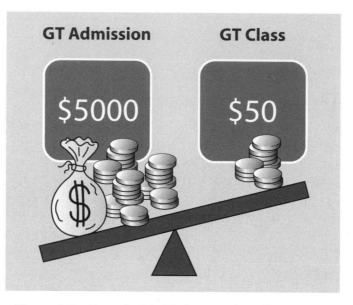

Figure 4.4   Example 4.1: GT class cost-benefit analysis.

To promote educational initiatives, management or your superiors will overlook systems and monitor using discrete accountability measures to track success. When determining whether the GT class was cost-effective or not, the accountability and success of your interdisciplinary teaching model may be as simple as using your admissions records to track recurrent admissions for one specific area before and after your intervention. The example in Figure 4.4 compares the per-person cost of a GT class taught by five core medical specialties when a patient receives a gastronomy tube to the cost of a GT-related admission. The comparison demonstrates a significant cost savings and successful program implementation.

Developing the Curriculum

After identifying your complex learning needs, the key players, the pathway of dissemination, and your budgetary needs, you will begin carefully orchestrating curriculum development. You will develop content with outcome measures in mind, relative to the target end-point in sight. Integrating the unique insight and perspectives of patients and caregivers may contribute to further enrichment of curriculum. Interconnecting curriculum development with content area for instruction requires five key factors:

- Literacy
- Cultural sensitivities
- Age
- Development
- Adaptability

Literacy

Create content commensurate with a 4th-grade reading level so it can be used across the continuum of literacy. This is challenging when you consider medical literacy in addition to the educational level of your audience, and visual aids are very helpful here (see Figure 4.5). *Medical literacy* refers to the knowledge caregivers have related to the medical aspects of their loved ones' care.

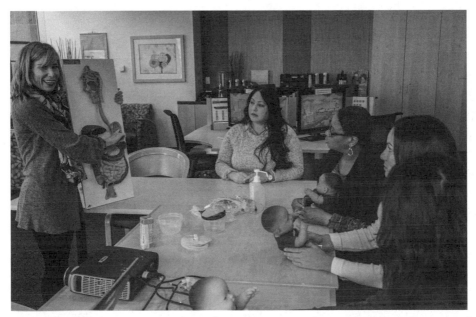

Figure 4.5   The instructor uses visual supports to supplement learning. Photograph courtesy of Christopher Stevens.

Cultural Sensitivities

Integrate participants' cultural considerations into the curriculum. For instance, when discussing the social rituals embedded in mealtime routines as part of a gastronomy class, create content general enough to apply across various cultures. All written and verbal content must reflect the continuum of prospective cultural sensitivities, with acknowledgment of potential healthcare disparities to facilitate equity.

Age

Knowing the learners' chronological and developmental age at the time of the learning opportunity is imperative. Curriculum for a set age group reflects who they are now and who they will become. The teaching moment may speak beyond this moment in time. Consider the questions that may arise after this teaching moment and provide guidance for troubleshooting. This may be done by tactically including information beyond the developmental age of the projected audience. For instance, for the pediatric GT tube class, include social implications in the occupational setting of adults. This may be an anticipated concern that may arise as a child develops or as a geriatric patient ages and therefore may be part of the original curriculum.

Development

You must also strategically formulate a content blueprint that is malleable enough to allow healthcare workers to refashion content when necessary. An individual learner's current level of socio-emotional and cognitive development may require you to adjust your delivery. This may also trigger the need to use more than one method of instruction, specific suggestions for which may be provided in your content. Integrate tools and guided practice with models to address and incorporate multiple learning styles.

Adaptability

Patients and caregivers who have developmental disabilities and/or sensory deficits require educational tools that facilitate learning based on their skillset. For example, use supplemental visual supports and models in larger sizes to compensate for individuals with visual impairments. The curriculum should be adaptable for individuals with cognitive-communication impairments. Provide notes to help the educator modify the curriculum for hands-on practice at a bedside or in a group. Illustrations and videos may also be readily accessible as part of the curriculum to serve as supplemental tools for the instructor if content delivery becomes a challenge. An individual learner may be "nonverbal," which alludes to either not being able to talk or having limitations with expressive communication that result in unsuccessful verbal communicative exchanges. If the curriculum encourages the instructor to ask participants to verbally return the information presented, probable modifications must be readily available.

Learning Needs Assessment

Begin curriculum development by discussing how to accommodate your patients' needs through a learning needs assessment. A list of constituents to address as part of your initial learning needs assessment is provided in Example 4.2.

Example 4.2: Learning Needs Assessment

Language

- How well do you speak English?
- Do you speak a language other than English?
- What is this language?
- What language do you feel most comfortable speaking with your doctor or nurse?
- In which language would you feel most comfortable reading medical or healthcare instructions?

Factors That Impact Learning and Care Management

- Are you deaf or do you have serious difficulty hearing?
- Are you blind or do you have serious difficulty seeing, even when wearing glasses?
- Do you have difficulty being understood when you talk?
- Do you have difficulty understanding others when they talk to you?
- Do you use assistive devices and tools for communication?
- Do you have serious difficulty concentrating, remembering, or making decisions?

The Caregiver Prefers Learning By

- Observation with return demonstration
- Verbal explanation
- Reading material
- Multimedia means
- Online
- Visually (pictures, drawings, and diagrams)

Reading/Math Skills Screen

- How often do you have someone help you read hospital instructions or other written material from your doctor or pharmacy?
- What is your highest grade level completed?

Readiness and Motivation to Learn About Care Management

- At this time, are you ready to learn about your child's problem and care:
  Yes   No
  If no, why not?_____

- At this time, do you want more information about what is needed to care for your child?
  Yes   No

Adapted from Hasnain-Wynia et al. (2007).

Building the Team

Curriculum development emerges through teamwork. Build your curriculum development team with a wide selection of content experts with a variety of expertise (see Figure 4.6).

Interprofessional collaboration encourages input from multiple backgrounds, areas of expertise, and perspectives. In addition, the balance between professionals and individuals involved in the patients' care heightens the wealth of information available (see Figure 4.7). When you're delegating curriculum roles, close communication during the initial stages will help you avoid replication of content and help to maintain continuity across the interprofessional collaboration.

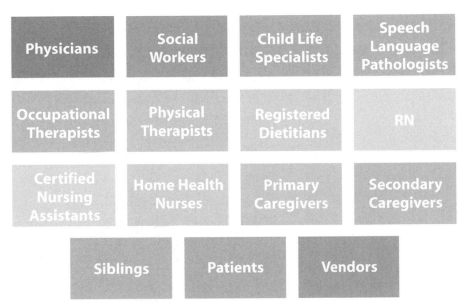

Figure 4.6   Interprofessional collaboration across disciplines.

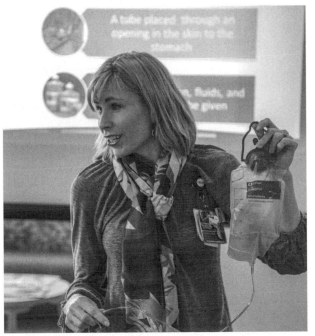

Figure 4.7   A registered dietitian describes the process of gavage feeding.
Photograph courtesy of Christopher Stevens.

Essential Considerations When Creating Your Interprofessional Education Strategies

Address Variability: There are many variables with any process. Considering different perspectives will optimize the success of your intervention, as what seems like a wonderful idea may in fact not be beneficial to your outcomes. Interdisciplinary insights easily identify challenges that you may face but also can become their own significant challenges. All perspectives and opinions need to be valued. People need to remain open to change to allow a new, improved process to develop.

Schedule for Convenience: When scheduling the intervention, prioritize the best times for your patients, their families, and caregivers. When you maintain a consistent and reliable class schedule, that empowers the community to spread the word, thereby optimizing greater participation. Assign a class coordinator to manage class logistics (see Figure 4.8).

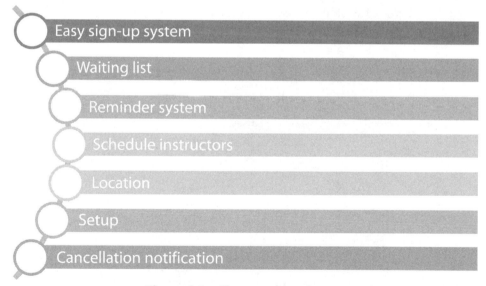

Figure 4.8   Class considerations.

Consider Staffing Needs: With an interdisciplinary team, scheduling a common time to meet becomes a difficult puzzle. Working in smaller groups or dividing into individual projects can often ease the pain. Consider the job descriptions of your interprofessional team (e.g., exempt vs. non-exempt employees) and the ability to allocate time toward the project. For example, non-exempt professionals may be able to schedule hours solely dedicated to providing education. Alternatively, exempt staff must build these activities around their scheduled patient care. If your institution has the financial support, then use it. Otherwise, utilize your cost-benefit analysis to demonstrate how time to create and implement your intervention will benefit the institution.

Provide Language and Cultural Services: Ensure that all of the patients and families can benefit from class instruction. Use interpreters and translated materials. This is imperative and necessary but also presents challenges.

Consider Varied Participation Styles: Attendees have their own style of participation (see Figure 4.9). Some are more inclined to interrupt, continue to talk, share personal examples, monopolize conversations, or possibly ask the same questions over and over again. The verbose participant may override the shy participant. In these circumstances, consider asking attendees to hold questions until the end of a section to ensure all information is provided. This prevents tangents and optimizes efficiency. If you find that the same question is being asked at multiple classes, edit your presentation to address that issue.

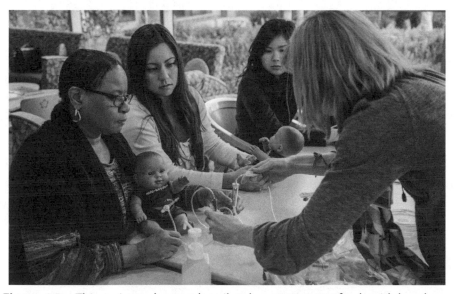

Figure 4.9   This registered nurse describes how to connect feeds with hands-on learning and guided practice. Photograph courtesy of Christopher Stevens.

Maintain Consistency: The hallmark of success lies in consistent delivery across healthcare workers. Observe your peers using the created education model as part of training before teaching.

Address Diversity: Keep in the forefront of your mind that you are interacting with audience members who come to you with varying levels of medical literacy, educational literacy, cultural and religious beliefs, gender identity, and possible cognitive impairments. You may find it to be a challenge at times to cater your word choice and inherently change the complexity of curriculum-based information to best meet the needs of your audiences. This is an example of when group instruction becomes a challenge for even the most experienced instructors. In some cultures, such as some Arabic and Hispanic groups, women look to the male in the family to make decisions. In reference to this example, these individuals tend to additionally be uncomfortable questioning authority (even asking a clarifying question), as this is not consistent with their cultural beliefs.

Be Sensitive to Stages of Grief and Loss: Your audience may consist of individuals in crisis, attempting to gather information to make informed decisions about their healthcare or that of a loved one. They are processing the emotional and social effects on their life, as well as the general physical care. Simplify instruction as much as possible and make on-the-spot adaptations when necessary. For example, during a gastronomy tube class, a caregiver may become emotional stating that their child is not ever going to be able to eat again. You should be empathetic while keeping the course on track through redirection. A sample response may be, "I realize you are receiving information that is difficult to process right now, which is why you are here to learn about gastronomy tubes. Hopefully this information will empower you to make that choice given this very difficult time."

Additionally, the geriatric population will pose new challenges pertaining to end-of-life decisions. For example, in a gastronomy tube class you may have three patients with very different experiences learning how to care for their g-tube (see Figure 4.10). As the educator, the language you choose, the education topics you focus on, and your empathy may need to be customized for each participant.

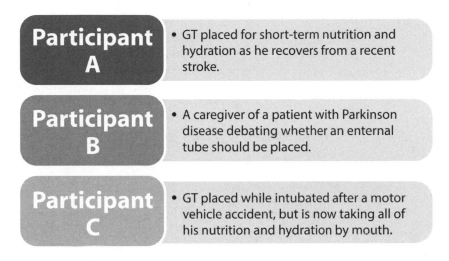

Figure 4.10   Example 4.3: Participant variability in one class.

Be Ready for Resistance to Change: The recipients of education may engage in an educational encounter with you with a preconceived opinion about the topic. They may have misconceptions gathered from television, social media, or their own imagination. They may experience learned helplessness and think, "I can't do this," even though they are completely competent and equipped to succeed. They are resistant to deviate from the reality that they have previously known and embraced. Anxieties may dissolve as a result of clarified misconceptions, opportunities to learn using a variety of teaching techniques to demystify concepts, and utilizing the audience members to bond through information exchange.

Make Room for Children: Many people have other children they are caring for who may need to come along with their parents. Sibling involvement can be a distraction for caregivers who may be juggling the role of supervisor and new learner. Depending on the siblings' age, literacy, and psychosocial adaptation, you may want to consider one-on-one teaching as opposed to group-based instruction. Siblings may not be in a phase of acceptance, and therefore, participation may be premature. In a pediatric setting, when holding group instruction, make sure you provide childcare services or prepare families so that they make the necessary alternative arrangements.

Document Appropriately: It is important to have ongoing documentation that demonstrates not only who and what was taught, but also the level of understanding and accuracy of return demonstrations. One goal could be to have an ongoing spreadsheet where this is evident, putting all education information on each topic in the same document.

Benefits of the Interprofessional Education Model

Putting into practice an interprofessional education model with standardized curriculum implementation imparts a multiplicity of benefits to staff, patients, and families:

- Preexisting curriculum (after initial creation) permits you to organize and be more comprehensive in your delivery of information.
- Using a guide illustrating and prioritizing specific talking points will significantly decrease variability in instruction between nurses and other specialists.
- Overlap of information, presentation of conflicting statements, or content delivery that confuses the patient or caregivers will decrease.
- Small group settings invite peer-to-peer sharing. Allowing a participant to teach empowers the attendees. Although the learning curve and medical literacy may vary from one to another, they can communicate on an equal platform as peers seeking similar knowledge. Peer-to-peer teaching fosters unsolicited conversations and interpersonal connections. Exchanges tend to be non-confrontational, and superiority will not be perceived among the participants.
- Consolidated learning, positive influential peer interactions, psychosocial support, and multiple nonmedical perspectives emerge.
- This education model provides participants with a hands-on experience, using all of their senses to listen, see, feel, and manipulate demonstrative models when applicable.
- Seeing that you are not alone in this scary new experience and that others are struggling or excelling at this endeavor is empowering to patients, families, and caregivers.
- The health system saves time and money, because teaching is done only once, information is not repeated, and healthcare outcomes improve.

- With the appropriate class, addressing patient, family, and caregiver questions along the way helps to see their understanding and clarify misconceptions. It also allows all in the group to benefit and learn. Seeing others ask questions may open up additional dialogue.

- Encouraging families to engage in the role of a teacher can foster unsolicited conversations and interpersonal connections. You will find that peer-to-peer learning is well received, as the platform for exchange tends to be non-confrontational. Because superiority will not be perceived among peers, neither party will feel threatened.

Evaluating the Intervention

Evaluating your intervention is imperative to demonstrating success, impact, and an effective process. Before you implement the program, reflect on the intervention process to examine potential problems such as adequacy of training and appropriateness of materials. Second, consider an impact evaluation to identify enabling and reinforcing factors. Feedback from patients, families, and healthcare workers may reveal very positive results that you might miss if you only evaluate the end result. Course evaluations typically measure impact by capturing the type of information listed here:

- Increased confidence
- Sense of pride
- Empowerment as a partner in care-giving and decision-making
- Motivation to learn more information
- Enhanced community partner knowledge

Finally, outcome measures provide statistical evidence of the intervention's impact. Carefully consider variable specificity, measurement precision, and sample size to ensure accurate results and the ability to detect change. Figure 4.11 provides some typical outcome measures.

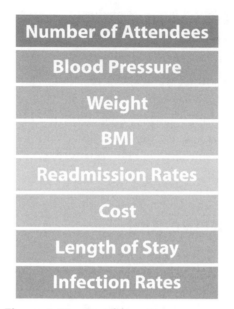

Figure 4.11   Possible outcome measures.

Conclusion and Key Points

Interprofessional education has evolved. It efficiently congregates diverse experiences, insight, and expertise to create a valued product that can potentially demonstrate fiscal success while improving the health of a multitude of patients. The healthcare system is changing. Outcomes are being prioritized and the responsibility is expanding profoundly from the physicians to all healthcare providers. In this sense, all healthcare providers are "obligated *to be* collaborative, *to know* and *to practice* collaboration to maximize health benefits and to create workplace environments that qualify as moral communities" (Ewashen et al., 2013, p. 326).

This chapter provided you with the tools to be, to know, and to practice interprofessional education. You journeyed through conceptualizing a complex learning need, building your team, designing your intervention, troubleshooting, and evaluating your efforts. Change is in your hands and you are capable of it. Recruit your team and make it happen today.

References

Chung, C. L. R., Manga, J., McGregor, M., Michailidis, C., Stavros, D., & Woodhouse, L. J. (2012). Interprofessional collaboration and turf wars: How prevalent are hidden attitudes? *The Journal of Chiropractic Education, 26*(1), 32–39.

Commodore-Mensah, Y., & Dennison Himmelfarb, C. R. (2012). Patient education strategies for hospitalized cardiovascular patients: A systematic review (structure abstract). *Journal of Cardiovascular Nursing, 27*(2), 154–174.

Ewashen, C., McInnis-Perry, G., & Murphy, N. (2013). Interprofessional collaboration-in-practice: The contested place of ethics. *Nursing Ethics, 20*(3), 325–335.

Hasnain-Wynia, R., Pierce, D., Haque, A., Hedges Greising, C., Prince, V., & Reiter, J. (2007). Health Research and Educational Trust Disparities Toolkit. hretdisparities.org accessed on 6/1/15.

Hjalmarson, H. V., Ahgren, B., & Kjölsrud, M. S. (2013). Developing interprofessional collaboration: A longitudinal case of secondary prevention for patients with osteoporosis. *Journal of Interprofessional Care, 27*(2), 161–170. doi: 10.3109/13561820.2012.724123

Indiana State Nurses Association. (2014, May/June/July). Independent study: Interprofessional collaboration: The IOM Report and more. *ISNA Bulletin*, 8–11.

Institute of Medicine (2013). Health Professions Education: A Bridge to Quality. Washington DC: National Academies Press.

Matziou, V., Viahioti, E., Perdikaris, P., Matziou, T., Megapanou, E., & Petsios, K. (2014). Physician and nursing perceptions concerning interprofessional communication and collaboration. *Journal of Interprofessional Care, 28*(6), 526–33.

Micklos, L. (2014). Transition and interprofessional collaboration in moving from pediatric to adult renal care. *Nephrology Nursing Journal, 41*(3), 311–316.

Mitchell, R., Paliadelis, P., McNeil, K., Parker, V., Giles, M., Higgins, I., … Ahrens, Y. (2013). Effective interprofessional collaboration in rural contexts: A research protocol. *Journal of Advanced Nursing, 69*(10), 2317–2326.

Rice, K., Zwarenstein, M., Conn, L. G., Kenaszchuk, C., Russel, A., & Reeves, S. (2010). An intervention to improve interprofessional collaboration and communications: A comparative qualitative study. *Journal of Interprofessional Care, 24*(4), 350–361.

Willumsen, E., Ahgren, B., Ødegard, A. (2012). A conceptual framework for assessing interorganizational integration and interprofessional collaboration. *Journal of Interprofessional Care, 26*(3), 198–204. doi: 10.3109/13561820.2011.645088

"A genuine leader is not a searcher for consensus but a molder of consensus."
—Martin Luther King, Jr., 1967

Advancing Patient and Family Education Through Interprofessional Shared Governance

Lori C. Marshall, PhD, MSN, RN
Marifel Pagkalinawan, RN, BSN, CPHON
Elsie Jalian, PharmD
Yvonne R. Gutierrez, MD, FAAP
Jennifer Ward, RN, BSN

OBJECTIVES

- Discuss the benefits of embedding the patient-family education processes into a shared governance structure.

- Explain the types of patient-family education needs that are best addressed through interprofessional collaboration.

Introduction

The idea of *shared governance* has evolved over many decades. Kanter's (1977, 1993) theory around structural empowerment is often cited for proponents of shared governance made popular by Porter-O'Grady (1996). The idea is that an individual employee will have a sense of empowerment if he feels he is part of the decision-making process in the institution. An empowered employee in turn will be more satisfied at work and hopefully more productive.

To empower an employee, we must allow him to be involved in key decisions that occur in the institution. The concept of shared governance is one in which employees are helping to make decisions. This differs from a more traditional governance structure in which management makes decisions that are then passed down to employees without much input from them.

Shared governance also brings accountability to employees. Because they are now involved in the decision-making processes for the institution, they care more about the outcome. They feel a responsibility in investing time to make the new policy or process successful. Healthcare has recognized the benefit of taking this a step further to add interprofessional collaboration, with a benefit of improved work products (Stutsky & Spence Laschinger, 2014; World Health Organization [WHO], 2010).

Interprofessional collaboration or *collaborative practice* is defined by the WHO (2010) as follows:

> *"Collaborative practice in healthcare occurs when multiple health workers from different professional backgrounds provide comprehensive services by working with patients, their families, carers, and communities to deliver the highest quality of care across settings.*
>
> *Practice includes both clinical and non-clinical health-related work, such as diagnosis, treatment, surveillance, health communications, management, and sanitation engineering."* (p. 11)

It is also important to consider the need for interprofessional collaboration to occur at a rapid pace as part of an "e-culture" (Kanter, 2001) through effective communication approaches, using communication technology connected by a shared decision-making structure (WHO, 2010). According to Kanter (2001), e-culture is a result of the Internet and the information age, which drives a new connectivity. E-culture is particularly important because it sets the stage for the types of communication tools used, strategies, and the speed at which people interact. It is a critical foundation of structural empowerment and interprofessional collaboration.

This chapter provides insights on why it is important to use an interprofessional shared-governance structure for patient and family education processes. Key partnerships and level of the structure are presented and include benefits, limitations, and tips for implementing these ideas.

Applying Shared Governance to the Healthcare System

Nursing-led, interprofessional shared governance is gaining momentum as an ideal mode of governance in large institutions, especially those that are Magnet-recognized facilities (Clavelle, Porter-O'Grady, & Drenkard, 2013). Nurses are the largest sector of the health professions and are in an amazing position to facilitate collaboration by the nature of their role. Health systems recognize that using the shared-governance model helps gain earlier buy-in from staff on new policies and procedures. As shared governance takes hold across more and more hospitals, it is vital to tap into this already existing mode of education and policy-making in order to move patient and family education (PFE) efforts forward and across a health system.

> **Definition 5.1:** *Magnet® Recognition. An organizational designation given by the American Nurses Credentialing Center (ANCC). Magnet organizations "serve as the fount of knowledge and expertise for the delivery of nursing care globally. Grounded in core Magnet principles, they will be flexible and constantly strive for discovery and innovation. They will lead the reformation of health care, the discipline of nursing, and care of the patient, family, and community."*
> *From the ANCC website: http://nursecredentialing.org/Magnet/ ProgramOverview/New-Magnet-Model*

The true essence of interprofessional shared governance is the involvement of staff—alongside physicians, pharmacists, social workers, dietitians, and other professions with leadership support—in key decisions for hospital policies and processes. There are a wide variety of models available and used successfully by many institutions, including hospitals. Most of them involve multiple committees or councils with specific jurisdiction and an overseeing/unifying committee.

You can see an example of such a structure in Figure 5.1. In a healthcare setting, each unit or work area would have a representative elected by that unit to sit on each council. The councils then have a member from each of the disciplines.

The responsibility of each member is two-fold:

- The first is to take information from the council back to their work area. This is usually accomplished by the members reporting back to their unit leadership group and/or staff meetings.
- The second responsibility is to bring concerns from their work area to the council for discussion and resolution.

Councils meet on a set schedule (monthly to bimonthly) and discuss agenda items that are brought to each council by their members or other concerned staff. The council will then vote or reach a consensus on the agenda item. Once this decision is made, it will be then disseminated to the various units of the hospital via that unit's representative on the council.

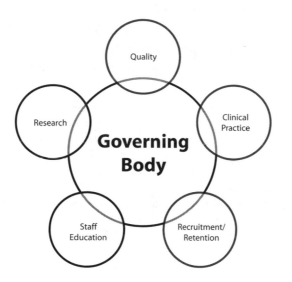

Figure 5.1   Common shared governance council or committee structure.

Optimizing PFE Exposure via Shared Governance

One model to explore is the use of an interprofessional hospital committee that includes members from all care settings and medical staff. This hospital-wide committee can broker the important relationships for success. Patient and family education endeavors should be linked to the interprofessional shared governance model if the health system has one. Ideal committees to join would be ones involving education, clinical practice, or quality. Those are the councils that usually are affected by PFE (patient-family education) initiatives.

Even if a hospital committee is present, patient and family education should be a sub-group in a relevant council such as clinical practice or staff development. It is also best to have the PFE committee chair or co-chair as members of relevant councils. There may be a few members of the PFE committee who are also council members. This solidifies the PFE group as a permanent member of the council.

Furthermore, the PFE should have a standing agenda spot at each meeting. This way, the PFE group will have the opportunity to present all their undertakings at the council meetings without having to vie for an agenda spot at each meeting. This consistent presence reiterates to the council members the importance of PFE.

Integration of the PFE into shared governance results in many benefits for the hospital and healthcare system. For one, you avoid duplication of tasks. With the presence of the PFE in the councils, there is a transparency of the committee's work. An overall awareness of the work that is being done by the PFE will prevent duplicate proposals from being drafted and worked on in the other councils.

With PFE proposals consistently present on the shared governance agendas, the work of the committee can flow through to the councils seamlessly. Without such incorporation into the council structure, PFE projects may get delayed in their appearance at council and subsequent approval for rollout.

One possible limitation to having the PFE present at council may be some delays due to disagreement on a policy or proposal from the council members. Because the council members are not members of PFE, they may not fully understand the impact the proposal may make and thus may slow down the process of the approval.

An important best-practice technique to implementing and collaborating in shared governance is to make sure the PFE members understand the process of the shared governance structure. Integrating PFE into shared governance will only be accepted and welcome if the PFE shows respect to their processes.

Health System/Hospital-Wide Approach

A system-wide approach requires connecting the PFE committee to the working groups, committees, disciplines, and councils of the organization, as shown in Figure 5.2. As a discipline, physicians should be considered critical collaborators. They are often outside of the council structure, which is why a hospital committee offers better support of the culture for this discipline.

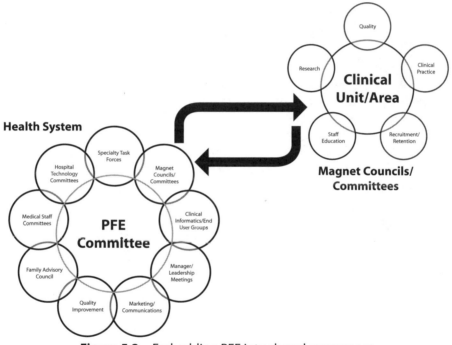

Figure 5.2   Embedding PFE into shared governance.

Physician Collaboration

Engaging physicians in interprofessional shared governance work is essential for the success of any patient-family education projects and activities. While it is safe to say all disciplines are important to a shared, collaborative governance process, you need to understand the challenges of organizing your physician colleagues and how to effectively engage them. In general, they cannot have the same sort of structure imposed on them as hospital staff. This is particularly true in academic or teaching medical centers.

"I think it has been so great to work as a multi-disciplinary team. It seems like having physicians involved in this process has helped to shape some of the education and throughput capabilities, keeping in mind our day-to-day bedside interactions with patients, which are unique to each care provider. We have an understanding of some of the challenges that we face with adequately educating our patients and preparing them for a smooth discharge. Additionally, the ability to use education tools, such as interactive patient care, to augment our bedside education /interactions with patients and families is exciting, especially surrounding important procedures, medication changes, discharge planning, and even just understanding who the doctors and nurses are that are caring for their child. Continuing physician involvement will help to educate medical staff on how to incorporate patient education in their daily practice."
–Physician at Hospital Medicine

For example, a physician's schedule may change from a clinic mode to hospital service mode and vary from month to month; thus, it is important to support flexibility with physician members on a hospital PFE committee. In addition, the physician's schedule for seeing patients may be tied to their division's productivity, making it harder to get away at certain times. The struggle for physicians is trying to balance unfunded activities with those necessary for physician funding.

Consider the following tips for working with physicians on your PFE committee:

- Provide a clear connection between the PFE work and how it will help support their role as doctors.
- Keep things short and focused; don't expect them to be available for long periods of time.
- Have a complete idea of what you need for them to do, i.e., their specific contribution.
- Keep communication concise; be sure to state what you need/want.
- Give reasonable deadlines.
- Look for ways you can support their work and patient care.

- Leverage their knowledge about hospital systems and processes.
- Give them opportunities to present and serve as leaders of their peer group.

We needed a physician champion! "One of the ways our hospital was able to actually get our PFE committee to move hospital-wide was by having a physician co-chair the committee. It was probably the most important step to making the efforts seem credible at a health system level. Through the partnership, we were not only able to be more effective in leading the work, we gained new understanding and appreciation for the physician's role—what mattered, how important they are to anything involving patient and family education. Looking back at what we've accomplished, well, it would not have been possible without their collaboration."
–Former co-chair of a hospital PFE committee

Patient Care Services Level

At the patient care services level, staff and management from all units and work areas benefit from being exposed to the same information at the same time.

Limitations may include inability of each work area to see the benefit for their or other work areas. Some council members' views may be shortsighted, preventing them from understanding the scope of the initiatives or the breadth of the outcome.

To truly execute PFE endeavors through shared governance, the PFE members must respect and utilize the structure and functioning of the shared governance model. For example, in this model, new initiatives must first be discussed in clinical practice council and then taken to education council. Initiatives that bypass the clinical practice council and go straight to the education council are rejected by that council. The council feels as if their procedure is not respected and thwarted. The members no longer feel empowered. They may feel disrespected. Initiatives that start this way are often sidelined or delayed. But those initiatives that take the proper course quickly go through the system and will have the backing of the council.

Unit/Area Level

If implemented correctly, PFE integration into collaborative governance will also be beneficial at the unit or work area level (Spence Laschinger, Read, Wilk, & Finegan, 2014) to connect clinical practice settings that care for the same patient populations. Using this broader lens enriches perspective, which makes standardization of content and shared approaches possible.

Since the feedback is bi-directional, information discussed in council will quickly be brought "home" to the unit. The council members and PFE members of the unit can together apply the new PFE process in the unit. Unit feedback about a process or issue is then brought back upwards and across the organization. In order for this to be an effective model, staff at the unit level must be aware of the importance of the PFE initiatives. Otherwise, those staff may be resistant to change and the process change proposed by the committee and council.

What Types of PFE Projects Use Shared Governance?

Many materials and endeavors from PFE can and should go through the shared governance structure. Examples of such items include the following handouts, documentation forms, anything used on an interactive care system and technology, classes, and lesson plans used for PFE.

PFE Handouts/Content

Any document that is used as a patient-education handout should use this structure. This is especially pertinent to material that will be used across the continuum of care and/or for common conditions and needs.

PFE Documentation Forms and Notes

Any document developed for the purpose of documenting patient and family education should also be taken the shared governance route. Because not all forms used to document PFE originate in a PFE committee, you would need a bi-directional process to reach all staff. Given that structure is already in place via the shared governance model, it would be best (and simplest) to employ that process.

Interactive Patient Care Content and Functionality

Content to be placed on your organization's interactive patient care system can also go through this process. Content changes may involve video education, educational and feedback functionality, and information to support transitions and transfer of care. (Refer to Chapter 7 for more details on IPC functionality.) Your hospital's interactive patient-care system must be seen as a discipline-neutral resource.

> *Physicians are invaluable partners to help spread change. "By asking MDs early on, we have been part of the process and already think-ing about how the tools can be used for education for our patients, we have been able to see how it will free up the nurses to concentrate on the important tasks that only they can do, we have been able to get our patients excited about the move and the empowerment that the system will bring, we have been able to share this idea with our colleagues around the country and they are jealous! And it brings the nurses and MDs together as partners in care—part of the same team—focused on the patient and family. This is how we should mod-el all activities in the hospital." –Physician of Pulmonary Medicine*

> *Shared governance helps when implementing a new interactive pa-tient care system. "Our hospital, from the recommendation of our PFE, decided to purchase an interactive patient care (IPC) system for our patient education and entertainment. Teaching this new system was a daunting endeavor that required a lot of coordination and plan-ning. The brunt of that task was laid on the shoulders of our PFE. The PFE in turn took the task to the education council and asked for help in educating. We got many volunteers. Together with these volunteers, we set up multiple teaching sessions that ultimately were able to dis-seminate the information to our entire staff."*
> *–PFE committee member*

Curricula and Classes

Any complex-care curricula or classes that are taught by nurses or other disciplines on every unit need to be developed using the interprofessional shared governance process. Regardless of the decentralized or centralized process used for the teaching, utilizing the shared governance model to develop it is ideal because it ensures the organization has one message being delivered to patients and family per topic. Examples of such classes are the ones taught in a Family Resource Center. The content can easily be developed using the shared governance structure.

Using a case example, let's explore how the process works when you combine all of the PFE needs using the interprofessional shared governance journey of a Central Vascular Catheter (CVC) class.

Start with the Idea

An idea might be discussed in the PFE committee and also by nurses teaching on units, the Family Resource Center (FRC), or in your infection control task force.

Identify Key Development Stakeholders

In order to roll out a comprehensive teaching tool, the team must engage and consider the following as partners:

- The bedside nurses
- CVC consultants
- Home health agencies (nurses and suppliers)
- Physicians
- Electronic documentation team
- The caregiver
- The patient

Identify the Councils/Committees Needed to Review, Approve, and Support the Efforts

It's important to identify all parties that should review and support the efforts:

- Patient and Family Education—Concept, handouts
- Clinical Practice—Content in lesson plans to match clinical practice
- Clinical Informatics User Group—Documentation
- Quality Council—Review class data and outcomes

- CVC Task Force—Experts in central line care
- Medical Staff Committees—Addressing clinical issues and link to medical practices
- Quality Improvement Groups—Connect with performance improvement initiatives.

Develop the Curriculum (Clinical Practice Council and PFE Committee)

Complex care patient and family education learning needs are best met by engaging multiple stakeholders to contribute to the formulation of a standardized curriculum. It should reflect the use of evidence-based practice that provides the best quality of education and evaluation. In the case of a CVC class, we might refer to the information from the Centers for Disease Control and Prevention (CDC) for information on central line–associated bloodstream infections (CLABSI) (2015). In determining, for example, how an institution using the shared governance model can influence the rate of its CLABSI from the patient-family education level, you would take several steps:

1. Gather data on the CLABSI rates from infection control groups or CVC groups.
2. Determine the staff who should form the initial core group of instructors to shape instruction, documentation, and evaluation. This would include experts in central line care, nurses who are directly involved in providing instruction to families in central line care, someone with experience in research and forms of evaluative process, and nurses who have previous experience in providing classes to caregivers in a Family Resource Center (FRC) setting.

Design PFE Documentation

To further expand participation in curriculum development, enjoin the experts in electronic documentation. With the electronic documentation team, design a PFE form that captures the experience of teaching and learning for each caregiver—learning needs, very specific knowledge and skills associated with PICC line flushes, method of teaching, evaluation, demonstrations, and return demonstrations—and provide a comments section. Seek the clinical practice council, as well, if the items documented provide a summary of skills and knowledge taught. Present a sample of the electronic PFE forms and seek feedback from an electronic documentation committee and clinical managers. For certain educational efforts closely tied to quality and outcomes, it is important to consider data collection needs from electronic documentation. This will be discussed in greater detail in Chapter 11. The data provides valuable information to further develop and revise the teaching plan.

For patients receiving complex care requiring a CVC, a physician might suggest adding the class as part of order sets even at new diagnosis. Adding a care plan related to CVC education would increase the bedside nurses' awareness of the need to send these families to a centralized class for education.

Create the Handouts

The language preferred by the caregiver for teaching should be determined at registration for CVC classes. Unless the educator has been certified as an interpreter in the preferred language, a form of video remote interpreting (VRI) or telephonic services can be used to assist in translating. Handouts should be made available in the languages predominant in the population of patients the facility caters to.

Update Interactive Patient Care to Support the Class

A video showing the PICC line or CVC care consistent with the practices at the facility can be loaded in the hospital's interactive patient care system or shown in the room using a DVD player. When appointments for teaching are made at intake, the staff at the FRC will ask the learner to watch the video. The goal is that repeated exposure to the process of caring for the CVC will increase retention. Furthermore, the caregivers can have the opportunity to absorb some of the material prior to the class and then also have the opportunity to ask questions at the centralized class.

Develop a Lesson Plan

Teaching central line care could initially be focused on caregivers who would need to learn the least amount of skills associated with a CVC when the patients go home. For example, they may only be required to flush a peripherally inserted central catheter (PICC line) daily. Introduce the idea to teach PICC line flushes to a patient-family education (PFE) committee to review and discuss its potential impacts and benefits. It would be worthwhile to mention a history of teaching success at a FRC. While the core group should have the primary decision on setting the standards for the curriculum, it is equally important to determine the hospital committees or councils that could judge the execution of the core group's work.

Once the PFE committee approves the idea, develop a teaching plan using current practice. Review existing bedside education and compare it to the hospital's policies and procedures. Conduct an informal interview of frontline staff regarding their insights and challenges in teaching PICC line flushes. Consult with CVC specialists.

When brainstorming for a plan of instruction, ascertain what can motivate and assist a caregiver to listen attentively to instruction and perform the skill well. You should:

- Determine the preferred language of instruction.
- Know any cultural issues that may arise.
- Let them know the importance of their role.
- Have complete materials available, including handouts.
- Provide enough time for practice, feedback, and empowerment.
- Encourage the caregiver to gain more confidence at the bedside by practicing on the patient.

Pilot Test the Curriculum

After drafting a lesson plan, the core group should perform a trial run with each other to determine the length of time for instruction and how much more time is required when interpretation is present. The trial should also include the materials listed. Find out what would drive a practical schedule to provide the class at the FRC and conduct a soft opening or pilot sessions with actual caregivers, both in English and another language. Adjust the length of class and coordinate the schedule with the FRC staff. Improve the lesson plan according to observations made in the soft opening/pilot session.

A system of shared governance demands a complex system of checks and balances and excellent communication skills. Invite CVC experts to witness a teaching session and to provide feedback. Presenting at committee or task force meetings not only advertises the program and ensures that teaching is congruent with clinical practice, but also assures them that the group is a full partner in the healthcare system's goals (in this case, decreasing CLABSI rates).

In cases where practice at the bedside or consumables such as caps or intravenous disposables change, bring these back to the team and enhance the curriculum and handouts when necessary. For example, it might be deemed necessary to emphasize oral hygiene, daily baths, and daily linen change not only while the patients are in the hospital, but also when they go home. These would need to be added to the curriculum.

Revise the Lesson Using a Rapid Feedback Process

In the journey to curriculum development and execution, you might find that other skills can be woven into the session, such as hand washing technique, clearly a key component in preventing infection and its spread. For example, educators might find it necessary to teach the S-A-S-H (saline-administration of medication/fluid-saline-heparin) technique without the administration of medication/fluid, because they are taught by the home health agencies. As well, there might be a need to expand the curriculum to include other populations with vascular access catheters such as Hickman line, Broviac, apheresis, and Med-Comp catheters. This requires new objectives to cover practicing dressing changes. Expanding classes may also mean increasing the number of classes from once a week to twice a week to provide more options for caregivers to attend the classes. Classes do not require that patients have a CVC inserted prior to the caregiver learning how to care for the CVC; for parent caregivers, it can help them make decisions about the insertion of the catheter (for example, suggesting the insertion of the PICC line on the right arm of a left-handed child).

Communicate the Plan Back Through the Councils

In order to establish accountability on the part of the educators, you must package a presentation to a quality improvement and safety council. This is also an important step to clarify roles of the bedside staff connected to the broader curriculum. The council unit representatives are expected to take this information back to their units in order to understand their role in the education process.

A PFE Policy Enhances Collaboration

A PFE policy is an invaluable tool that guides and connects interprofessional collaboration work across the health system. Not only does it spell out the philosophical underpinnings of how your health system views learners, but it also aligns the PFE activities across the organization down to the patient level.

Please be sure to check what is already in place for your health system. In some cases, a policy is in place but could use some enhancements to strengthen its role in shaping the PFE process. While a health system has a generally accepted format, there are certain categories that you should make sure are addressed in the PFE policy.

Important policy elements include:

- Have an organizational philosophy about patient and family education.
- Specify the role of patients and families as learners. How does the health system view the learners? This sets the stage for the tools, resources, and learning environment made available to them.
- Organize the policy from high level down the staff level and specify the roles and responsibilities at each level:
    - Hospital-wide PFE committee
    - Clinical or patient care
    - Unit or area level
    - Staff level
- Develop staff or countrywide mandates to support continuance education.
- Provide information on how learning needs for patients and families are determined.
- Develop core competencies of staff who provide patient and family education.
- Have a process for evaluating the effectiveness and impact of patient-education activities.
- Have a reporting mechanism for PFE activities.

Conclusion and Key Points

It is critical to acknowledge everyone's contributions to the meaningful development of patient family education. Patient-family education needs that are best addressed through interprofessional collaboration include handouts, content, curricula, and classes, including decisions regarding interactive patient care systems that support patient education. There are several important benefits of having PFE as part of a shared governance structure. Shared governance and structural empowerment are linked to nurses having higher perceptions of a culture of safety (Armstrong & Laschinger, 2006), improvement outcomes of care (Spence Laschinger, Read, Wilk, & Finegan, 2014), and greater satisfaction with work (Spence Laschinger, Almost, & Tuer-Hodes, 2003).

It is important to know the roles of each council, committee, and stakeholder in order to establish the collaborative network that helps build needed cooperation, communication, and trust (Stutsky & Spence Laschinger, 2014). A challenge of leading health system PFE efforts is aligning every aspect of the work so it supports forward motion. We recommend that you use a plan to organize the efforts. This enables your organization to create the shared mental model around the work.

References

Armstrong, K., & Laschinger, H. (2006). Structural empowerment, Magnet® hospital characteristics, and patient safety culture: Making the link. *Journal of Nursing Care Quality, 21*(2), 124–132.

Centers for Disease Control (2015). CLABSI information page. Website accessed from http://www.cdc.gov/HAI/bsi/bsi.html

Clavelle, J. T, Porter-O'Grady, T., & Drenkard, K. (2013). Structural empowerment and the nursing practice environment in Magnet® organizations. *The Journal of Nursing Administration, 43*(11), 566–573.

Kanter, R. M. (1977). *Men and women of the corporation.* New York, NY: Basic Books.

Kanter, R. M. (1993). *Men and women of the corporation* (2nd ed.). New York, NY: Basic Books.

Kanter, R. M. (2001). *Evolve: Succeeding in the digital culture of tomorrow.* Boston, MA: Harvard Business Press.

King, M. L. (1967). A genuine leader is not a searcher for consensus but a molder of consensus. Speech Domestic Impact of the War. November 1967, National Labor Leadership Assembly for Peace.

Porter-O'Grady, T. (1996). More thoughts on shared governance. *Nursing Economic$, 14*(4), 254–255.

Spence Laschinger, H., Read, E., Wilk, P., & Finegan, J. (2014). The influence of nursing unit empowerment and social capital on unit effectiveness and nurse perceptions of patient care quality. *JONA The Journal of Nursing Administration, 44*(6), 347–352.

Spence Laschinger, H., & Wong, C. (1999). Staff nurse empowerment and collective accountability: Effect on perceived productivity and self-rated work effectiveness. *Nursing Economics, 17*(6), 308–316, 351.

Spence Laschinger, H., Almost, J., & Tuer-Hodes, D. (2003). Workplace empowerment and Magnet® hospital characteristics. *Journal of Nursing Administration.* 33 (7/8). pp 410–422.

Stutsky, B. J., & Spence Laschinger, H. (2014). Development and testing of a conceptual framework for interprofessional collaborative practice. *Health and Interprofessional Practice, 2*(2), eP1066.

World Health Organization (WHO). (2010). *Framework for action on interprofessional education & collaborative practice* (WHO/ HRH/HPN/10.3). Retrieved from http://whqlibdoc.who.int/hq/2010/WHO_HRH_HPN_10.3_eng.pdf

Maximizing Knowledge-Transfer: Tools and Technology

*"Simulation is a technique—not a technology—to replace
or amplify real experiences with guided experiences that
evoke or replicate substantial aspects of the real world in
a fully interactive manner."*
–David M. Gaba, 2004, p. i2

Use of Simulation for Patient and Caregiver Education

Michelle Kelly, RN, MN, BSc, PhD
Lori C. Marshall, PhD, MSN, RN
Cathrine Fowler, RN, RM, BEd, MEd, PhD

OBJECTIVES

- Describe the most common approaches in using simulation for patient and caregiver education.

- Identify the key elements required for an effective patient or caregiver education simulation experience.

- Explain the benefits and limitations of simulation-based learning for enhancing self-care management.

- Develop a plan to implement at least one simulation approach into an existing patient- or caregiver-education curriculum to enhance efficacy for self-care management.

Introduction

Simulation as a contemporary educational technique has been enthusiastically embraced over the last 15 years within the healthcare education and practice areas. Drawing on experiences from aviation, mining, and the military, rehearsing "situations" within healthcare simulations appears to confer benefits for subsequent clinical encounters (Cook et al., 2012). Traditionally, simulation has been associated with cardiopulmonary resuscitation (CPR) and resuscitation techniques. With technological enhancements of task trainers and mannequins, the breadth and application of simulation within healthcare has expanded dramatically. Much of the research to date around the benefits of simulation has focused on skill acquisition and accuracy (e.g., surgical techniques) (Al-Kadi et al., 2012). Emerging research is adding different perspectives about how simulation: prepares students for clinical practice (McGrath, Lyng, & Hourican, 2012; Rochester et al., 2012), improves teamwork and communication skills (Frengley et al., 2011; Miller, Crandall, Washington, & McLaughlin, 2012), and influences patient outcomes (Zendejas, Brydges, Wang, & Cook, 2012). Within nursing simulations, researchers are turning their attention toward the "thinking" elements of practice to determine how such learning experiences help nurses manage subsequent clinical encounters (Lapkin, Levett-Jones, Bellchambers, & Fernandez, 2010). Further, those who practice and evaluate healthcare simulation are increasingly focusing on the educational (pedagogical) aspects to ensure an evidence-based approach to this learning strategy based on sound, relevant frameworks (Berragan, 2011; Schaefer et al., 2011).

In addition to ensuring skill competency, simulation scenarios increasingly focus on aspects of patient safety and quality care (Cant & Cooper, 2010) and the holistic elements of clinical practice (Disler, Rochester, Kelly, White, & Forber, 2013). Contemporary simulations often incorporate the use of highly technical mannequins and are carried out either within purpose-built facilities in hospital or education settings, or delivered *in situ*—for example, within an actual hospital bed space. Irrespective of the type of setting, a unique feature of simulation (when delivered according to recommended guidelines) is the *experiential* nature of the learning experience; that is, drawing from and building on existing experience and facilitating the learner to actually experience the situation (Arthur, Levett-Jones, & Kable, 2013; Jeffries, 2005). If a blend of all three perspectives of learning is harnessed into simulations—that is, cognition, emotional, and social—the impact will be greater.

In addition to triggering the cognitive or thinking aspects of practice as a scenario (or any learning activity) unfolds, well-planned simulations can elicit *emotional responses* in participants, particularly when decisions about "patient" care are time-critical (Endacott, Kidd, Chaboyer, & Edington, 2007). Illeris believes that:

> *"The character of the learning results with respect to usefulness and durability, that is in which situation it may be recalled and how long it may be remembered by the learner, will be closely connected with how the emotional dimension has been functioning as part of the entire process." (2002, p. 20)*

Such considerations for developing and delivering simulation experiences are relevant regardless of whom the participants will be. One of the elements of practice yet to be fully explored with regard to simulation is in *patient and caregiver education*. Although this could be considered within the realm of "conversation-focused" simulations—for example, mental health scenarios/developing therapeutic communication skills (Orr, Kellehear, Armari, Pearson, & Holmes, 2013) and breaking bad news (Park, Gupta, Mandani, Haubner, & Peckler, 2010)—different participants and contexts of the scenario require added considerations.

Instead of healthcare students and clinicians being the participants, *patients and care-givers* with varied experiences of the health sector and degrees of health literacy are the focus of the learning encounters. Aspects such as age, cultural background, language, and level of dexterity also need to frame the particular approach within the simulation teaching activity for positive outcomes and to help the patient/caregiver manage and maintain healthcare needs. The level of support, guidance, and feedback should be *individually tai-lored* to the cognitive and physical capacities of the caregiver and patient.

An important element of patient and caregiver education is confirming knowledge and developing or supporting self-belief for skill transfer, which are critical components to enable self-care management. Many things influence knowledge-transfer, including the fear of making mistakes or hurting a loved one when providing care. Becoming aware of caregivers' anxieties, values, beliefs, and experiences is an important first step when using a strengths-based approach for teaching clinical procedures (what have they experienced previously together, and what has helped or hindered these interactions). Creating a set-ting of mindfulness for the caregiver (and those modeling and teaching the procedures) is an equally important aspect within a step-wise approach for improving caregivers' confidence in skill technique *and* in how to engage and interact with the recipient of care. *Mindfulness* is a particular way of paying attention, to help people cope with everyday life or deal with stressors (Shapiro & Carlson, 2009). Notwithstanding these broader concepts, ensuring procedures are delivered using safe, reliable techniques is paramount in preventing infections, injury, or additional complications. Drawing from traditional healthcare simulation practices, this chapter will outline strategies to engage and enable caregivers in learning how to provide safe care to their family members using a step-wise approach. Considerations related to the age continuum of both caregivers and patients, their level of cognition, dexterity, and so on will be discussed. The chapter also addresses misperceptions on what constitutes an effective simulation task trainer for patient-family education.

Framework for Healthcare Simulations

The intent of this section is to highlight and refer you to information and literature that has shaped contemporary healthcare simulation practice. David M. Gaba, who is considered a pioneer in contemporary healthcare simulation, published a seminal piece of work in 2004 that provided a vision and range of considerations for designing, integrating, and delivering simulations (see Table 6.1). These 11 dimensions for healthcare simulation continue to shape and influence simulation practices today.

Table 6.1	Gaba's 11 Dimensions for Healthcare Simulations
Dimension	**Focus**
1	The purpose and aims of the simulation activity
2	The unit of participation in the simulation
3	The experience level of simulation participants
4	The healthcare domain in which the simulation is applied
5	The healthcare disciplines of personnel participating in the simulation
6	The type of knowledge, skill, attitudes, or behavior addressed in simulation
7	The age of the patient being simulated
8	The technology applicable or required for simulations
9	The site of simulation participation
10	The extent of direct participation in simulation
11	The feedback method accompanying simulation

Source: Gaba, 2004.

Another frequently cited work is a systematic review undertaken by Issenberg and colleagues which sought to determine the features and uses of high-fidelity medical simulations that facilitated learning (Issenberg, McGaghie, Petrusa, Gordon, & Scalese, 2005). Their examination of 109 articles that focused on effective learning resulted in a list of

10 "conditions" that contribute to effective learning in medical education. A *selection* of these conditions relevant to the context of patient/caregiver education is listed here:

- Provide feedback during the simulation learning experience.
- Ensure that learners repetitively practice skills on the task trainer.
- Ensure that learners practice with increasing levels of difficulty.
- Ensure that learning on the simulator occurs in a controlled environment.
- Provide individualized learning on the simulator task trainer.
- Clearly define outcomes and benchmarks for the learners to achieve.

These "conditions for effective learning" complement Gaba's "dimensions" (Table 6.1) and have informed simulation practices, in particular considerations about the learning environment and the range of activities related to the learner's background and level of experience. However, specific educational frameworks or pedagogy are not openly featured in either of these simulation-training frameworks. Although arising from medical origins, these 11 dimensions and 10 conditions have applications across all health disciplines, as well as for patient/caregiver education.

Concurrently, Jeffries (2005) developed a nursing-focused framework for designing, implementing, and evaluating healthcare simulations. His framework, now used internationally, features characteristics to be mindful of with regard to the teacher, student, and educational practices in the context of the simulation (specifically the design characteristics), as well as the learning outcomes.

More recently, a variety of general educational frameworks that shape simulation pedagogy has been raised in the literature to link learning with practice. Examples include: sociocultural frameworks, such as communities of practice (White, 2010); sociomaterial perspectives (Hopwood, Rooney, Boud, & Kelly, 2014); and the concept of informal learning (Hager & Halliday, 2006).

Although listing these frameworks might seem very academic, the features of and approaches to learning outlined in these frameworks aim to help educators appreciate issues to be mindful of and understand how to engage learners for best outcomes. In essence, learning is a social activity, and people learn from participating and observing others, including teachers. Also, what people gain from participating in a hands-on activity is more than what we plan, because there is often additional unanticipated, unplanned, or opportunistic learning, which has ongoing effects as people apply their newfound techniques in the context of providing patient care. It's important that you're aware of these unintended consequences when you're reconnecting with caregivers and patients on subsequent occasions, such as refresher sessions or follow-up in the home.

Terminology Used in Healthcare Simulations

Only the terminology specifically relevant to this chapter is raised in Table 6.2. More extensive glossaries in this field exist and continue to emerge as healthcare simulation matures. A short discussion follows.

Table 6.2	Terminology Used in Healthcare Simulations
Term	*Meaning*
Artifacts	Generally refer to tools, equipment, or general content within the environment that are used to perform an action (in this case a clinical procedure) or set the scene. Examples are catheters, intravenous cannulas, gastric tubes, syringes, etc.
Task trainer	A "body part" made of plastic, silicone, or another material to practice specific clinical skills or tasks. Examples include urinary catheter models, and arms to practice inserting intravenous cannulas. Another range of trainers is available in computer or virtual format, some with a "feeling" (haptic) capability to give feedback to the users when they push or pull too hard. Virtual trainers are used for inserting intravenous cannulas or performing virtual surgical techniques, for example.
Manikin/ mannequin	Usually refers to specifically designed simulators that resemble the human form. Full body mannequins are the common meaning of this term. The level of technical capability refers to the sophistication of the simulator, the control mechanisms, and the features. For example, if the mannequin is connected to a gas supply, pulses can be created and felt at representative points on the mannequin, and chest rise and fall is also possible. Speaking through the mannequin is possible using prerecorded sound files or in real time by an educator, to increase the interactions with learners and level of realism.

Fidelity	Previously, this term was used exclusively to describe the simulator (mannequin) as in the degree of realism it portrayed (high-, medium-, or low-fidelity human patient simulator). Nowadays, also describes the simulation environment or the experience. For example, a low-technology piece of equipment may be used within a highly authentic environment and with the addition of moulage (sights, sounds, and smells) to create a high-fidelity experience for the learner.
Briefing and debriefing	These terms represent the preparation and feedback phases which bookend the simulation experience. The intent is to ensure learners are entering the simulation experience with a level of context to enable engagement and realistic responses, while the debriefing phase aims to trigger reflection on simulation events through open-ended questions, guiding discussion, and reflection among the participants.
In-situ simulation	When the learning experience takes place in the actual environment such as a hospital bed, room, or unit. The benefit here is that learners have access to the exact equipment and spaces used in everyday practice rather than enacting a scenario in a different environment with different equipment.
Hybrid simulators	In this context, a task trainer or other artifact is incorporated with a person (actor, peer) so that realistic human responses and reactions are made possible, but learners are undertaking a procedure or task on the trainer. An example here is inserting a urinary catheter into a trainer placed on a treatment bed with a person seated on a stool at the head of the bed and drapes positioned as such to give the illusion the two are connected (see Roger Kneebone and colleagues' research and publications [2001; 2002; 2006] for further detail).

Healthcare Simulation Modalities and Practices

Clinical skill rehearsal with task trainers or models made from straw, clay, or plastic have been used for centuries to prepare students for practice across the health disciplines (Owen, 2012). Contemporary skills training is also possible using virtual and computer-generated simulation modalities, which allow learners to improve technique, reduce errors, and improve their times and scores (Stirling, Lewis, & Ferran, 2014). Often a final report or score sheet provides data and feedback about the user's performance.

The advent of full-bodied *mannequins* aimed to extend learning beyond "the task" to encompass more of the person in providing care (Herrmann, 2008). Improvements in technology in the last 20 years have led to more sophisticated human mannequins that can reproduce a range of physiological features and allow for vocal responses that enhance the level of interaction and realism of the experience. However technical the equipment, the critical "human factors" are not yet fully represented in the simulation mannequins. Aside from the equipment in the bed, the environment and ways of setting the scene influence the level of participant engagement and the emotional elements of learning (Hopwood et al., 2014).

Simulation Scenarios with Mannequins, Hybrids, or Task Trainers

Most often, simulation scenarios based on real patient cases (particularly adverse events) can be enacted and involve two or more participants, representing a team-based approach to patient care. Scenarios often begin with patient handover/handoff, and then events unfold that participants respond to. The scenario finishes at a defined point of time according to the learning objectives; review of performance follows, which may include audio-visual footage from the simulation. The latter element, debriefing, provides an opportunity for participants to raise questions and clarify concepts. A well-structured and facilitated debriefing can enrich the simulation learning experience (Dreifuerst, 2009; Neill & Wotton, 2011).

Role plays, which have a long history within healthcare education, have been incorporated into simulation strategies, often with actors or trained volunteers to portray the patient. These "patients" require direction about their role, their relevant health background, and the allowed scope of their responses in order to "control" the planned experience of the simulation participants and to achieve the intended learning outcomes (McAllister et al., 2013a; Nestel, Groom, Eikeland-Husebo, & O'Donnell, 2013). Benefits of using simulation role play include more authentic performances—and hence more authentic learner experiences—and genuine feedback from the "patients" about how they were treated within the encounter (Bokken, Linssen, Scherpbier, van der Vleuten, & Rethans, 2009). This format provides additional perspectives about clinical interactions not easily obtained through other training methods. In addition, rehearsing conversations about self-care before the need to undertake these in healthcare settings is beneficial. Caregivers and patients can learn how to frame discussions and respond appropriately to healthcare providers to develop or preserve a position of self-management.

A different form of role play is the use of silicone masks as with Mask-Ed (KRS simulation) to portray specific characters (McAllister, Searl, & Davis, 2013b). Described as the educator within the mask, interactions with learners who only see the "character" become more authentic as responses to student questions from the masked educator can be focused to the specific situation. This approach is essentially a blend of role play and hybrid simulation modalities. A benefit here is the human touch, which is not currently possible with other simulators or commercial mannequins.

Irrespective of the modality, core principles of how people learn, what they bring to the situation, and ways of maximizing engagement and feedback need to be incorporated into learning experiences. Recommended approaches to using healthcare simulations are applied to the patient/caregiver simulation educational strategies; they provide examples of low-tech effective interventions.

There are recommended standardized simulation practices in place for planning and delivering healthcare simulations (Arthur, Levett-Jones, & Kable, 2013; Jeffries, 2005), including staff training and certification (see the Society for Simulation in Healthcare website at the end of the chapter). However, this should not deter those who wish to extend patient and caregiver education to incorporate simulation techniques. Indeed, patient education has a long history, particularly in nursing. Key points to remember and incorporate in educational sessions have been raised earlier in this chapter. Additional aspects to consider are:

- The amount of time for the session and timing with regard to patient-discharge plans
- The ratio of learners to teachers
- The frequency of sessions, or the need to repeat session
- When to increase the level of complexity and decrease the level of support (the so-called "scaffolding of learning")
- Using clear explanations of the reasons for and importance of the procedure
- Emphasizing critical points (e.g., hand washing, storage of opened gastric feeds, and so on)

You may also want to consider that you can "layer the learning," that is, build on existing experiences and use an audio-visual clip or digital app as a reminder of key procedural points or as a "just-in-time" refresher.

Different Approaches (and Key Elements) to Caregiver Education

There are increasing requirements to provide simple to complex care in the home as a means of reducing the cost of medical care and improving outcomes for patients and their caregivers in terms of readmission to hospital (Naylor, Aiken, Kurtzman, Olds, & Hirschman, 2011). This home-care focused approach to healthcare is supported by the growing sophistication of simulations, which create significant opportunities to help caregivers learn to provide necessary medical interventions, and to troubleshoot and manage emergency events. For example, parents who have children with acute or chronic illnesses requiring at-home interventions are a key group who will potentially benefit from using simulation activities to gain confidence and competence. The use of simulations provides a supportive environment for caregivers to safely practice a skill, gain confidence, and build competence. Simulations allow caregivers to experience first-hand the application of an intervention and explore the difficulties they may encounter in their home situations. They also begin to understand the potential risks of home care and how to manage these safely. The use of simulation provides a space to voice their fears and anxieties, especially if they are concerned about inflicting pain on their loved one or if they are unsure about the patient's capacity to manage self-care; for example, self-administration of insulin injections.

The outcomes of any caregiver or patient education session are multiple. The first outcome involves the development of confidence and competence to independently and safely complete the necessary clinical task or intervention. The second outcome is to ensure the caregiver and/or patient can translate the learning into their home and family situation. The third outcome is to problem-solve unexpected issues or events that challenge the successful completion of the intervention. For example, consider a child's rapidly changing development—these changes can overwhelm a parent if not understood (So et al., 2014). Finally, address when and where the caregiver or patient can seek additional support and advice. Across the age continuum, there are several issues to consider that assist in the development, teaching, and implementation of clinical skills (see the following sidebar).

Considerations (Across the Age Continuum) for Caregiver and Patient Education

Considerations about the patient:

- Age and temperament
- Health status: acute or chronic illness or disorder
- Potential for pain/discomfort
- Potential to exacerbate illness or inflict damage mentally or physically to the patient
- Anticipated, often rapid, developmental (children) and cognitive (adults) changes

Considerations about caregivers:

- Emotional state
- Level of confidence and dexterity
- Knowledge and experience of managing the patient's illness/disorder
- Literacy level including numeracy, comprehension, and health literacy
- Cultural beliefs and requirements
- Available family and community support networks (whom they can call for help)
- Anticipated cognitive changes and physical capabilities

The Learning Approach

A crucial first step in patient and caregiver education is the development of a collaborative working relationship among the caregiver, patient, and health professional that enables knowledge and information sharing. This provides an opportunity for *co-learning,* "… joint inquiry which requires the mutual acceptance of each other's points of reference and appreciation of what each party brings to the inquiry" (Ospina, Godsoe, & Schall, 2001, p. 3). Collaboration requires developing an explorative environment that draws on the caregiver's and/or the patient's knowledge about the patient and the illness, their experience with managing the illness, and contextual factors that include the home environment and family support (Fowler, Lee, Dunston, Chiarella, & Rossiter, 2012).

Referring back to the PPFEM in Chapter 1, simulation serves as an important aspect of learning in healthcare, as shown in Figure 6.1. The mode of simulation appropriate for the patient and caregiver will depend on their previous experiences with the healthcare system. A particular educational focus may need to be around *learning to negotiate health and care needs* so the respective simulation modes, as illustrated in Figure 6.1, are recommended based on the PPFEM-HSA presented in Chapter 1. Teaching a skill or intervention to a caregiver or patient goes beyond instruction and allowing practice. It requires a much more comprehensive approach that builds the collaborative relationship. You must avoid a checklist approach to competency assessment.

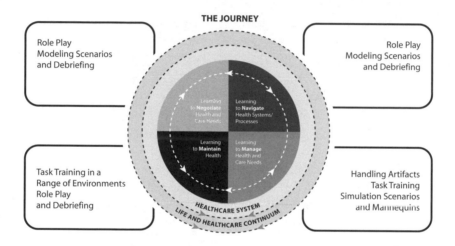

Figure 6.1   Recommended simulation modes to support patient-caregiver learning.

The first step, development of the collaborative relationship, is facilitated by using a strengths-based approach that requires the health professional to shift from being the expert to joining with the caregiver and patient to co-produce knowledge (Fowler et al., 2012). This co-productive approach creates a situation in which the caregiver's knowledge is a significant learning resource for the interaction and enables a feedback loop to check feasibility of knowledge and skills transfer into the home situation (Lee, Dunston, & Fowler, 2012). In most situations, this approach enables the successful transfer of skills-development as it builds on and extends what the caregiver and/or patient already know and can do (Mahan & Stein, 2014). It also facilitates a culturally sensitive approach and a fit with the home situation, because learners need to identify how it will apply to their lives (Mahan & Stein, 2014).

Educators frequently use a *four-step cyclical process* to support skills development when using task trainers and other forms of simulation. These steps include:

1. **Gaining the learner's attention.** This includes allowing the parent or child to handle the equipment. For children, it's important to allow them to use the artifacts in creative, often unintended ways.

2. **Explaining and demonstrating the skill.** Not only demonstrating the skill, but explaining the steps being taken. The caregiver or patient might ask questions or require additional clarification.

3. **Allowing the learner to perform the skill.** While this is occurring, avoid intervening unless asked for assistance by the caregiver or patient. If you do intervene, encourage the caregiver or patient to maintain control of the equipment and gently guide their hands. Provide verbal encouragement.

4. **Providing feedback.** It is important to focus on the caregiver's or patient's strengths. Ask the caregiver or patient how they thought they did during the practice. What do they need to focus on next time?

Steps 2 and 3 of this cycle can be repeated several times until the learner has successfully performed the task. Once the caregiver or patient has successfully performed the task, avoid asking them to keep repeating the task. Learning a new skill can be stressful and tiring, so it is better to stop when peak performance has been achieved, rather than allow a deteriorating performance to be the parent's or child's final memory of the learning session.

The choice of simulation activity, whether a task trainer or sophisticated mannequin, depends on the task or learning experience that is required. If the task is complex, breaking it down to a series of simpler tasks can support and facilitate learning and build confidence and self-belief (see Table 6.3).

Step	Simulation Technique	Intent
	Table 6.3 A Step-Wise Approach to Blending Simulation Education for Caregivers and Patients	
1	Provide exposure to and opportunities to handle artifacts.	Depending on level of willingness, provide a sample gastric tube or other catheter for a hands-on experience; helps to demystify the procedure, satisfy curiosity, and build confidence.
2	Practice on-task trainers.	Rehearse the motor skill until there is a degree of comfort and control, but not perfection. Stop once the caregiver has successfully achieved the skill rather than repeating numerous times, which can lead to performance deterioration.
3	Embed the skill into a clinical simulation scenario incorporating a mannequin.	You're widening the context to include how to approach the situation and deal with multiple aspects around an episode of care (e.g., a crying baby, interruptions, and doing the skill in different environments, etc.). This way, caregivers experience common disruptions and learn how to manage and troubleshoot these challenges or events.
4	Finally, rehearse the skill on the patient while still in a hospital/healthcare facility.	Support and guidance can be offered relative to a realistic context; the caregiver experiences the most realistic situation possible prior to undertaking the procedure in the home setting.

Interspersed between these steps is awareness of the important role that feedback and demonstration or modeling the procedure has on improving the caregiver's self-efficacy. Incorporating perspectives from teachers and caregivers who have greater expertise in the relevant field provides context and direction and improves confidence in self-belief in "mastering" the procedure at hand.

An integral part of supporting a caregiver to learn a task or intervention is ensuring that the patient management plan is achievable within the context of the caregiver's family and home life. Simulation learning activities must be framed using the right approach and be based on multiple factors, as discussed earlier in this chapter. Figure 6.2 brings to bear the interplay between the patients and their caregivers based on the patient's age/developmental level and capacity for self-care.

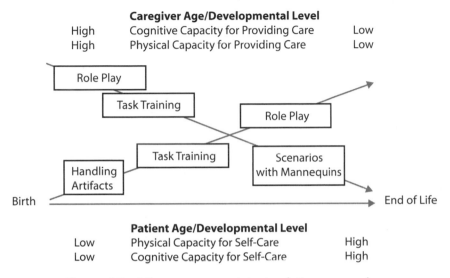

Figure 6.2   Life span-appropriate simulation approaches.

Simulation makes it possible for caregivers to learn clinical techniques or skills without having to first practice on themselves or a family member/child. This decreases the fear and concerns that can make it difficult for caregivers and patients to concentrate on and learn the required motor skills. Indeed, the motor skill is one component of learning how to, for example, deliver gastric feeding through a tube. For pediatrics and the elderly, knowing how to engage with the learning task, being attuned to the optimal times for embarking on the task, and having the confidence to manage what unfolds are equally important concepts for success. Confidence and self-belief are required for managing the requisite task in the first instance, and in the context of the home setting, to adapt their approaches to suit the environment and situation.

Use the PPFEM (Chapter 1) "story" to build a plan and assess the patient and the caregiver:

- Are there adequate physical resources available to complete the task or intervention?
- Do they have access to money to buy additional equipment?

- Does the caregiver have the support of the family to manage the task or intervention at home?

- Do they know where to and/or when to call if they have concerns about the task or intervention?

- Do they have someone to act as a backup person who can learn to do the task or intervention if they are unavailable due to illness, work, or other events?

Practical Approaches for Using Simulations for Patient and Family Education

This section provides a review of the types of simulation approaches and artifacts best used for patient and family education and explains the different ways they can be used to support self-care management. We give our insights on their benefits and limitations. You might remember using a paper plate, a doll, or an IV arm board to serve as a way to teach peripherally inserted central catheters (PICC) or central line care. For certain clinical conditions, such as asthma, the tools become more concrete: a metered dose inhaler, spacer, peak flow meter, or nebulizer can be used during training. Several types of simulation resources are used for patient and family education when they need to learn complex skills that are "under the skin" or when they need to know how to respond based on certain conditions. When you finish reading this chapter, we challenge you to improve your patient education by choosing at least one self-care management skill that you or your organization teaches that would be improved by using a simulation strategy.

Commercial Training Models

Although commercial training models such as SimMan/Baby are more commonly used when training healthcare providers, they are readily available for purchase and have benefits for patient and family education. When commercial training resources are used for task training, they require the use of artifacts to complement the simulation experience. Examples of artifacts include urinary catheters, feeding tubes, and dressing/wound care supplies.

Application considerations for commercial training models:

Benefits	Limitations	Best Uses
Readily available for purchase	Costly	CPR
No time involved in developing, designing, or making	Require replacement parts and servicing	Wound care
	Wide range of product quality	Catheter care
Provide an authentic learning experience—high fidelity		Ostomy care
	Usually only have one available, making it harder for groups	Central line care
One training model can support multiple task training needs		Nasogastric tube insertion
	Require dedicated storage space	Tracheostomy
Total body represented	Need staff with specific expertise in using computer-driven trainers or mannequins	Injections
Create context of parts of the body (trainers made for one part of the body)		Positioning
		Transfer skills (e.g., bed to chair)
Mannequins: physiologic and vocal capabilities	Must clear tubes or bladders of fluid after each use	Application of braces or hardware
	Medical tapes may not adhere to trainer or mannequin skin	Role play/scenario-based simulation
	Range of skin tones and appearance limited	
	Varied design and material quality	

Commercial training tools are used most commonly with patients and families for CPR education. Depending on volume and frequency of training, you will need two to four mannequins for a CPR class (see Figure 6.3). The standard ratio is one instructor to six learners. A health facility caring for varied age ranges will need infant, child, and adult mannequins. Also consider the population served and consider whether you need both male and female models.

Commercial training tools also serve as a resource for scenario-based training and role play, whether in individual or group learning experiences. Examples of classes where a mannequin would be used include scenarios involving an earthquake, fire safety, and first aid.

Selection considerations for commercial training models:

Durability	*Infection Control*	*Replacement Part Considerations*
Skins may tear if used for puncture	Specific cleaning requirements (replace lungs/airways)	Moderately priced
Mixed materials (cloth with plastic or rubber parts) may be hard to clean/sanitize	Use a mask with filter for air/mouth breathing	Ongoing costs need to be accounted for within a budget
Rubbery skins mark easily		Availability of parts
Need to be replaced every few years		Costs of upgrades
Cleaning chemicals can break down skins		
Predicted number of classes and people handling the mannequins		
Site for training—bed, floor, bench (setting up and packing away equipment)		
Skins weaken with exposure to fluids		

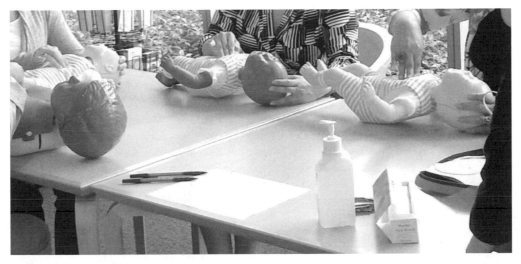

Figure 6.3   Commercial training tools include CPR manikins.
Photo courtesy of Lori Marshall.

Adapted Trainers

An adapted trainer (see Figure 6.4) involves purchasing dolls or certain types of mannequins to make task-training models. This includes "tinkering," which is modifying existing models/resources and creating a hybrid trainer for use as a standardized skills trainer.
These types of resources require the use of artifacts to complete the simulation experience.

Application considerations for adapted trainers:

Benefits	*Limitations*	*Best Use*
Readily available for purchase	Some time involved in developing, designing, or making	Complex care skills such as:
Moderately priced		Ostomy care
Provides an authentic learning experience—high fidelity	Must be shared by learners for group instruction	Central line care
	Requires more storage space	Nasogastric tube insertion
Less costly than high-end commercial sim trainer	Difficult to see the other side of the tube or line	Injections
Light and dark skin tones available	Range of skin tones and appearance	Suctioning

TIP

How to incorporate adapted trainers into a class. An adapted trainer is good for providing context or a reference point to the body, and they come in a variety of skin tones, age ranges, and genders. During the class, the RN educator can use it at the start of a class to discuss a general concept, such as a central line. The RN educator can also cover safety and securing a line or tube. Given the cost of dolls and adaptive trainers, it is not feasible to have more than one or two available for teaching. It is also important to be culturally sensitive when selecting dolls and mannequins so they represent the diversity of the patients and families at your organization. Specifically, provide varied ages and appropriate skin tones for learners.

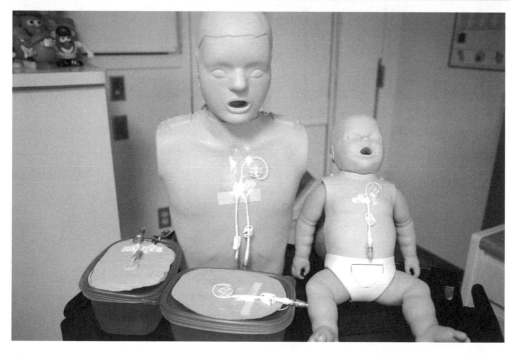

Figure 6.4   Adapted and custom-made trainers are moderately priced yet high-fidelity learning tools. Photo courtesy of Lori Marshall.

Selection considerations for adapted trainers:

Durability	Infection Control	Cost of Replacement Parts
Skins may tear when used for punctures	Wipe using manufacturer recommended solution	Moderately priced
Rubbery skins mark easily		
Need to be replaced every few years		
Cleaning chemicals can break down skins		

Custom-Made Task-Training Models

These are solely used for skills-based learning, with groups of patients and caregivers. They require the use of artifacts to complete the simulation experience (see Figure 6.5).

Application considerations for custom-made task-training models:

Benefits	Limitations	Best Use
Good for focused, complex skill learning	Require design and creativity	Tracheostomy care
Can be made in larger quantities so each learner has her own	Require time to make	Central line care
	Part of the model must be made off-premises due to the use of oven for curing clay	Gastrostomy tubes care
Authentic hands-on experience		G-J tube
		J-tube
Lower cost	Require fine and gross motor skills	Injections
		Dressing changes
		Wound irrigation

A training model costs approximately $4 and requires 1 hour of labor to make each one. These models last about 7 years or more depending on care and thickness of "skins." They require occasional remounting of the "skin" to the container. This high-fidelity learning experience is a low-cost, high-yield way to educate groups.

These task trainers permit concurrent instruction of up to 10 learners at a time. For a single focused topic class, we use the American Heart Association (2010) instructor guidelines with a training ratio of 1:6 (one RN patient-family educator to six learners). We have found that for classes such as central line care where there can be four different lines, 1:4 is better. The custom-task trainers provide opportunities to see what an artifact such as a central line or gastrostomy tube looks like on the other side. They are best used for learners 7 years of age/developmental age level and older who are able to follow directions. Learners need to manipulate artifacts; they require fine and gross motor skills.

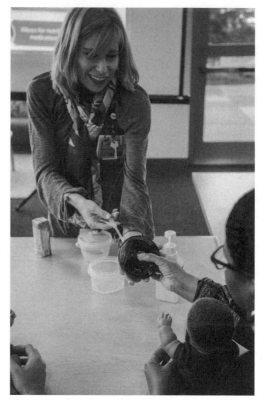

Figure 6.5   These kinds of trainers require fine and gross motor skills.
Photo courtesy of Christopher Stevens.

These task-training models were designed so that each learner had her own practice set up and could carry out all care management needs such as cleaning, dressing change, or instilling fluids as with medication administration or feeding regimes. Caregivers feel the sensation of flushing lines, unclamping a feeding line, then feeling and seeing the liquids going faster or slower with gravity.

Custom-made task-training models are constructed with non-toxic polymer clay shaped and molded to look like a gastrostomy or tracheostomy stoma with surrounding skin, or skin with an entry site for a PICC/CVC. To ensure a multicultural look, is it recommended to choose clay in several skin tones such as pink/beige, tan, and dark brown. Models with stomas can be lined with red color clay for a more realistic look. Models are mounted onto a round plastic food storage container lid that twists onto the small container. A class training set is 10 models for each of the classes.

Learners then complete each of the learning tasks using their model. The model design accommodates use of liquids on the "skin" to simulate cleaning for skin care. Additionally, because the models have a container that can be easily disconnected from the "skin," it permits practicing using liquids (water or normal saline). This is important for medication administration in both GT and central line care, as well as feeding through a gastrostomy tube.

Selection considerations for custom-made task-training models:

Durability	Infection Control	Cost of Replacement Parts
Skins lasts 7 years or longer; container may need to be replaced	Hard cured surface cleans easily with an antimicrobial wipe	Minimal cost to make additional skins or purchase containers
Skins need to be reattached to the container every few years	Containers easy to rinse and dry after use with liquids	
Resist marks		
Skins hold color over time		

Role Play with Standardized Scenarios

A well-designed role play is useful to teach critical thinking, responses, or changing perspectives. Role plays are also useful to strengthen confidence for communication exchanges among patients, caregivers, and healthcare providers (see Figure 6.6). Role play can serve as a way to develop self-awareness of emotional or physical reactions to situations.

Application considerations of role plays:

Benefits	Limitations	Best Use
Flexible to a variety of needs	Some time involved in developing, designing, or making	Recognition of symptoms or changes in the patient in order to act
Provide an authentic learning experience	May elicit strong emotional reactions	Development of coping ability and skills to navigate healthcare journey
Encourage culturally and linguistically appropriate learning	Require a quiet space to conduct so the audio is not competing with other noise	Development of skills to communicate with healthcare providers
	Less authentic when in a hospital setting	Reinforce behavior changes
	Cannot cover all possible scenarios or situations	Adopt new coping skills
		When patient is ready to go home
		First call back or follow-up appointment

Role playing with a scenario is useful for a variety of ages, starting with children 5 years of age/developmental level, depending on the context and content complexity of the role play. This is useful for teaching parenting skills, behavior management, mental health, stress reduction, and coping skills. In general, caregivers can rehearse difficult conversations with the aim of empowering them to negotiate the healthcare system and communicate with healthcare providers.

Tapping into *somatic knowledge* (knowledge beyond words) is important and becomes the key to mainstream patient education and an important program aspect. For example, consider a first-time parenting program. The instructor can talk about what it is like to walk the floor with a crying baby at 2 a.m. This is not like the real feeling of being awakened during sleep and hearing the crying. To gain the emotional reaction and bodily response, a better approach is to use an audio recording of a crying baby while holding a baby mannequin. A commercial version is available; see Figure 6.7.

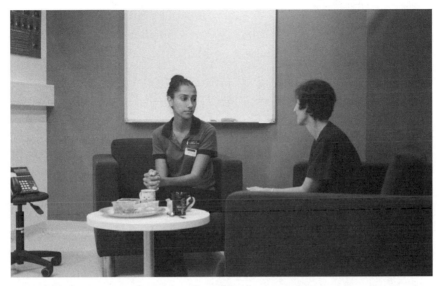

Figure 6.6   Role plays, as illustrated here, can include conversations with a clinician and a student nurse. Photo courtesy of Michelle Kelly.

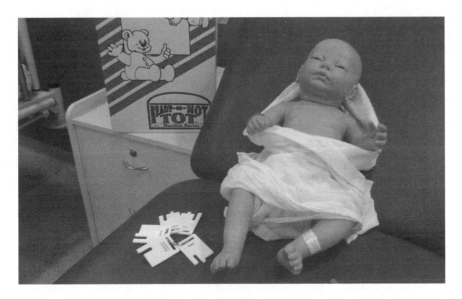

Figure 6.7   *Ready or Not Tot*: Lifelike baby with a range of vocal keys that insert into the toy's back. The baby can be happy, can cry continuously, etc.
Photo courtesy of Michelle Kelly.

It is also possible to use a crying sim baby as part of a group learning experience. For example, ask the parent holding the baby to pass it to another parent. As each parent provides a strategy, continue to pass the sim baby around the group. Participants will identify a much greater number of strategies.

Once the sim baby is no longer crying, ask the parents:

- What might the baby have experienced during this period of crying? How might the baby have felt? What needs might the baby be trying to tell them? What strategies identified during this activity would the parents feel comfortable using?

- How did it feel to hold this crying baby and not be able to settle or calm it? What might be some actions that parents take when frightened and exhausted that could be dangerous for a baby? What might they need as a parent if their baby had a prolonged period of crying?

As mentioned previously in the chapter, role play can be effective to help educate patients and families on navigating communication exchanges and interactions with healthcare providers. When debriefing is added to role play, it can support learning aimed at maintaining health and wellbeing by permitting the learner to try out approaches and adopt new behaviors.

Conclusion and Key Points

As a nurse, you should consider adding simulation to your patient-family education routines. Simulation can serve as an important foundation for knowledge-transfer and for helping to develop self-regulated learners. Task-training devices do not need to be expensive to be effective. They need to have a design relevant to the skill being taught and the flexibility to accommodate a spectrum of care needs related to a topic. Many believe that a high-fidelity/high-impact learning experience can yield better outcomes, reduce readmissions, and create greater caregiver-awareness of how care should be delivered. The challenge is to now demonstrate and prove these assumptions.

Websites

Simulation professional groups:

Society for Simulation in Healthcare (SSH): http://www.ssih.org/

International Nursing Association for Clinical Simulation and Learning (INACSL): http://www.inacsl.org/i4a/pages/index.cfm?pageid=1

Australian Society for Simulation in Healthcare (ASSH), a specialist community of Simulation Australasia:
http://www.simulationaustralasia.com/divisions/about-assh

Society in Europe for Simulation Applied to Medicine (SESAM):
http://www.sesam-web.org/

International Network for Simulation-based Pediatric Innovation, Research, and Education (INSPIRE): http://inspiresim.com/

Global Network for Simulation in Healthcare:
http://139.173.32.21:8080/ (under construction)

http://www.ssih.org/News/articleType/ArticleView/articleId/1590/

References

Al-Kadi, A. S., Donnon, T., Paolucci, E. O., Mitchell, P., Debru, E., & Church, N. (2012). The effect of simulation in improving students' performance in laparoscopic surgery: A meta-analysis. *Surgical Endoscopy and Other Interventional Techniques, (26)*11, 3215–24.

American Heart Association (AHA) (2010). Basic Life Support (BLS) For Healthcare Providers Instructor Manual. American Heart Association.

Arthur, C., Levett-Jones, T., & Kable, A. (2013). Quality indicators for the design and implementation of simulation experiences: A Delphi study. *Nurse Education Today, 33*(11), 1357–1361. doi: 10.1016/j.nedt.2012.07.012

Berragan, L. (2011). Simulation: An effective pedagogical approach for nursing? *Nurse Education Today, 31*(7), 660–663. doi: 10.1016/j.nedt.2011.01.019

Bokken, L., Linssen, T., Scherpbier, A., van der Vleuten, C., & Rethans, J. (2009). Feedback by simulated patients in undergraduate medical education: A systematic review of the literature. *Medical Education, 43*(3), 202–210. doi: 10.1111/j.1365-2923.2008.03268.x

Cant, R., & Cooper, S. (2010). Simulation-based learning in nurse education: Systematic review. *Journal of Advanced Nursing, 66*(1), 3–15. doi: 10.1111/j.1365-2648.2009.05240.x

Cook, D. A., Brydges, R., Hamstra, S., Zendejas, B., Szostek, J., Wang, A., ... Hatala, R. (2012). Comparative effectiveness of technology-enhanced simulation versus other instructional methods: A systematic review and meta-analysis. *Simulation in Healthcare, 7*(5), 308–320.

Disler, R., Rochester, S., Kelly, M. A., White, H., & Forber, J. (2013). Delivering a large cohort simulation—Beginning nursing students' experience: A pre-post survey. *Journal of Nursing Education and Practice, 3*(12), 133–142. doi: 10.5430/jnep.v3n12p133

Dreifuerst, K. T. (2009). The essentials of debriefing in simulation and learning: A concept analysis. *Nursing Education Perspectives, 30*(2), 109–114. doi: 10.1043/1536-5026-030.002.0109

Endacott, R., Kidd, T., Chaboyer, W., & Edington, J. (2007). Recognition and communication of patient deterioration in a regional hospital: A multi-methods study. *Australian Critical Care, 20*(3), 100–105. doi: 10.1016/j.aucc.2007.05.002

Fowler, C., Lee, A., Dunston, R., Chiarella, M., & Rossiter, C. (2012). Co-producing parenting practice: Learning how to do child and family health nursing differently. *Australian Journal of Child and Family Health Nursing, 9*(1), 7–11.

Frengley, R., Weller, J., Torrie, J., Dzendrowskyj, P., Yee, B., Paul, A., … Henderson, K. (2011). The effect of a simulation-based training intervention on the performance of established critical care unit teams. *Critical Care Medicine, 39*(12), 2605–2611. doi: 10.1097/CCM.0b013e3182282a98

Gaba, D. (2004). The future vision of simulation in healthcare. *Quality and Safety in Health Care, 13*(S1), i2–i10. doi: 10.1136/qshc.2004.009878

Hager, P., & Halliday, J. (2006). *Recovering informal learning: Wisdom, judgement and community* (Vol. 7). Dordrecht, Netherlands: Springer.

Herrmann, E. (2008). *Remembering Mrs Chase.* Retrieved from NSNA website: http://www.nsna.org/Portals/0/Skins/NSNA/pdf/Imprint_FebMar08_Feat_MrsChase.pdf

Hopwood, N., Rooney, D., Boud, D., & Kelly, M. A. (2014). Simulation in higher education: A sociomaterial view. *Educational Philosophy and Theory.* Advance online publication. doi:10.1080/00131857.2014.971403

Illeris, K. (2002). *The three dimensions of learning: Contemporary learning theory in the tension field between the cognitive, the emotional and the social.* Roskilde, Denmark: Roskilde University Press.

Issenberg, S. B., McGaghie, W., Petrusa, E., Gordon, D., & Scalese, R. J. (2005). Features and uses of high-fidelity medical simulations that lead to effective learning: A BEME systematic review. *Medical Teacher, 27*(1), 10–28. doi: 10.1080/01421590500046924

Jeffries, P. (2005). A framework for designing, implementing, and evaluating simulators used as teaching strategies in nursing. *Nursing Education Perspectives, 26*(2), 96–103.

Kneebone, R., & ApSimon, D. (2001). Surgical skills training: Simulation and multimedia combined. *Medical Education, 35*(9), 909–915. doi: 10.1046/j.1365-2923.2001.00997.x

Kneebone, R., Kidd, J., Nestel, D., Asvall, S., Paraskeva, P., & Darzi, A. (2002). An innovative model for teaching and learning clinical procedures. *Medical Education, 36*(7), 628–634.

Kneebone, R., Nestel, D., Yadollahi, F., Brown, R., Nolan, C., Durack, J., … Darzi, A. (2006). Assessing procedural skills in context: Exploring the feasibility of an Integrated Procedural Performance Instrument (IPPI). *Medical Education, 40*(11), 1105–1114.

Lapkin, S., Levett-Jones, T., Bellchambers, H., & Fernandez, R. (2010). Effectiveness of patient simulation manikins in teaching clinical reasoning skills to undergraduate nursing students: A systematic review. *Clinical Simulation in Nursing, 6*(6), e207-e22.

Lee, A., Dunston, R., & Fowler, C. (2012). Seeing is believing: An embodied pedagogy of "doing partnership" in child and family health. In P. Hager, A. Lee, & A. Reich (Eds.), *Practice, learning and change: Practice-theory perspectives on professional learning* (pp. 267–276). Heidelberg, Germany: Springer.

Mahan, J., & Stein, D. (2014). Teaching adults—Best practices that leverage the emerging understanding of the neurobiology of learning. *Current Problems in Pediatric and Adolescent Health Care, 44*, 141–149.

McAllister, M., Levett-Jones, T., Downer, T., Harrison, P., Harvey, T., Reid-Searl, K., … Calleja, P. (2013a). Snapshots of simulation: Creative strategies used by Australian educators to enhance simulation learning experiences for nursing students. *Nurse Education in Practice, 13*(6), 567–572. doi:10.1016/j.nepr.2013.04.010

McAllister, M., Searl, K. R., & Davis, S. (2013b). Who is that masked educator? Deconstructing the teaching and learning processes of an innovative humanistic simulation technique. *Nurse Education Today, 33*(12), 1453–1458. doi:10.1016/j.nedt.2013.06.015

McGrath, M., Lyng, C., & Hourican, S. (2012). From the simulation lab to the ward: Preparing 4th year nursing students for the role of staff nurse. *Clinical Simulation in Nursing, 8*(7), e265–e72.

Miller, D., Crandall, C., Washington, C., & McLaughlin, S. (2012). Improving teamwork and communication in trauma care through in situ simulations. *Academic Emergency Medicine, 19*(5), 608–12.

Naylor, M, Aiken, L., Kurtzman, E., Olds, D., & Hirschman, K. (2011). The importance of transitional care in achieving health reform. *Health Affairs, 30*(4), 746–754.

Neill, M., & Wotton, K. (2011). High-fidelity simulation debriefing in nursing education: A literature review. *Clinical Simulation in Nursing, 7*(5), e161–e168.

Nestel, D., Groom, J., Eikeland-Husebo, S., & O'Donnell, J. (2011). Simulation for learning and teaching procedural skills: The state of the science. *Simulation in Healthcare, 6*(7), S10–S13. doi: 10.1097/SIH.0b013e318227ce96

Orr, F., Kellehear, K., Armari, E., Pearson, A., & Holmes, D. (2013). The distress of voice-hearing: The use of simulation for awareness, understanding and communication skill development in undergraduate nursing education. *Nurse Education in Practice, 13*(6), 529–535. doi:10.1016/j.nepr.2013.03.023

Ospina, S., Godsoe, B., & Schall, E. (2001, November). Co-producing knowledge: Practitioners and scholars working together to understand leadership. *International Leadership Association Conference*. Miami, FL.

Owen, H. (2012). Early use of simulation in medical education. *Simulation in Healthcare, 7*(2), 102–16.

Park, I., Gupta, A., Mandani, K., Haubner, L., & Peckler, B. (2010). Breaking bad news education for emergency medicine residents: A novel training module using simulation with the SPIKES protocol. *Journal of Emergencies, Trauma & Shock, 3*(4), 385–388. doi: 10.4103/0974-2700.70760

Rochester, S., Kelly, M. A., Disler, R., White, H., Forber, J., & Matiuk, S. (2012). Providing simulation experiences for large cohorts of 1st year nursing students: Evaluating quality and impact. *Collegian, 19*(3), 117–24.

Schaefer, J., Vanderbilt, A., Cason, C., Bauman, E., Glavin, R., Lee, F., & Navedo, D. (2011). Literature review: Instructional design and pedagogy science in healthcare simulation. *Simulation in Healthcare, 6*(7), S30–S41. doi:10.1097/SIH.0b013e31822237b4

Shapiro, S., & Carlson, L (2009). *The art and science of mindfulness: Integrating mindfulness into psychology and the helping professions.* Washington, DC: American Psychological Association. Retrieved from http://dx.doi.org/10.1037/11885-000

So, S., Rogers, A., Patterson, C., Drew, W., Maxwell, J., Darch, J., … Pollock-BarZiv, S. (2014). Parental experiences of a developmentally focused care program for infants and children during prolonged hospitalization. *Journal of Child Health Care, 18*(2), 156–167.

Stirling, E., Lewis, T., & Ferran, N. (2014). Surgical skills simulation in trauma and orthopaedic training. *Journal of Orthopaedic Surgery and Research, 9*(126). doi: 10.1186/s13018-014-0126-z

White, C. (2010). A socio-cultural approach to learning in the practice setting. *Nurse Education Today, 30*(8), 794–797. doi: 10.1016/j.nedt.2010.02.002

Zendejas, B., Brydges, R., Wang, A., & Cook, D. (2012). Patient outcomes in simulation-based medical education: A systematic review. *Journal of General Internal Medicine, 28*(8), 1078–89. doi:10.1007/s11606-012-2264-5

Supporting Knowledge-Transfer Through Interactive Patient Care

David Wright, MPH
Lori C. Marshall, PhD, MSN, RN
Ellen Swartwout, PhD, RN, NEA-BC

OBJECTIVES

- Discuss current challenges in patient education.
- Explain the role of education in activating patients to manage and maintain desired health status and advance patient-care outcomes.
- Describe the role of technology in expanding the utility and effectiveness of patient education.

Introduction

"There isn't enough time." "The patient is too old, too sick to understand." "I don't have the resources." "How do I know the education I provide is effective?"

These are common concerns and questions expressed today by nurses, especially when it comes to the need to support patient education. Despite the uncertainties and the challenges you face in education, its role could not be any more important today, particularly as our healthcare system transitions from an episodic treatment to a population health management model of healthcare delivery and management.

Inpatient admissions are declining and length of stay is shorter, making the need for education greater (Weiss & Elixhauser, 2014). The cost of care continues to rise, resources and providers' time is limited, but the demand for longitudinal care management is increasing as our population ages and the prevalence of chronic disease grows (Ernst & Young, 2014; The Advisory Board Company, 2013).

Few will challenge that our current healthcare delivery model is unsustainable. Transformation must be more than a buzzword or term used in our strategic plans. The transformation we need will occur when the care-management model moves the locus of control for health status to the health consumer, to the patient and her family. Patients supported by their families and caregivers must take greater interest and responsibility in understanding, managing, and controlling their health in order to stay ahead of the impending trends.

This shift in control begins with being more effective at engaging, empowering, and activating patients by educating them. Nursing professionals must use education as a tool and core component in care management. Education is a dynamic resource that is measureable and configurable based on what you know about the patient and his family. As a nursing professional, you are often responsible for selecting the patient-family education approach.

This chapter will deepen your understanding of patient engagement and interactive patient care concepts and provide examples of how patient engagement tools can enrich the quality and consistency of the education you provide. Additionally, it will provide examples on how to leverage technology for promoting the development of self-regulated learners, which leads to greater involvement in care decisions and participation in care.

The Current State of Education

For years, education has been something we get to if there is time or we treat it as a passive activity, often done through printed teaching materials provided to the patient. This paradigm exists regardless of the care setting. An increasing number of healthcare systems are employing educators to advance the quality and reach of patient education. The question is whether this approach is scalable, cost-efficient, and effective in creating patient understanding of their condition, medications, care plan, and lifestyle changes needed to yield the outcomes you seek.

All will agree that when patients complete and understand the education they are given, they are prepared and empowered to succeed in their journey to heal and improve their health status. The question today must be: Does the education the patients receive result in heightened adherence with their care plan and motivate them to manage and maintain their own health?

Patient engagement and, in particular, activation is critical to transforming the cost and the outcomes of our current care delivery methods. Patient engagement requires that we empower them with the tools and resources to enable them to accept and keep the responsibility to own and manage their health. We cannot properly empower patients without patient-specific education that is demonstrably understood through teach-back methods. The patients must respond to what they have learned.

The Challenge Ahead in Empowering and Educating Patients

Healthcare organizations are tasked with using different strategies to achieve the *Triple Aim* of healthcare (The Institute for Healthcare Improvement [IHI], 2015; Berwick, 2008). Experts consider patient and family engagement to be of great importance to improving these healthcare outcomes. The Agency for Healthcare Research and Quality (AHRQ) reported that research shows that more engaged patients can lead to better outcomes in quality and safety (AHRQ, 2013).

> **Definition 7.1:** *IHI Triple Aim. "A framework developed by the Institute for Healthcare Improvement that describes an approach to optimizing health system performance. It is IHI's belief that new designs must be developed to simultaneously pursue three dimensions, which we call the "Triple Aim":*
>
> > *Improving the patient experience of care (including quality and satisfaction)*
> >
> > *Improving the health of populations*
> >
> > *Reducing the per capita cost of health care (IHI, 2015)*

In a study that evaluated the patient activation measure (Hibbard & Greene, 2013), key outcomes included:

- Reduction in average length of stay
- Increased compliance with treatment plans
- Lower lab values for patients with diabetes or high cholesterol

The nurse holds a prominent role in actively involving patients and their families with their care (Sofaer & Schumann, 2013). Nurses have the ability to empower, engage, and activate patients to become partners in care and ultimately be a part of their care outside of the healthcare setting (Pelletier & Stichler, 2014). Patient and family education is one of the best resources nurses and the healthcare team has to empower patients with the knowledge and tools necessary to be effectively involved in their care and to improve self-management of their condition or health status.

The Collaborative Approach

Effective patient and family engagement requires a shift in the role of the nurse and healthcare team from unidirectional care providers to a more collaborative approach with patients (Coulter, 2012). A greater focus on patient and family engagement necessitates shared decision-making among patients, families, and clinicians. Because collaboration is crucial to shared decision-making among patients, families, and clinicians, it is necessary to first understand what is important to the patient, and then use that knowledge to collaboratively determine the next steps in their healthcare journey (Elwyn et al., 2013).

A more collaborative approach to care management requires time and attention from the nurse and healthcare team when resources are limited and patients have higher acuity, shorter stays, and greater expectations. When the patient and family have a solid understanding of their condition and care plan, the time spent by the care team with the patient is more efficient and effective. Therefore, it is important to leverage education to establish a baseline of patient understanding regarding their condition and care plan. With that in place, the nurse's time with the patient is spent evaluating comprehension and competency and reinforcing what is important for the patient and family to know and use in self-care management. A greater proportion of the nurse's time with the patient is focused on shared decision-making and care planning, based upon what is learned about the patient's level of understanding from their education and their resulting level of activation.

Effective patient education is fundamental to patient and family activation. It is also a resource used by care providers to optimize their interaction and time spent with the patient and their family. The key is to ensure that the educational approach is specific, delivered in a way and at a time best received by the patient, and structured to ensure maximum comprehension and retention.

Delivering effective education begins with a collaborative assessment of the patient's readiness to learn and the most effective learning style and time for each patient. Before completing that assessment, however, take the time to understand the patient's readiness and likelihood to engage in their care. The more likely and able the patient and/or family is to engage in their care, the more ready they will be to receive and comprehend the education needed to establish a baseline of understanding about their condition and care plan. You need advanced skills and corresponding tools, such as the Patient Activation Measure (PAM) (Hibbard Stockard, Mahoney, & Tusler, 2004), to first assess the patient's activation level and readiness to learn, and then to leverage that knowledge in developing a care plan that is specific to the patient, their needs and goals (Hibbard et al., 2004).

Addressing Patient Diversity Through Effective Education Planning

The role of education in care delivery and management is more important now than ever before. The challenge is to understand and accommodate for the many different factors that influence the effect of education on patient and family engagement. Cultural diversity, socioeconomic influences, and increased demands on staff make education planning and delivery more challenging. Healthcare teams face many barriers to effective patient-family education, including access to appropriate content, the time to provide the education and assess comprehension, and nursing experience and skill in effectively planning and delivering education. Education is a continual process requiring ongoing planning, evaluation, and adaptation strategies based on how the patient responds. It requires strong critical thinking skills to assess the best method, approach, timing, and content for teaching and preparing patients to care for themselves based on what you know and have learned about the patient. To effectively educate, you must understand the patient's ability to comprehend what is taught and his ability to use that knowledge to manage their own health status.

Patient and family engagement begins with patient education. The challenge for nurses and healthcare teams is to determine how to provide the education in the most efficient and effective way. Technology can be a highly effective conduit to help engage patients through education and self-management activities to enhance health.

Delivering Interactive Patient Care: The "How To" of Patient Engagement

The words "patient engagement" have become a central theme in conversations about transformative work among most healthcare providers. Although it is a common point of discussion, many report a lack of strategy or methodology to effectively engage their patients.

> *"Interactive patient care (IPC) has emerged as a care-delivery method that effectively engages and empowers patients to control their health status. IPC is based on the premise that a more engaged patient and family will have a better experience and better outcomes" (Bozic et al., 2013; Cook et al., 2013; Hibbard & Greene, 2013).*

Fundamentally, IPC empowers patients through education, resources, and skill building. Education is a common, yet essential part of IPC. IPC is not limited to any one care setting. It is most effective as a cross-continuum model of care delivery, particularly as we move to a more population health–centered approach to care management. As a core component of IPC, education (whether overt or implicit) plays a role in every aspect of care delivery regardless of care setting.

Education in an IPC delivery model is different from today's most common practice. IPC requires that an education plan be developed prospectively for and with the patient, whether in the inpatient or ambulatory setting, or in continuing-care management at home or work. The education plan, as a core component of IPC, is developed to be patient-specific based on condition(s), literacy level, cognitive ability, and a clinician-assessed capacity for engagement and activation. With a plan in place, you will be better prepared to provide education in a deliberate and scheduled way throughout the stay or visit rather than at the point of departure. Education should be sequential and additive and should be paced based upon a measured level of activation and progressive comprehension.

Delivering Purposeful Education

Interactive patient education requires different processes, content, and skill. It requires the nurse to shift her mindset away from viewing the educational process as a "task" and toward viewing it as a core component of the patient's care plan and regimen. As discussed in earlier chapters, education should be purposeful, continuous, and a common thread in every care-plan or visit-plan for a patient. You must customize appropriate and careful content selection to the patient's needs (literacy, cultural appropriateness, and level of engagement). Interactive patient education requires continual evaluation. In your ongoing evaluation, consider whether the education you planned and provided is preparing and empowering the patient to proactively manage his/her health. Have you developed the education plan with cross-continuum care management in mind, providing consistency of content, progressive teaching, and long-term education planning across all care settings?

A more interactive care delivery model provides a strong platform to treat education as a dynamic and cost-effective resource for healthcare quality and safety improvement. When education is viewed as a tool or resource to activate the patient rather than a task to be completed, the power of patient understanding, the influence of knowledge gained on patient adherence, and, ultimately, outcomes are significantly positive.

Consider the following example of interactive patient education as a tool to prevent falls.

CASE EXAMPLE

Fall Prevention

There are many different methods to prevent patient falls. There is no one "silver bullet" or solution to stop or minimize falls. Consider the impact of educating patients about their risk of falling, educating them about how they can prevent a fall, and then reminding them throughout their care about their role and what they (as engaged participants) must do to remain safe from falling. Consider empowering the patient and her family to control her risk of falling through effective and continuous education. Regardless of the setting, a fall is costly, often requiring additional treatment or preventable emergency-department visits. Creating patient awareness and providing the tools to help the patient remain safe—to prevent a fall at home or in the hospital through education—is more likely to result in fewer falls and ultimately lower healthcare costs (Albert and Shelton, 2015). Interactive patient-facing pathways, like the example in Figure 7.1, can be used to guide a learner through a set of related experiences that lead to a more informed patient (or caregiver). The example starts with a patient self-assessment that creates awareness about the risk of falling. The pathway then automatically delivers video education about falls and how to prevent them. The learning is then reinforced by continued self-assessments and reminders to the patient. For example, the pathway may also include a visual reinforcement on the system so the patient/family remembers he is at risk at all times. This type of pathway enables the nurse to forge a more meaningful learning partnership with the patient and family, where the emphasis is to clarify and verify knowledge-transfer rather than complete a task.

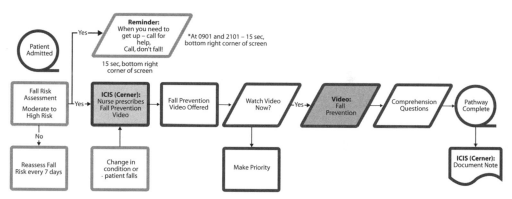

Figure 7.1   Example of an automated fall-prevention workflow available through IPC technology. Courtesy of GetWellNetwork, Inc.

Designing an Interactive Patient Education Program

An interactive patient education program must be designed around the goal of patient and family empowerment. The end goal is to provide the patient with the knowledge, tools, and skills to take control of her own healing and/or health status. Effective education requires a prospective plan. The plan should include the teaching method you've chosen based on how the patient and family will best receive, comprehend, and retain the knowledge and skills needed to manage their condition and/or health status. You should design the education plan with an approach, schedule, and content that are sensitive to the patient's needs and status.

The interactive patient education plan must be sensitive to cultural diversity, cognitive and physical limitations, socioeconomic status, and—importantly—the patient's level of engagement. You should select content with any cultural sensitivity in mind and at a review or reading level that is appropriate for the level of health and educational literacy of the patient. The development of the education plan must be deliberate, focused, and based on the clinician's assessment of the patient's ability to engage and participate in his own care. The patient's readiness to learn and level of engagement and activation should influence the depth, frequency, and pace of education delivered.

When designing the plan, follow a structure that ensures consistency in process and result. For example, a commonly accepted approach to structuring an education plan is to use the *Tell-Show-Do-Practice-Review* structure to organize the plan (Addelston, 1959). This structure provides an efficient approach to education, yet ensures that the care team consistently employs the important elements of effective education. Table 7.1 provides an example of how this structure is used to plan and deliver education about pediatric asthma.

Table 7.1   Tell-Show-Do-Practice-Review Framework for Education Planning

Pediatric Asthma Education

Tell	Inform patient and/or parents of new diagnosis of asthma
	Discuss importance of education and explain how to prevent flare-ups
	Assess patient/family readiness for education and determine level of activation through discussion
	Share educational resources and education plan for patient and caregivers
Show	Prescribe patient-specific videos on IPC technology tool
	Plan the method and time of delivering education based on what you know about the patient and their level of engagement
	Ensure that patient views and completes the videos you have prescribed
	Teach the signs and symptoms to watch for to prevent flare-ups
	Teach how to use nebulizer

continues

Table 7.1	Tell-Show-Do-Practice-Review Framework for Education Planning (continued)

Pediatric Asthma Education

Do	Complete and discuss daily assessment of signs and symptoms present at bedside with patient and caregivers
	Patient and caregivers perform use of nebulizer when taught by nurse
Practice	Patient and caregiver independently practice use of nebulizer at bedside
	Patient and caregiver practice use of nebulizer upon rounds
	Patient and caregiver complete self-check of any signs and symptoms and report to nurse daily
Review	Assess understanding and competency each day using teach-back methods
	Post discharge, patient and caregiver discuss challenges with use of devices and in managing condition with physician; additional education prescribed during the clinic visit as needed
	At home, patient and/or caregiver watch newly prescribed videos from their physician to support better achievement of lifestyle changes needed to manage the patient's health status through mobile IPC technology

Once the education plan is established, the nurse's role is to ensure that the patient completes it. Effective education requires selecting the right content and the best method of delivery, assessing patient comprehension, and testing the patient's ability to teach back and/or demonstrate competency.

Where Does Technology Fit in Patient Education?

Patient engagement and meaningful use of clinical information systems are important components for the achievement of healthcare quality (Davis, Schoenbaum, & Audet, 2005). Clinical integration systems have been critical in fulfilling desired patient outcomes and value-based purchasing in clinical care (Grauman, Graham, & Johnson, 2012).

Consumers of healthcare are using technology in ways never imagined before. Patients enter the healthcare system with information about their condition and are afforded choice in determining their healthcare path (Wassan et al., 2012).

Technology has become a tool used to help educate and engage patients in their care. It is important to note, however, that technology alone cannot create the shift in care delivery from nurses *caring for* to *partnering with* patients and families. The role of the nurse and healthcare team will continue to emerge. Using technology as an instrument to enhance patient engagement through IPC is a critical aspect in activating patients as true partners in their own care (Aruffo, 2014; Bernabeo & Holmboe, 2013).

Studies have shown that technology solutions are effective approaches to improve care quality, because they can be used to help patients become active partners in their healthcare journey. In a study with cardiac surgery patients, those subjects who used an electronic platform and mobile devices during their recovery with a personalized plan of care had a reduced length of stay and an increased likelihood to be discharged to home independently (Cook et al., 2013). In another study, when patients actively engaged in their care through technology as a part of quality improvement initiatives, they reported better outcomes and satisfaction, especially related to transparency and information sharing (Roseman, Osborne-Stafsnes, Amy, Boslaugh, & Slate-Miller, 2013).

Interactive patient education requires more time to prepare, complete, and evaluate at a time in healthcare when resources are scarce and time is precious. An IPC technology platform can serve as a cost-effective and efficient means of providing meaningful, patient-specific education at all points of care across the continuum, requiring less time from providers and more opportunity for patients and their families to benefit from the education. IPC technology has been in use for more than a decade. The technology enables the kind of interactive care referenced in this chapter and throughout this book. Today, cloud-based IPC technology solutions provide easy access to prescribed education anytime and anywhere. Caregivers utilize IPC technology as the platform to prescribe, deliver, and evaluate the effect of patient education. In fact, patient education is a common element among a variety of functionality available through IPC technology.

IPC technology enables a more consistent, efficient, and continuous approach to education. IPC leverages point-of-care and continuing-care (at home or work) resources accessible by patients, their family/caregivers, and their care providers through easy to navigate, real-time interactive tools that are prescribed based upon the priority needs of the patient. See Figure 7.2.

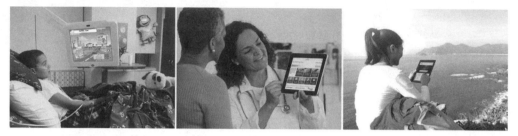

Figure 7.2 These photos show how IPC technology is commonly used in different care settings such as the hospital, the clinic, and the home. Photos courtesy of GetWellNetwork, Inc.

These devices are used on hospital televisions, tablets in the ambulatory care center and physician offices, and on any Internet-capable computer or smart device anywhere; patients and their families may access a host of interactive care tools designed to empower the patient and keep her engaged with their care plan. IPC technology provides an easy-to-use platform to educate the patient on her condition, medications, care plan, tests and procedures, and lifestyle changes to improve her health status. The flexibility offered through technology supports the need to address and accommodate for cultural sensitivity, and for physical, literacy, and cognitive limitations in the education process. See Figure 7.3.

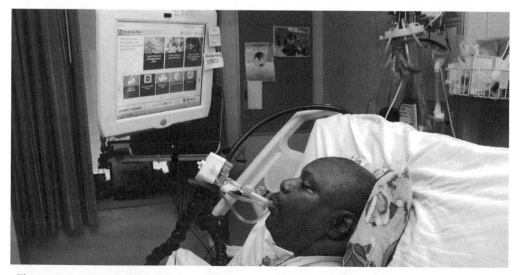

Figure 7.3 IPC is a powerful engagement tool for those who require Assistive Adaptive Communication technology. Photo courtesy of GetWellNetwork, Inc.

Typically, IPC solutions are customized to the individual patient based on what you know about him. It starts with the basic information about the patient such as name, age, and care environment (inpatient, clinic, emergency department, or home). This occurs through an interface that pulls data from the admission, discharge, and transfer system (often called ADT). Augmentative and alternative communication (AAC) is discussed in detail in Chapter 10.

Using Health Level Seven (HL7) interfaces with various health information technology (HIT) systems, including the Electronic Health Record, an IPC technology platform can receive data such as medication orders, patient diagnosis, and treatment plans to automatically and dynamically initiate patient-specific educational interventions at appropriate points throughout the patient's stay in a hospital. The interactive capabilities of IPC technology also allow for reminders to patients regarding medications, doctor appointments, and the need to complete daily signs and symptoms checks at home or at work using cloud-based mobile technology. The interactive nature of an IPC technology platform allows for real-time intervention and monitoring of patient status and progress from ongoing patient response and feedback (see Figure 7.4).

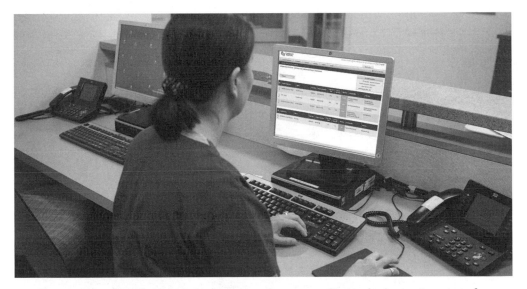

Figure 7.4   *Meaningful use* is a term you hear regarding today's requirements for health information technology and use of systems such as IPC. Photo courtesy of GetWellNetwork, Inc.

IPC technology serves as one type of data integrator that allows for information exchange between nurses and other healthcare providers. It provides a data set that you may use to make changes and adaptations to the patient's care plan.

The bi-directional interface capabilities of IPC technology platforms leverage data to automatically trigger prescribed interventions based on data values and interpretation, as well as providing real-time evaluation of the effectiveness of these educational interventions. As a nurse, you might be asked to join a clinical informatics workgroup to design interfaces between HIT systems, such as your EHR and the IPC platform, with the goal of automating clinical interventions and documentation. The resulting interface enables you to capture data that is useful to gauge a patient's progress and involvement with their learning. Participation in these design groups allows you to evaluate current clinical processes and redesign workflows to optimize both effectiveness and efficiency of processes.

IPC technology can enable a new level of workflow efficiency and effectiveness for nurses, particularly when it comes to educating the patient. For example, a well-known, leading provider of IPC technology solutions offers a unique workflow technology that automates patient care processes. These workflows, called *Patient Pathways,* can be triggered by the caregiver, by a prescription or diagnosis in the electronic health record, and/or through data feedback from the patient—either the patient's response (such as comprehension of education received) or the patient's progression or completion of a care (see Figure 7.5).

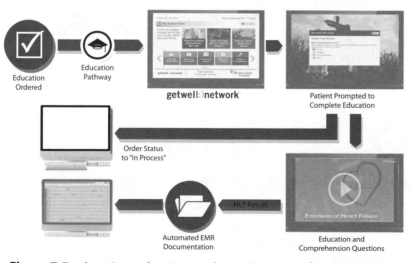

Figure 7.5   A patient education pathway. Courtesy of GetWellNetwork, Inc.

Creating Evidence-Based Patient Pathways

IPC solutions such as GetWellNetwork have established evidence-based *Patient Pathways* that cross the care continuum by providing continuity of information, education, and intervention, regardless of the patient's location. This type of IPC platform provides a customized educational experience and adaptable resource in the hospital, physician's office, ambulatory clinic, and at home through a health system or through the provider's patient portal.

The IPC platform supports self-regulated learning by making education available at a time that is right for the patient and/or family. Because IPC crosses the care continuum, it promotes continuity of a health system's educational messaging. In addition, IPC technology can assist with reinforcement and remediation of learning.

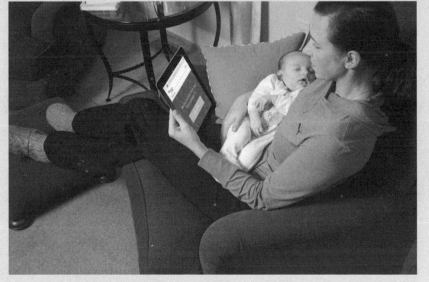

Photo courtesy of GetWellNetwork, Inc.

IPC technology is designed to be easy for the patient and family to navigate, with ready access to resources they need to understand their condition and treatment plan. It places education at the center of the patient's interactive care experience and empowers the patient to own the process, supported by her nurse and care team as needed. IPC technology provides a user experience that prioritizes patient learning through resources, reminders, and prompts, and it leverages tools that provide repetition and encouragement for the patient (see Figure 7.6).

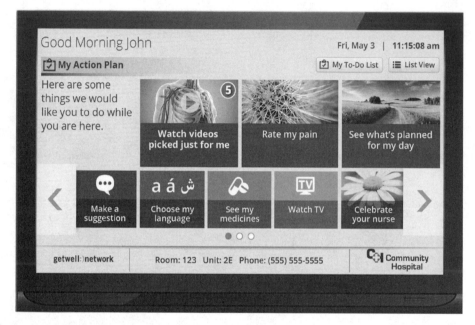

Figure 7.6   Example of the user experience as seen from an adult in an inpatient setting. Courtesy of GetWellNetwork, Inc.

What Are the Impacts and Benefits of Interactive Patient Education?

Can effective, interactive patient education truly contribute to transforming the healthcare system? Worldwide, healthcare providers are committed to meeting the *Triple Aim*. The well-known target of improving the quality, safety, and cost of healthcare is the foundation of strategy for the great majority of healthcare providers globally. Although it is not a panacea, patient and family engagement is now recognized to be one of the most critical elements of our strategy leading to the needed transformation of our healthcare system and the achievement of the triple aim (IHI, 2015).

Patient and family engagement occurs when patients have the "tools" to manage their health within an agreed-upon care plan specific to their needs. That care plan should include adequate and appropriate patient-specific education. With today's shorter lengths of stay and higher acuity patient encounters, clinicians often report having insufficient time to provide needed education, let alone assess patient readiness, literacy, and/or comprehension. More often than not, clinicians must rely on printed materials and a high-level review of the materials on the day of discharge or at the end of a visit. Particularly with chronic conditions, there is too much information for anyone—let alone an ill patient—to be able to comprehend in enough detail to influence patient activation or patient understanding of what their care plan is and how to care for themselves outside the episode of care. The result is that patients do not make the needed changes or fail to adhere (at least long-term) to their prescribed care plan. This issue results in high readmission rates, falls at home, and unnecessary physician office or emergency-department visits.

One of the primary goals of IPC is to equip and empower patients and their families with information, knowledge, and skills to care for themselves and carry out their care plan—to control their own healthcare journeys. As shown in Figure 7.7, IPC helps patients progress through the four core PPFEM-HSA (Chapter 1) areas of learning; in turn, a nurse's role is to ensure the knowledge and skills are obtained and the patient is competent to apply them in his daily life. IPC is dynamic and supports a learner across the healthcare continuum.

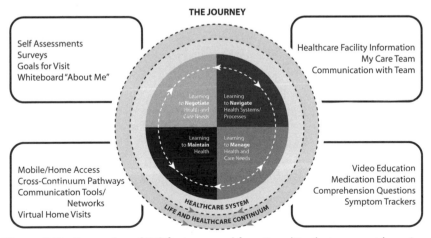

Figure 7.7 Examples of IPC features and functionality that support learning.

As discussed earlier in this chapter, effective interactive patient education occurs when we first establish an educational plan with the patient and family, outlining the what, how, when, and why of their educational needs. A truly interactive patient care experience begins at the entry into any point of care, inpatient, ambulatory, or at-home visit or a check-in call from a case manager. With the tools, automation, and interoperability available through IPC technology, educating the patient can be so much more effective in building patient motivation to care for himself because he feels equipped to do so. Particularly with chronic conditions and behaviors that influence health risk and are estimated to impact most of the costs of care within our delivery system (Centers for Disease Control and Prevention [CDC], 2015), patients need to receive education progressively and in a way that will most benefit each individual.

Interactive patient education is a way to involve patients and families as active participants in managing their care, their safety, and ultimately their healthcare outcomes. Consider the possibility that we too often assume the patient knows or is competent in how to care for himself outside the episode of care—especially if he has been living with a disease or condition for some time, or if he does not ask questions. There are several excellent examples of new ways to teach and engage patients through education, such as "Ask Me 3" (National Patient Safety Foundation [NSPF], 2015), or innovative ways of leveraging shift-change communication to engage the patient with teach-back. Therefore, the most important aspects of educating for impact is plan, readiness, right time, right method, and partnering with the patient to examine or inspect what they know and what they have learned.

When applied in that way, interactive patient education can be highly effective at improving patient-care outcomes regardless of setting. Further, having continued access to educational resources and/or the ability to "prescribe" new or additional education in a progressive plan—or because of changes in condition—is key to leading the patient through a healthier journey.

Conclusion and Key Points

We are at a change point in healthcare. The current delivery and cost model is not sustainable. Transformation is needed in order to improve healthcare quality, safety, and service experience at a much lower cost. Patient engagement and education are fundamental elements needed to create that transformation. Patient education is a core ingredient for building and sustaining the skills and tools and the level of patient activation needed to empower and engage patients in managing their health. It is a core requirement in transforming our approach to healthcare delivery.

Patient education is not a one-time act. It requires a longitudinal view based on a deliberate assessment of the needs of the patient. It should not be one more task that must be done before completion of the visit with the physician or call with the care manager. It should be more than a discharge-preparation requirement. Patient education is core to cross-continuum care management of patients and their families, and so it must be designed and delivered in a way that progressively improves the health status of a patient through empowerment and engagement.

An IPC technology platform can be a valuable resource for nurses and educators, providing the tools needed to plan, deliver, and evaluate the impact of education on the patient's level of activation, and to yield a resulting improvement in the patient's health status over time.

As nurses and healthcare professionals, we must work to transform a model of care delivery that we know is not scalable or sustainable long-term. Thus, your call to action must be to leverage the value of education in a way that fundamentally and sustainably shifts the locus of control for health status to patients, empowering them to be more effective in managing their health status.

References

Addelston, H. (1959). Child patient training. *Fortnightly Review of the Chicago Dental Society, 38*(7), 27–29.

The Advisory Board Company 2013 Research Brief: Three Key Elements for Successful Population Health Management. Retrieved from http://www.advisory.com/research/health-care-advisory-board/studies/2013/three-elements-for-successful-population-health-management

Aruffo, S. (2014). *Can technology drive sustainable patient engagement?* Retrieved from http://www.dorland-health.com/dorland-health-articles/CIP_0213_17_TeachToolsxml

Bernabeo, E., & Holmboe, E. S. (2013). Patients, providers, and systems need to acquire a specific set of competencies to achieve truly patient-centered care. *Health Affairs, 32*(2), 250–257.

Berwick, D., Nolan, T. W., & Wittington, J. (2008). The Triple Aim: Care, health and cost. *Health Affairs, 27*(3), 759–769.

Bozic, K. J., Belkora, J., Chan, V., Youm, J., Zhou, T., Dupaix, J., … Huddleston, J. (2013). Shared decision making in patients with osteoarthritis of the hip and knee: Results of a randomized controlled trial. *The Journal of Bone and Joint Surgery, 95-A*(18), 1633–1639.

Centers for Disease Control and Prevention (CDC). (2015). Retrieved from http://www.cdc.gov/chronicdisease/overview/index.htm

Cook, D. J., Manning, D. M., Holland, D. E., Prinsen, S. K., Rudzik, S. D., Roger, V. L., & Coulter, A. (2012). Patient engagement: What works? *Journal of Ambulatory Care Management, 35*(2), 80–89.

Davis, K., Schoenbaum, S. C., & Audet, A. M. (2005). A 2020 vision of patient-centered primary care. *Journal of General Internal Medicine, 20*(10), 953–957.

Deschamps, C. (2013). Patient engagement and reported outcomes in surgical recovery: Effectiveness of an e-health platform. *Journal of the American College of Surgeons, 217*(4), 648–655.

Elwyn, G., Barr, P. J., Grande, S. W., Thompson, R., Walsh, T., & Ozanne, E. M. (2013). Developing CollaboRATE: A fast and frugal patient-reported measure of shared decision making in clinical encounters. *Patient Education and Counseling, 93*(1), 102–107.

Ernst and Young 2014: Health Industry Post: News and analysis of current issues affecting health care providers and payers; Population Health Management: A strategy for success in the new age of accountable care. Retrieved from http://www.ey.com/Publication/vwLUAssets/Health_Industry_Post_population_health_management/$FILE/Health_Industry_post.pdf

Grauman, D. M., Graham, C. J., & Johnson, M. M. (2012). 5 pillars of clinical integration. *Healthcare Financial Management, 66*(8), 70–77.

Guide to Patient and Family Engagement in Hospital Quality and Safety. June 2013. Agency for Healthcare Research and Quality, Rockville, MD. Retrieved from http://www.ahrq.gov/professionals/systems/hospital/engagingfamilies/guide.html

Hibbard, J. H., & Greene, J. (2013). What the evidence shows about patient activation: Better health outcomes and care experiences; fewer data on costs. *Health Affairs, 32*(2), 207–213.

Hibbard, J., Stockard, J., Mahoney, E., & Tusler, M. (2004). Development of the Patient Activation Measure (PAM): Conceptualizing and measuring activation in patients and consumers. Health Services Research, *39*(4), Part I. 1005–126.

The Institute for Healthcare Improvement (IHI). (2015). The IHI Triple Aim. Retrieved from http://www.ihi.org/engage/initiatives/TripleAim/Pages/default.aspx

National Patient Safety Foundation (NPSF). (2015) Ask Me 3. Retrieved from http://www.npsf.org/?page=askme3

Pelletier, L. R., & Stichler, J. F. (2014). Ensuring patient and family engagement: A professional nurse's toolkit. *Journal of Nursing Care Quality, 29*(1), 1–5.

Roseman, D., Osborne-Stafsnes, J., Amy, C. H., Boslaugh, S., & Slate-Miller, K. (2013). Early lessons from four 'aligning forces for quality' communities bolster the case for patient-centered care. *Health Affairs, 32*(2), 232–238.

Sofaer, S., & Schumann, M. J. (2013). *Fostering successful patient and family engagement: Nursing's critical role.* Washington, DC: National Alliance for Quality Care. Retrieved from http://www.naqc.org/WhitePaper-PatientEngagement

Wassan, J. H., Forsberg, H. H., Lindblad, S., Mazowita, G., McQuillen, K., & Nelson, E. C. (2012). The medium is the (health) measure: Patient engagement using personal technologies. *Journal of Ambulatory Care Management, 35*(2), 109–117.

Weiss, A. J. (Truven Health Analytics), & Elixhauser, A. (AHRQ). (2014). Overview of hospital stays in the United States, 2012. (HCUP Statistical Brief #180). Rockville, MD: Agency for Healthcare Research and Quality. Retrieved from http://www.hcup-us.ahrq.gov/reports/statbriefs/sb180-Hospitalizations-United-States-2012.pdf

"Peering succeeds because it leverages self-organization—a style of production that works more effectively than hierarchical management for certain tasks."
–Don Tapscott, 2010

Using Telehealth to Support Patient and Family Education

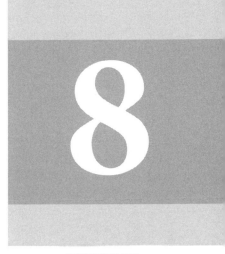

Alberto E. Tozzi, MD
Orsola Gawronski, RN, MSN
Emanuela Tiozzo, RN, MSN

Introduction

This chapter provides a practical application of how telehealth is used to increase self-care management and support population health. The chapter will also include a review of current methods and related benefits. We will provide examples of innovative self-monitoring and planning tools such as mobile apps, symptom trackers, and interactive remote assessment tools.

The time needed for introducing innovations in healthcare is far longer than in other disciplines. For example, it takes nearly 20 years from discovery to introduce a new therapy into a consolidated clinical path. However, this scenario is likely to rapidly change due to some unrestrainable forces that have been rising in recent years. One is the increase in technology adoption and connectivity among individuals at an extremely fast pace. Connectivity has favored the spread of knowledge in several domains and of technology itself. Its logical consequence is an improvement in participation in health processes by citizens, putting a strong pressure on healthcare systems to better address patients' needs.

OBJECTIVES

- Describe the types of telehealth tools commonly used to support self-care management.
- Discuss how telehealth supports patient and family engagement with population health management resources.
- Explain the benefits and limitations of each method based on the learning and self-care management objectives.
- Develop a plan to implement at least one telehealth method that can be incorporated into a telehealth program to support self-care management.

More than ever, patients today have a high control of their home environment, of their clinical and body parameters, and ultimately of their health. This is thanks to technological applications embedded in cell phones, in wearable tools, and in home appliances and other instruments. This context poses risks and opportunities. Medical knowledge is available to anybody through open tools available on the Web. The success of Massive Online Open Courses (MOOC) underlines how people in every corner of the world are willing to increase their knowledge in different disciplines, including medicine, beyond the limits of formal education. It is quite obvious that patients are particularly interested in their health and that they are increasingly more confident with medical concepts and sometimes do a correct diagnosis by themselves. In extreme situations, a do-it-yourself approach can be disastrous if a solid partnership with a medical doctor does not exist. On the other hand, having patients pursuing the objective of maintaining good health and successfully treating their diseases is a treasure that healthcare must not waste.

With the spread of connectivity, communication among patients, families, and physicians has become more intense and frequent. Organizational and budget constraints exert a strong pressure to keep patients out of hospitals as much as possible if they have mild diseases or if they are convalescent. Recovery at home is the thing that patients may want most; however, medical counseling, monitoring of clinical parameters, and treatment are basic patients' needs, even in the home environment. With the simplicity of a phone call, any person can now establish a video communication with doctors or nurses, monitor and send their clinical parameters to a health provider, and receive signals and alerts that deserve medical interventions. Hospitals and healthcare are moving ultimately to patients' homes, and it is not surprising that this is associated with better outcomes.

Telehealth plays a pivotal role in this scenario and creates a number of advantages that are easily recognized. The usual processes of diagnosis and treatment can be sped up, because relevant information is not dependent on a face-to-face encounter between patient and physician. This leads to improved short- and long-term outcomes, and to a decrease of patients' discomfort and travel time to healthcare providers. We can improve healthcare especially in remote areas, where traditional face-to-face visits are rarely obtained.

One of the most important consequences of widespread telehealth adoption is a strong impulse toward patient-centered healthcare. Connection between health providers and patients greatly improves patients' self-management. Providers' feedback allows all involved to adjust decisions that patients make for their health. Moreover, health literacy, indicated as an important objective for quality-of-care improvement, is strongly favored by telehealth. Finally, telehealth has the important potential to represent a tool for changing lifestyles more effectively than other interventions.

Consumer health electronics has played a central role in adopting telehealth solutions. Contrary to what one might expect, a high pressure for using telehealth and telemonitoring is coming from patients. In general, the wide availability of tools embedded in smart phones or on the Web has caused a strong expectation from the public, who consider telehealth solutions natural. As a matter of fact, patients and their families are almost always willing to accept telehealth solutions.

What Is Telehealth?

You can find several definitions of telehealth in scientific publications and online. We have provided one such definition here.

> **Definition 8.1:** *Telehealth: The use of electronic information and tele-communications technologies to support long-distance clinical health-care and provide patient and professional health-related education.*

You can apply the use of technology for remote communication embedded into the concept of telehealth to a number of clinical situations, depending on the information being exchanged. Telehealth may include the following:

- **Video visits**: Patients are remotely examined with the help of simple video cameras and with additional sensors that allow them to transmit clinical information such as blood glucose levels, blood pressure, cardiac auscultation, otoscopy, urinalysis, and so on. In these encounters, the patient and the doctor are in different locations.

- **Remote monitoring**: Some patients, due to chronic conditions or due to the need to obtain an accurate diagnosis, may be strictly monitored with simple devices such as glucometers, blood pressure monitors, cardiac implanted devices, spirometers, etc. Data from these devices is automatically transmitted to a health center, which can continuously detect alert signals and promptly implement interventions.

- **Self-management tools**: Telehealth increases patient autonomy. For patients undergoing remote monitoring of clinical parameters, software applications, often available on a smart phone, can recognize their personal trends in the monitored clinical parameter. Decision tools apply simple algorithms to this data to provide patients with appropriate recommendations about management and therapy.

- **Online support groups**: Online communities of patients represent a real and solid support for some types of patients. These communities not only discuss their personal experiences, but often provide fine-grained and specific advice about management and therapy, especially regarding chronic diseases.

Terminology Used in Telehealth

Terminology used in telehealth includes a number of terms that are often used interchangeably. A brief list of commonly used terms is shown in Table 8.1.

Table 8.1   Terminology Used in Telehealth

Term	Meaning
eHealth	Healthcare practice supported by electronic processes and communication. The term encompasses a range of services such as electronic health records, telemedicine, consumer health informatics, mHealth, etc.
mHealth	Practice of medicine and public health supported by mobile communication devices—such as mobile phones, tablet computers, and PDAs—for health services and information. mHealth is generally intended as a segment of eHealth. It may include collecting community and clinical health data; delivering healthcare information to practitioners, researchers, and patients; real-time monitoring of patient clinical parameters; and directly providing care.

Remote monitoring or telemonitoring	Type of ambulatory healthcare in which patients use mobile medical devices to perform a routine test and send the test data to a healthcare professional in real time, or continuously monitor a clinical parameter. Remote monitoring includes devices such as glucose meters for patients with diabetes and heart- or blood-pressure monitors for patients receiving cardiac care.
Teleconsultation	Consultation between a provider and specialist at distance using either store-and-forward telemedicine or real-time videoconferencing.
Telemedicine and telehealth	Telemedicine is the use of medical information exchanged from one site to another via electronic communications to improve patients' health status. Closely associated with telemedicine is the term *telehealth,* which is often used to encompass a broader definition of remote healthcare that does not always involve clinical services. Videoconferencing, transmission of still images, eHealth including patient portals, remote monitoring of vital signs, continuing medical education, and nursing call centers are all considered part of telemedicine and telehealth. Telemedicine is not a separate medical specialty. Products and services related to telemedicine are often part of a larger investment by healthcare institutions in either information technology or the delivery of clinical care. Telemedicine encompasses different types of programs and services provided for the patient. Each component involves different providers and consumers.
Telenursing, telehealth nursing, nursing telepractice	The delivery, management, and coordination of care and services provided via telecommunications technology within the domain of nursing.

Telehealth and eHealth use the Internet to store and transmit information globally. As of today, Western countries have a high prevalence of people who have access to the Internet at home (70% of adults in the United States; 85% in the U.K.). Most people in these countries own a cell phone (over 90%). Although the frequency of technology use is much lower, there is an increasing trend toward its adoption in developing countries as well. Wide access to digital technologies provides a preferential channel to transmit information and the opportunity to access educational sessions on health behaviors and procedures. Predictors for technology adoption include higher education, higher income, and lower age.

Telehealth, leveraging the Internet's characteristics, has the potential to overcome some of the barriers of face-to-face programs, such as the need for frequent visits, which may involve time away from family and work, as well as travel expenses. Moreover, online resources can be accessed at any time, and telehealth has the potential to reach larger numbers of individuals at a much lower cost than face-to-face treatment.

Telehealth can also deliver health education aimed at behavior change. Health education online "packages" may have extensive, relevant educational content that may be tailored to the individual's needs. Flexibility of online content and virtual tools are added values compared with traditional print educational tools. In fact, Internet-based interventions may provide a wide range of techniques for behavior change, such as aids to goal setting, planning, self-monitoring, skill and knowledge building, reminders, and peer social support. These elements also promote partnering with health professionals.

Telehealth nursing is rapidly emerging in several health systems seeking to improve their efficiency. Indeed, nurses who adopt telecommunications and health technologies, such as audio, video, or remote data collection, are already providing telehealth nursing. Telehealth nursing may be applied for patient remote monitoring, home consultations, patient triage, patient counseling, and patient education to decrease emergency-room accesses and to manage clinical paths. Through telehealth consultations, patients get in contact with nurses to discuss emerging symptoms, medication management, or other issues, such as how to change a dressing. Some areas of nursing practice include TeleICU, Teletriage, Teletrauma, Telestroke, Telepediatrics, Telemental Health, Telecardiology, Telehomecare, Telerehabilitation, and Forensic Telenursing.

Evidence Supporting Efficacy of Telehealth in Improving Outcomes

Despite the fact that some have invoked telehealth as a magic solution to improve the efficiency of healthcare processes, there is much debate due to the paucity of scientific studies documenting its impact. Indeed, we do not have the large amount of scientific studies on effectiveness of telehealth as we do for drugs and medications. Moreover, the very high speed of technology improvement creates problems in repeating studies with the same telehealth intervention for comparison.

Table 8.2 provides information on the benefits you can expect from telehealth implementation.

Table 8.2 Benefits Expected from Telehealth Implementation	
Indicator	*Mechanism*
Reduced mortality	Early recognition of health problems, especially in critical and chronic patients, and early intervention
Reduced hospitalization	Reduction of acute episodes in chronic patients; telehealth can decrease hospitalizations due to stricter monitoring and better recognition of subclinical episodes
Increased quality of life	Patients feel more attention and satisfaction from the healthcare process because of better connection and direct involvement
Early detection of exacerbations	Strict and frequent monitoring and recognition of subclinical episodes
Personalized interventions	Targeted interventions tailored to context and characteristic of patient's illness, behavior, understanding of symptoms, and psychosocial/home situation
Patient empowerment, education, behavioral reinforcement, and motivation	Information tailored to individual patient's need and directly delivered to the home of the patient, reinforcing behavioral change; positive feedback and personalized approach may increase patient's motivation in relation to their treatment
Improved access to care	Patients may access healthcare services at any distance from the provider
Improved efficiency of nursing tasks	Nurse utilization improves by limiting avoidable hospitalizations and primary care face-to-face interventions
Reduced costs	Impact on direct costs due to improvement of care but also on indirect costs by limiting time away from home and travel for patients and providing timely interventions to multiple patients at the same time

Despite the paucity of studies, a recent meta-review including 31 reviews found that 65% of examined eHealth and telehealth interventions were effective or cost-effective, or promising (Elbert et al., 2014).

Regarding specific disciplines, a domain for telehealth application is emergency medicine in pre-hospital care, where real-time communication is expected to improve outcomes. Stroke management has been one of the areas where telehealth studies have been most frequent. Stroke management may benefit from telehealth solutions to speed up the administration of thromboplasminogen activator in acute ischemic stroke, which should be given within 3 to 4.5 hours from onset of symptoms (Adams et al., 2007; del Zoppo, Saver, Jauch, & Adams, 2009; Hacke et al., 2008). An additional impact of telehealth is in the review of brain CT when the point of care is in an underserved area (Demaerschalk et al., 2012). It seems clear that adoption of telehealth in these cases increases the number of consultations, although short-term and long-term mortality are similar compared with a face-to-face model of care (Chowdhury, Birns, Rudd, & Bhalla, 2012; Demaerschalk, Raman, Ernstrom, & Meyer, 2012; Pedragosa et al., 2009; Zaidi et al., 2011).

Trauma represents another case in which telehealth may be beneficial, especially to manage major incidents. Telehealth interventions in this area include improved access to consultation with experts (especially during disasters), teleradiology, and assessment of burns (Ashkenazi et al., 2007; Benner, Schachinger, & Nerlich, 2004; Duchesne et al., 2008). In general, telemedicine seems to have a positive impact on mortality and hospital costs (Duchesne et al., 2008; Saffle, Edelman, Theurer, Morris, & Cochran, 2009) and leads to a decrease of hospital admissions when used for referral in acute burns (Wallace, Smith, & Pickford, 2007).

ST elevation myocardial infarction is recommended to be treated with reperfusion within two hours of medical contact (Lassen, Bøtker, & Terkelsen, 2013). Telemedicine-equipped ambulances have been effective in expediting referral to percutaneous coronary intervention of patients with ST elevation myocardial infarction and reducing mortality (Sanchez et al., 2011; Terkelsen et al., 2005; Zanini et al., 2008).

Remote monitoring of chronic patients is an important application for telehealth. Type 1 diabetes is one of the fields where self-monitoring of blood glucose leads to better control of the disease and to better values of Hb A1C (Greenwood, Young, & Quinn, 2014).

Interestingly, educational interventions coupled with self-monitoring seem to be associated with the best outcomes (Greenwood, Young, & Quinn, 2014).

A meta-analysis of 12 RCTs comparing home blood-pressure monitoring with usual care showed significant improvement of blood-pressure control and reduction of both SBP and DBP, and a modest but significant increase in use of antihypertensive medications (Omboni & Guarda, 2011).

A recent review of six randomized controlled trials examined remote management versus standard clinic follow-up of inflammatory bowel disease (Huang, Reich, & Fedorak, 2014). The results suggested that remote management through telehealth resulted in variable improvements in quality of life, clinic visits, relapse rates, and hospitalization rates.

Another review suggested that digital self-management of asthma shows promise, with evidence of beneficial effects on some outcomes (Morrison et al., 2014). An additional review documented the benefits of telemonitoring in management of chronic diseases (Bashshur et al., 2014). Positive impacts have been measured in hospital admissions or readmissions, length of stay, and emergency-department visits for congestive heart failure, stroke, and chronic obstructive pulmonary disease. The review also observed reductions in mortality (Bashshur et al., 2014).

Patients' Attitudes About Using Technologies for Health

Internet access represents a basic requirement for implementing telehealth. Because Internet penetration differs by world region, most experiments have been conducted in developed countries. Internet use can therefore represent a useful indicator for you to use to assess the potential use of telehealth in your health system or patient population. A snapshot of the number of Internet users and percentage of the resident population with access to Internet in 2014 is reported in Figure 8.1 (Miniwatts Marketing Group, 2014).

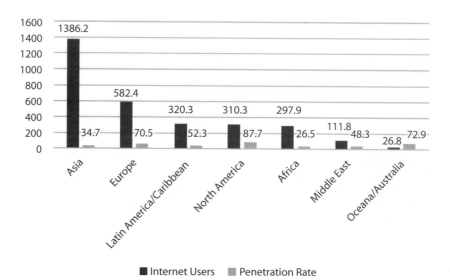

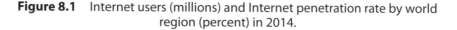

Figure 8.1   Internet users (millions) and Internet penetration rate by world region (percent) in 2014.

Use of technology for health in U.S. residents has been described by the Pew Research Center through a series of studies. Some of the most significant findings are reported here.

A high proportion of U.S. adults go online to search for health information, and nearly one-third to try to make a diagnosis by themselves through the Web (see Figure 8.2) (Fox & Duggan, 2013). People mostly start by using a Web search engine, while only a minor percentage of them start from health information specialized sites (Fox & Duggan, 2013). Almost half of them thought, after reading online, that they needed a medical consultation (Fox & Duggan, 2013). Moreover, 41% of persons who made a diagnosis by themselves stated that a medical professional partially or completely confirmed it (Fox & Duggan, 2013). Among individuals included in the study, the use of the Internet as a tool for diagnosis was more frequent in women, younger people, and those individuals with a higher socioeconomic level (Fox & Duggan, 2013).

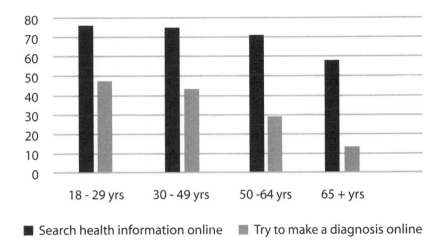

Figure 8.2   Percentage of U.S. adults searching for health information online and looking online for a diagnosis, by age group. Adapted from Pew Research Center (2013).

Tracking health has become easy with the introduction of commercial devices that allow users to monitor some simple parameters simply using a cell phone. A significant proportion of U.S. adults track some aspects of their health, such as weight, diet, exercise routine, blood pressure, blood sugar, sleep patterns, headaches, or some other health indicator (Fox, Duggan, & Purcell, 2013).

From a study conducted in 2013 on more than 3,000 adults living in the United States, nearly four out of ten, mostly between 30 and 64 years old, are caring for an adult or child patient (Fox et al., 2013). Caregivers are much more likely than non-caregivers to consult online reviews of drugs, go online for a diagnosis, participate in online social networks for health purposes, and gather other health information online (Fox et al., 2013).

Among caregivers, 39% are responsible for drug administration for a patient, but only 7% use websites or apps for support in these activities. On the other hand, 87% of caregivers in the United States own a cell phone, and 37% of them have used it to look for health information online (Fox et al., 2013).

> **NOTE**
>
> It's important to consider older people and investigate their confidence in using technology. Indeed, the elderly represent a significant portion of chronic-disease sufferers and deserve great medical attention that can potentially be managed through telehealth.

A recent survey shows that the proportion of older people who go online decreases from 74% in the 65 to 69 years age group to 37% in those older than 80 (Smith, 2014). However, Internet use does increase constantly over time in this age group. The challenges for using technology in this segment of the population are quite obvious, especially considering difficulties in reading. Moreover, older individuals do not frequently believe that using the Internet may be beneficial for their health (Smith, 2014). Finally, older persons often need assistance when using a new technology. Nonetheless, an interesting finding of the aforementioned study is that nearly one-third of older adults use online social networks (Smith, 2014).

In general, attitude toward use of technologies varies according to age, gender, and education level. Because this observation suggest that certain segments of the population have better opportunities to adopt technological solutions, telehealth programs should be tailored to patients' needs and attitudes.

Connecting Telehealth, Education, and Self-Care

The improvement and refinement of digital tools have opened the door to the development of personalized models that may be adapted to specific clinical targets. The current potential allows healthcare providers to not only monitor patient personal information, but also to integrate patient data with population and environmental data.

The integration of data creates the opportunity for knowledge-based, decision support systems. These systems may enhance the effectiveness of interventions guiding prescriptions when directed to clinicians, and improving behaviors, compliance to therapy, and referral to health service in case of need, when applied to patients.

Indeed, several diseases may be prevented or better monitored and managed with the direct participation of patients. Telehealth may facilitate self-management of chronic or complex diseases to empower patients. The expected benefit is self-management of disease and improvement of patients' quality of life and lifestyle.

In essence, telehealth and telemonitoring become powerful tools for you to educate patients and their families. Their impact is not limited to routine actions, such as taking medications regularly, improving lifestyles, or monitoring vital signs, but also includes the sharing of notions from evidence-based guidelines that should promote health and autonomy. Especially for chronic patients, telehealth is useful to patients to recognize symptoms of exacerbation of their disease in a timely manner, thus prompting them to contact their health provider.

An important case study in self-management of chronic diseases has been recently published in the field of hypertension management. In this clinical trial, patients at high risk of cardiovascular events were offered self-monitoring tools and decision aids to self-titrate treatments (McManus et al., 2014). Patients in the intervention group were instructed to self-monitor their blood pressure with a validated monitor and to follow a specific algorithm to adapt their therapy to blood-pressure trends. Patients were also instructed to seek medical advice when measured values were too high or too low. The intervention in this trial was successful in that patients assigned to self-management of hypertension achieved a better control compared with those assigned to usual care (McManus et al., 2014).

Another interesting study showed that e-learning is effective in improving the attitude of patients and their families in managing health issues. In this study, the authors implemented an e-learning module to teach a group of parents how to recognize infantile hemangiomas and when to request a medical consultation. The results suggested a high concordance between dermatologists and parents after the e-learning interventions (de Graaf et al., 2014).

Web-Based Resources and Apps

Web interventions may even be created with the interaction of patients themselves. Lifeguide (www.lifeguideonline.org) is an initiative focused on the development of online tools for behavior change addressing several health issues. Some of the Web interventions have been designed to be interactive, thus representing at the same time a resource for education and self-care.

The American Heart Association has developed a Web-based interactive communication tool called Heart360 (http://www.heart360.org), based on Microsoft's HealthVault (www.healthvault.com), a personal health record platform. Heart360 is designed to facilitate the information exchange between patients and their providers, and to promote patient engagement in disease management. Patients learn how factors such as blood pressure, physical activity, cholesterol, glucose, weight, and medications affect their health while individually monitoring those factors. Shah et al. are also conducting a clinical trial to compare the efficacy of a monthly nurse telephone interaction with a Web-based interaction supported by Heart360 (Shah et al., 2011).

A clinical trial focused on a Web intervention for weight reduction, including a self-monitoring component in which a Web-based maintenance intervention was the experimental treatment. Participants exposed to the Web intervention regained less weight at 18 months compared with participants randomized to a self-directed control condition. The difference did not persist at 30 months. This observation may suggest that social support may be particularly important for maintenance of weight loss (Svetkey et al., 2008).

Available studies regarding telehealth in pediatrics concern usability or feasibility rather than providing solid evidence on effectiveness. For example, it is well known that telehealth interventions in the adult population with type 1 diabetes can improve glycemic control, reduce the number of hospital admissions, and increase patient satisfaction (Polisena et al., 2009). Although evidence of impact in pediatrics is much poorer, a study about telephone-based interventions for teens with poorly controlled type 1 diabetes resulted in a statistically significant decrease of Hba1C in the intervention group (Lehmkuhl et al., 2010).

Internet interventions for adolescents with type 1 diabetes have been described in literature (Mulvaney, Rothman, Osborn, Lybarger, & Wallston, 2011b; Mulvaney, Rothman, Wallston, Lybarger, & Dietrich, 2010). Their main educational goal was to support problem-solving and coping skills. The interventions used peer interaction about adherence problem-solving through a forum and social comparison of responses or weekly educational sessions previously administered face-to-face (Mulvaney et al., 2010, 2011b). Mobile technology is increasingly used to provide feedback about data that the adolescents upload to an app, whether via text messaging or short prompts. Active feedback or interaction with the provider is a relevant characteristic of the most effective programs (Mulvaney et al., 2011a).

> **NOTE**
>
> There is evidence that telehealth programs for adolescents should include the involvement and support of significant others, families, and peers. It is still not clear how this can be obtained. Networking between adolescents with chronic disease may be challenging and require careful monitoring to avoid negative behaviors and inappropriate sharing of information. Increasing adolescent participation in defining telehealth interventions will favor patient-centered choices (Harris, Hood, & Mulvaney, 2012).

A series of interventions may be delivered through apps. Indeed, the Apple store alone accounted for 75 billion app downloads in mid-2014 (Statista, 2015).

Several apps have been developed for weight control and nutrition, although most of them are tools for monitoring diet and/or weight, while few seem to contain structured training in weight-loss strategies. In the light of published evidence (Acharya, Elci, Sereika, Styn, & Burke, 2011; Burke et al., 2011, 2012; Thomas & Wing, 2013), patients trying to lose weight should be encouraged to use these devices instead of paper diaries. The proliferation of wearable sensors may facilitate monitoring weight-related behaviors, although research on the best way to use smartphones to induce a behavior change is still extremely limited (Thomas & Bond, 2014).

Apps for chronic diseases are available. One app for chronic kidney disease, for example (Renal Trkrr), is a comprehensive tool enabling an individual with chronic kidney disease to record her dietary intake, track her renal function (by user input), and communicate with her healthcare providers (by inputting providers' email addresses) (Diamatidis & Becker, 2014).

There are many online resources to support behavior change and self-management. The National Diabetes Education Program (NDEP, n.d.) has published a series of online resources (videos, podcasts, presentations, webinars, fact sheets, and self-management tools) available to providers and patients. Most of them are free of charge. Some examples of these online resources for patient education and self-care are listed in Table 8.3.

Table 8.3	Online Resources for Behavior Change from the National Diabetes Education Program (NDEP)	
Web Program	*URL and Promoting Agency*	*Content*
American Association of Diabetes Educators (AADE) System	American Association of Diabetes Educators http://www.diabeteseducator.org/ProfessionalResources/AADE7/A7S.html	System directed to diabetes nurse educators to facilitate patient goal-setting Transmission of patient self-assessments Group education management Tracking online services provided Annual fee requested
Better Choices, Better Health: Diabetes	National Council on Aging (NCOA) https://diabetes.selfmanage.org/bcbhds/SignUp	Six-week online workshop to promote self-management skills and techniques Tips and tools to create and track weekly plans to improve health Blood sugar, food, medication, and exercise monitoring Group discussions
EX: A new way to think about quitting smoking	EX http://www.becomeanex.org/	Modules on how to beat personal triggers Learn about addiction and how to build a personal support system
Prevent Choices	Omada Health https://preventnow.com/	16-week online program oriented to manage food habits, increase activity levels, prepare for maintenance, and reinforce healthy habits Curriculum based on an NIH-sponsored clinical trial

SugarStats	SugarStats https://sugarstats.com/	Free tool Online blood sugar tracking Community groups and meetings Discussion forums Personal statistics sharing with others
Virtual Lifestyle Management	DPS Health https://geha5info.vlmservice.com/	Online version of the Diabetes Prevention Program Interactive weekly lessons Goal setting, planning, and support through electronic messaging Free platform
Weight Watchers Online*Plus*	Weight Watchers https://welcome.weightwatchers.com/	Real-time support from expert coaches Resources for activity tracking Community groups Recipes and digital resources for meal planning

The Role of Social Networks in Patient and Family Education

Patients are increasingly changing their approach to healthcare. Moving away from a paternalistic model, patients are becoming more willing to be more informed about their own health, to have access to their clinical information, to want better hospital services, and to participate in communities of peers. Susannah Fox, at that time leading the Pew Research Institute, suggested that social networks "… widen the network of people we can talk with, increase the velocity of these conversations, inject them with more source material, allow to archive contents, and make them searchable" (Fox, 2013 August 8).

A study on families of patients with rare diseases showed that participating in online social networks increased the likelihood of talking with physicians, was perceived as useful for recognizing a diagnosis, and improved the management of the disease (Tozzi et al., 2013).

Several examples of social networks for patients exist. One of the prototypes of these online communities is PatientsLikeMe, a social network originally focused on contacts among patients with rare chronic diseases (Wicks et al., 2010). This community allows patients to share their own clinical information on a dedicated platform to provide clear visual information on clinical trends. An outstanding additional feature is sharing side effects of prescribed drugs. Interestingly, the level of detail of information regarding side effects is much higher than that commonly reported in information sheets. Such a social network takes advantage of contacts with peers for discussing not only medical issues, but also practicalities, and for finding psychological support.

Regarding the use of drugs, side effects, and perceptions of patients, a nice example of a social network with a focused scope is represented by Treato (www.treato.com). This platform allows patients to access areas of discussions about perceived efficacy and side effects of drugs. The very high number of comments posted allows patients to draw precise pictures of what to expect from a certain medicine and possibly to intercept safety alert signals.

There is also a tendency to use social networks as a replacement of communication means including emails, especially among young people. As a matter of fact, they use social networks like Facebook to stay updated out of the hospital, to check medications, and to meet people from the same hospital, possibly with the same disease (van der Velden & El Emam, 2013).

Finally, social networks are not only being passively used by patients as a mechanism of support. A new profile of activated patients using technologies for their health is rising: the e-patient. These patients are not only willing to engage in the management of their health, but can also actively cooperate with physicians to find out relevant information, as exemplified in the passionate book by the e-patient Dave deBronkart (deBronkart & Topol, 2013).

Planning an Intervention

Planning for a successful intervention in telehealth education should take into account existing evidence, theory, and the opinions of potential users. Evidence should be both quantitative and qualitative to explore what behavior-change intervention is most clinically effective or cost-effective, and to include users' viewpoints on behavior change interventions and reasons for adherence. Theory may inform what factors are key for behavior change.

First, identify key behaviors that users need to perform, such as lifestyle changes. Second, explore the way through which a digital intervention will be delivered: specific computer platforms, smartphones, or text messages. Computer programming allows you to provide detailed information that may be tailored in multiple sessions. These may be accessed at the user's pace and time. On the other hand, smartphones are more accessible, because people usually carry them wherever they go. Smartphones may also have sensors that may provide information on location (GPS) or mood change (voice sensors) (Bradbury, Watts, Arden-Close, Yardley, & Lewith, 2014). Text messages may provide very brief information with the advantage of having increased access to the widest range of individuals.

To define an intervention plan, it is useful to explore with stakeholders which intervention characteristics are acceptable and easy to use. Digital interventions developed without the involvement of users are less likely to be effective (van Gemert-Pijnen et al., 2011). Involving users through focus groups and iterative testing may improve their acceptance and increase the likelihood that their objectives for healthcare and prevention are met.

Next, the team will have to consider what is feasible and prioritize according to time and staffing resources.

Once the intervention is active, usability should be tested. This is an iterative process in which barriers to use are identified and managed through continuing change; satisfaction with or acceptability of the intervention is also evaluated. There are several methods for usability testing: think-aloud interviews, retrospective interviews, or a feasibility study. Think-aloud interviews are done by the researcher during a few sessions of the intervention. They are effective in identifying potential problems as the intervention is carried out, allowing for prompt changes related to differentiated instruction (DI) content or other issues that may arise. Retrospective interviews are important to describe users' experiences, what they liked or did not like about it, and to elicit suggestions for improvement. Both these interviews may provide useful data that is complementary to understand the usability of and satisfaction with the intervention.

Feasibility studies, in order to test the processes of carrying out an intervention and implementation studies, may follow.

NOTE

It is often unclear what makes a digital intervention effective. What is consistent among different reviews on asthma self-management is that using multiple behavior-change techniques seems to be more effective than single strategies (Morrison et al., 2014).

An Example: Pain Management in Surgical Children

Internet-based interventions have been developed to improve pain management and self-care. Most studies in this field compare Web clinical visits and peer interventions to usual care. There is limited but promising evidence on the effectiveness of Internet-based peer support programs on the improvement of pain intensity, activity limitations, and self-management; limited but promising evidence that social networking can reduce pain in children and adolescents; and insufficient evidence on Internet-based clinical support interventions (Bender, Radhakrishnan, Diorio, Englesakis, & Jadad, 2011). A total of 283 pain-related apps accessible on the Web were reviewed by de la Vega & Miró (2014), but none have published evidence on their usability, effectiveness, or user's satisfaction. Most patient-oriented apps describe pain and are a support for assessment and medication tracking. Very few focus on alternative ways of coping with pain (de la Vega & Miró, 2014). Pain apps can be valuable tools to educate patients on post-operative or chronic pain assessment and management and to track pain measurements.

In 2014, the Bambino Gesù Children's Hospital developed a post-operatory pain app for patients who underwent minor day surgeries. Those patients were subject to undetected pain, particularly during the first 48 post-surgical hours while at home. Before the project, the usual patient's post-surgical contact with the provider was during a follow-up visit 7 days after surgery or a random telephone call by a surgical nurse.

As Bambino Gesù Children's Hospital invested in pain-prevention activities through a project called "Hospital Without Pain," the target became patient/family empowerment and greater participation in their child's care. The objective was to provide patients and families with a tool to screen and transmit data on their child's post-operative pain to the surgical staff to receive prompt feedback on pain management (see Figure 8.3).

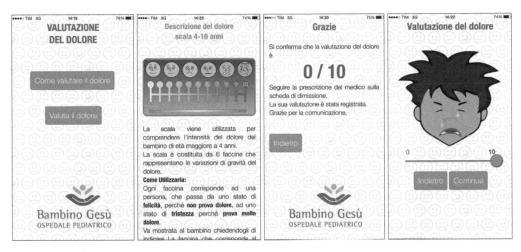

Figure 8.3   Pain management application screens for home assessment. Courtesy of Bambino Gesù IRCCS. Designed by Riccardo Ricci.

Parents that agreed to use the app were educated on the use of pain assessment scales (Visual Analogue Scale, Numeric Rating Scale, and FLACC), assessment timing, and the app's functions before discharge. Patients and/or parents were prompted to assess and register the child's pain at 24 hours, 5 days, and 30 days from the surgery, as well as any time the child presented with pain.

The project involved the following steps:

1. Develop a consensus on methods for home pain assessment, family education, information for families/patients on pain management, timing of the app's prompts, and nursing intervention for patients with moderate or severe pain.

2. Have a multidisciplinary discussion on the development of the pain app, involving clinical staff, nursing educators, telemedicine specialists, research mentors, and patients.

3. Train clinical staff on telehealth pain tools.

4. Screen patients and acquire informed consent.

5. Educate patients and families on pain assessment, pain management, and app use.

6. Enroll patients, manage data, and perform follow-up calls by a pain nurse.

7. Analyze satisfaction surveys for content and intervention review.

Almost all patients/families to whom the app was proposed agreed to use it, and 85% of the families enrolled were very satisfied. Patients with rated pain greater than 4 were contacted by a telehealth pain nurse for clinical support. Out of 547 patients enrolled so far, 42 (7.7%) registered pain greater than 4 and were successfully managed.

Conclusion and Key Points

The ultimate goal of telehealth should be to improve quality of care. As a matter of fact, telehealth interventions can greatly impact the clinical approach to vulnerable patients. On the other hand, telehealth is not only for exchanging clinical data, but also for communicating to patients information relevant to their health and educating them about management of their disease and prevention. It is well recognized that a significant fraction of searches on the Internet is about health topics. Telehealth provides a unique opportunity to educate patients and their families during consultations but also to suggest to them how to select the most accurate information that they may find on the Web. Improved health literacy is associated not only to better care, but also to better patients' autonomy. This principle is particularly important for patients with chronic diseases, which need long-term monitoring, and for patients whose contacts with healthcare centers are frequent.

Tools for remote monitoring of patient clinical parameters also give the opportunity to collect a very large quantity of information that usually remains unrecognized. Whether this data will be suitable to drive straightforward therapeutic decisions is still a matter of debate, and analytical approaches for long-term telemonitoring are an object of research. However, it seems obvious that continuous monitoring allows timely detection of abnormalities in monitored clinical parameters and implementation of appropriate interventions.

Another important effect of wide use of telehealth is an improvement of continuity of care. With particular emphasis on chronic patients, telehealth represents an extraordinary tool to accompany patients during the journey through their disease, independently of the health provider. This observation has extremely important implications that can be reflected in the organization of healthcare systems.

A likely scenario of an ideal patient who can fully take advantage of telehealth solutions may be as follows. Physicians may prescribe to a patient with a chronic disease not only lab tests or medications, but also participating in an online Web community of patients or downloading a tailored app. The app will provide patients with high-quality information about their disease, will allow them to track their disease, will track how medications are performing, will sync with some wearable devices, and will give a snapshot on how the patients are performing based on past data. All recorded data will be transparent to the patient's physician. Among educational resources, patients will be provided with online interactive video tutorials to improve their skills in specific procedures for their disease. Instead of making a new appointment for a new visit in person, the physician will program multiple contacts through a mobile phone videoconference with a nurse responsible for patient coaching. A televisit in which patients will transmit information on their vital signs may be programmed as well.

Finally, it is important for you to embrace telehealth and telemedicine not only as a way to address the issues relevant to improved access to healthcare, but also as an important means of empowering patients, giving them and their families more autonomy, supporting their decisions, and improving their health literacy level.

References

Acharya, S. D., Elci, O. U., Sereika, S. M., Styn, M. A., & Burke, L. E. (2011). Using a personal digital assistant for self-monitoring influences diet quality in comparison to a standard paper record among overweight/obese adults. *J Am Diet Assoc, 111*(4), 583–588. doi: 10.1016/j.jada.2011.01.009

Adams, Jr., H. P., del Zoppo, G., Alberts, M. J., Bhatt, D. L., Brass, L., Furlan, A., … Wijdicks, E. F. (2007). Guidelines for the early management of adults with ischemic stroke: A guideline from the American Heart Association/American Stroke Association Stroke Council, Clinical Cardiology Council, Cardiovascular Radiology and Intervention Council, and the Atherosclerotic Peripheral Vascular Disease and Quality of Care Outcomes in Research Interdisciplinary working groups: The American Academy of Neurology affirms the value of this guideline as an educational tool for neurologists. *Stroke, 38*(5), 1655–1711.

Antheunis, M. L., Tates, K., & Nieboer, T. E. (2013). Patients' and health professionals' use of social media in health care: Motives, barriers and expectations. *Patient Educ Couns, 92*(3), 426–431. doi: 10.1016/j.pec.2013.06.020

Ashkenazi, I., Haspel, J., Alfici, R., Kessel, B., Khashan, T., & Oren, M. (2007). Effect of teleradiology upon pattern of transfer of head injured patients from a rural general hospital to a neurosurgical referral centre. *Emergency Medicine Journal, 24*(8), 550–552. doi: 10.1136/emj.2006.044461

Bashshur, R. L., Shannon, G. W., Smith, B. R., Alverson, D. C., Antoniotti, N., Barsan, W. G., … Yellowlees, P. (2014). The empirical foundations of telemedicine interventions for chronic disease management. *Journal of Telemedicine and Telecare, 20*(9), 769–800. doi: 10.1089/tmj.2014.9981

Bender, J. L., Radhakrishnan, A., Diorio, C., Englesakis, M., & Jadad, A. R. (2011). Can pain be managed through the Internet? A systematic review of randomized controlled trials. *Pain, 152*(8), 1740–50. doi: 10.1016/j.pain.2011.02.012

Benner, T., Schachinger, U., & Nerlich, M. (2004). Telemedicine in trauma and disasters–From war to earthquake: Are we ready? *Studies in Health Technology and Informatics, 104,* 106–115.

Bradbury, K., Watts, S., Arden-Close, E., Yardley, L., & Lewith, G. (2014). Developing digital interventions: A methodological guide. *Evidence-Based Complimentary and Alternative Medicine, 2014*(2014). doi: 10.1155/2014/561320

Burke, L. E., Conroy, M. B., Sereika, S. M., Elci, O. U., Styn, M. A., Acharya, S. D., … Glanz, K. (2011). The effect of electronic self-monitoring on weight loss and dietary intake: A randomized behavioral weight loss trial. *Obesity, 19*(2), 338–44.

Burke, L. E., Styn, M. A., Sereika, S. M., Conroy, M. B., Ye, L., Glanz, K., … Ewing, L. J. (2012). Using mHealth technology to enhance self-monitoring for weight loss: A randomized trial. *American Journal of Preventative Medicine, 43*(1), 20–6. doi: 10.1016/j.amepre.2012.03.016

Chowdhury, M., Birns, J., Rudd, A., & Bhalla, A. (2012). Telemedicine versus face-to-face evaluation in the delivery of thrombolysis for acute ischaemic stroke: A single centre experience. *Postgrad Medical Journal, 88*(1037), 134–137. doi: 10.1136/postgradmedj-2011-130060

de Graaf, M., Knol, M. J., Totté, J. E., van Os-Medendorp, H., Breugem, C. C., & Pasmans, S. G. (2014). E-learning enables parents to assess an infantile hemangioma. *J Am Acad Dermatol, 70*(5), 893–898. doi: 10.1016/j.jaad.2013.10.040

de la Vega, R., & Miró, J. (2014). mHealth: A strategic field without a solid scientific soul: A systematic review of pain-related apps. *PLoS One, 9*(7), e101312. doi: 10.1371/journal.pone.0101312

deBronkart, D., & Topol, E. (2013). *Let patients help!* Create Space.

del Zoppo, G. J., Saver, J. L., Jauch, E. C., & Adams, H. P. (2009). Expansion of the time window for treatment of acute ischemic stroke with intravenous tissue plasminogen activator. *Stroke, 40,* 2945–2948.

Demaerschalk, B. M., Raman, R., Ernstrom, K., & Meyer, B. C. (2012). Efficacy of telemedicine for stroke: Pooled analysis of the Stroke Team Remote Evaluation Using a Digital Observation Camera (STRokE DOC) and STRokE DOC Arizona telestroke trials. *Telemed Journal and E-Health, 18*(3), 230–237. doi: 10.1089/tmj.2011.0116

Demaerschalk, B. M., Vargas, J. E., Channer, D. D., Noble, B. N., Kiernan, T. E., Gleason, E. A., … Bobrow, B. J. (2012). Smartphone teleradiology application is successfully incorporated into a telestroke network environment. *Stroke, 43*(11), 3098–3101. doi: 10.1161/STROKEAHA.112.669325

Diamantidis, C. J., & Becker, S. (2014). Health information technology (IT) to improve the care of patients with chronic kidney disease (CKD). *BMC Nephrology, 15*(7). doi:10.1186/1471-2369-15-7

Duchesne, J. C., Kyle, A., Simmons, J., Islam, S., Schmieg, Jr., R. E., Olivier, J., & McSwain, Jr., N. E. (2008). Impact of telemedicine upon rural trauma care. *The Journal of Trauma, 64*(1), 92–97. doi: 10.1097/TA.0b013e31815dd4c4

Elbert, N. J., van Os-Medendorp, H., van Renselaar, W., Ekeland, A. G., Hakkaart-van Roijen, L., Raat, H., … Pasmans, S. G. (2014). Effectiveness and cost-effectiveness of ehealth interventions in somatic diseases: A systematic review of systematic reviews and meta-analyses. *Journal of Medical Internet Research, 16*(4), e110. doi: 10.2196/jmir.2790

Fox, S. (2013, August 8). Accessed at http://susannahfox.com/2013/08/03/peer-to-peer-health-care-is-a-slow-idea-that-will-change-the-world/

Fox, S., & Duggan, M. (2013, January 15). Health online 2013. *Pew Research Center*. Retrieved from http://pewinternet.org/Reports/2013/Health-online.aspx

Fox, S., Duggan, M., & Purcell, K. (2013, June 20). Family caregivers are wired for health. *Pew Research Center*. Retrieved from http://pewinternet.org/Reports/2013/Family-Caregivers.aspx

Greenwood, D. A., Young, H. M., & Quinn, C. C. (2014). Telehealth Remote Monitoring Systematic Review: Structured Self-monitoring of Blood Glucose and Impact on A1C. *Journal of Diabetes Science and Technology, 8*(2), 378–389.

Hacke, W., Kaste, M., Bluhmki, E., Brozman, M., Dávalos, A., Guidetti, D., … Toni, D. (2008). Thrombolysis with alteplase 3 to 4.5 hours after acute ischemic stroke. *New England Journal of Medicine, 359*(13), 1317–1329. doi: 10.1056/NEJMoa0804656

Harris, M. A., Hood, K. K., & Mulvaney, S. A. (2012). Pumpers, skypers, surfers and texters: Technology to improve the management of diabetes in teenagers. *Diabetes Obes Metab, 14*(11), 967–72. doi: 10.1111/j.1463-1326.2012.01599.x

Huang, V. W., Reich, K. M., & Fedorak, R. N. (2014). Distance management of inflammatory bowel disease: Systematic review and meta-analysis. *World Journal of Gastroenterology, 20*(3), 829–42. doi: 10.3748/wjg.v20.i3.829

Lassen, J. F., Bøtker, H. E., & Terkelsen, C. J. (2013). Timely and optimal treatment of patients with STEMI. *Nature Reviews Cardiology, 10*(1), 41–48. doi: 10.1038/nrcardio.2012.156

Lehmkuhl, H. D., Storch, E. A., Cammarata, C., Meyer, K., Rahman, O., Silverstein, M. D., … Geffken, G. (2010). Telehealth behavior therapy for the management of type 1 diabetes in adolescents. *J Diabetes Sci Technol 4*(1), 199–208.

Magnezi, R., Bergman, Y. S., & Grosberg, D. (2014). Online activity and participation in treatment affects the perceived efficacy of social health networks among patients with chronic illness. *J Med Internet Res, 16*(1), e12.

McManus, R. J., Mant, J., Haque, M. S., Bray, E. P., Bryan, S., Greenfield, S. M., … Buckley, D. (2014). Effect of self-monitoring and medication self-titration on systolic blood pressure in hypertensive patients at high risk of cardiovascular disease: The TASMIN-SR randomized clinical trial. *JAMA, 312,* 799–808.

Miniwatts Marketing Group. (2014). *Internet world stats.* Retrieved from http://www.internetworldstats.com/stats.htm

Morrison, D., Wyke, S., Agur, K., Cameron, E. J., Docking, R. I., Mackenzie, A. M., … Mair, F. S. (2014). Digital asthma self-management interventions: A systematic review. *Journal of Medical Internet Research, 16*(2), e51.

Mulvaney, S. A., Hood, K. K., Schlundt, D. G., Osborn, C. Y., Johnson, K. B., Rothman, R. L., & Wallston, K. A. (2011a). Development and initial validation of the barriers to diabetes adherence measure for adolescents. *Diabetes Res Clin Pract, 94*(1), 77–83. doi: 10.1016/j.diabres.2011.06.010

Mulvaney, S. A., Rothman, R. L., Osborn, C. Y., Lybarger, C., & Wallston K. A. (2011b). Self-management problem solving for adolescents with type 1 diabetes: Intervention processes associated with an Internet program. *Pat Edu Couns, 85,* 140–142.

Mulvaney, S. A., Rothman, R. L., Wallston, K. A., Lybarger, C., & Dietrich, M. S. (2010). An internet-based program to improve self-management in adolescents with type 1 diabetes. *Diabetes Care, 33*(3), 602–604. doi: 10.2337/dc09-1881

National Diabetes Education Program (NDEP). (n.d.). *Diabetes HealthSense.* Retrieved from http://ndep.nih.gov/resources/diabetes-healthsense/index.aspx?terms=48

Omboni, S., & Guarda, A. (2011). Impact of home blood pressure telemonitoring and blood pressure control: A meta-analysis of randomized controlled studies. *American Journal of Hypertension, 24*(9), 989–98.

Pedragosa, A., Alvarez-Sabin, J., Molina, C. A., Sanclemente, C., Martín, M. C., Alonso, F., & Ribo, M. (2009). Impact of a telemedicine system on acute stroke care in a community hospital. *Journal of Telemedicine and Telecare, 15*(5), 260–263.

Pew Research Center (2013). Internet & American Life Project. Health Online. Accessed at http://www.pewinternet.org/2013/01/15/health-online-2013/

Polisena, J., Tran, K., Cimon, K., Hutton, B., McGill, S., & Palmer, K. (2009). Home telehealth for diabetes management: A systematic review and meta-analysis. *Diabetes, Obesity and Metabolism, 11,* 913–930.

Saffle, J. R., Edelman, L., Theurer, L., Morris, S. E., & Cochran, A. (2009). Telemedicine evaluation of acute burns is accurate and cost-effective. *The Journal of Trauma, 67,* 358–365.

Sanchez-Ross, M., Oghlakian, G., Maher, J., Patel, B., Mazza, V., Hom, D., … Klapholz, M. (2011). The STAT-MI (ST-Segment Analysis Using Wireless Technology in Acute Myocardial Infarction) trial improves outcomes. *Journal of the American College of Cardiology, 4*(2), 222–227. doi:10.1016/j.jcin.2010.11.007

Shah, B. R., Adams, M., Peterson, E. D., Powers, B., Oddone, E. Z., Royal, K., … Bosworth, H. B. (2011). Secondary Prevention Risk Interventions Via Telemedicine and Tailored Patient Education (SPRITE): A randomized trial to improve postmyocardial infarction management. *Circ Cardiovasc Qual Outcomes, 4,* 235–242.

Smith, A. (2014). Older adults and technology use. Pew Research Center. Retrieved from http://www.pewinternet.org/2014/04/03/older-adults-and-technology-use/

Stanton, A. L., Thompson, E. H., Crespi, C. M., Link, J. S., & Waisman, J. R. (2013). Project connect online: Randomized trial of an internet-based program to chronicle the cancer experience and facilitate communication. *J Clin Oncol, 31,* 3411–3417.

Statista. (2015). *Cumulative number of apps downloaded from the Apple App Store from July 2008 to October 2014 (in billions).* Retrieved from http://www.statista.com/statistics/263794/number-of-downloads-from-the-apple-app-store

Svetkey, L. P., Stevens, V. J., Brantley, P. J., Appel, L. J., Hollis, J. F., Loria, C. M., … Aicher, K. (2008). Comparison of strategies for sustaining weight loss: The weight loss maintenance randomized controlled trial. *Journal of the American Medical Association, 299*(10), 1139–48. doi: 10.1001/jama.299.10.1139

Tapscott, D. (2010). *Wikinomics: How mass collaboration changes everything.* New York, NY: Portfolio.

Terkelsen, C. J., Lassen, J. F., Nørgaard, B. L., Gerdes, J. C., Poulsen, S. H., Bendix, K., … Andersen, H.R. (2005). Reduction of treatment delay in patients with ST-elevation myocardial infarction: Impact of pre-hospital diagnosis and direct referral to primary percutaneous coronary intervention. *European Heart Journal, 26,* 770–777.

Thomas, J. G., & Bond, D. S. (2014). Review of innovations in digital health technology to promote weight control. *Curr Diab Rep, 14*(5), 485. doi: 10.1007/s11892-014-0485-1

Thomas, J. G., & Wing, R. R. (2013). Health-e-call, a smartphone-assisted behavioral obesity treatment: Pilot study. *JMIR Mhealth Uhealth, 1*(1), e3.

Tozzi, A. E., Mingarelli, R., Agricola, E., Gonfiantini, M., Pandolfi, E., Carloni, E., … Dallapiccola, B. (2013). The internet user profile of Italian families of patients with rare diseases: A web survey. *Orphanet Journal of Rare Diseases, 8*(76). doi: 10.1186/1750-1172-8-76

van der Velden, M., & El Emam, K. (2013). "Not all my friends need to know": A qualitative study of teenage patients, privacy, and social media. *J Am Med Inform Assoc, 20*(1), 16–24. doi: 10.1136/amia-jnl-2012-000949

van Gemert-Pijnen, J. E., Nijland, N., van Limburg, M., Ossebaard, H. C., Kelders, S. M., Eysenbach, G., & Seydel, E. R. (2011). A holistic framework to improve the uptake and impact of eHealth technologies. *J Med Internet Res, 13*(4), e111.

Wallace, D. L., Smith, R. W., & Pickford, M. A. (2007). A cohort study of acute plastic surgery trauma and burn referrals using telemedicine. *Journal of Telemedicine and Telecare, 13*(6), 282–287.

Wicks, P., Massagli, M., Frost, J., Brownstein, C., Okun, S., Vaughan, T., … Heywood, J. (2010). Sharing health data for better outcomes on PatientsLikeMe. *J Med Internet Res, 12*(2), e19.

Zaidi, S. F., Jumma, M. A., Urra, X. N., Hammer, M., Massaro, L., Reddy, V., … Wechsler, L. R. (2011). Telestroke-guided intravenous tissue-type plasminogen activator treatment achieves a similar clinical outcome as thrombolysis at a comprehensive stroke center. *Stroke, 42,* 3291–3293.

Zanini, R., Aroldi, M., Bonatti, S., Buffoli, F., Izzo, A., Lettieri, C., … Ferrari, M. R. (2008). Impact of pre-hospital diagnosis in the management of ST elevation myocardial infarction in the era of primary percutaneous coronary intervention: Reduction of treatment delay and mortality. *Journal of Cardiovascular Medicine, 9,* 570–575.

"The two words 'information' and 'communication' are often used interchangeably, but they signify quite different things. Information is giving out; communication is getting through."
–Sydney J. Harris

Maximizing Knowledge-Transfer Using Language Assistance

Lori C. Marshall, PhD, MSN, RN
Regina Little, BA, IS
Andrew Bielat, BS, BA
Victor Collazo, NIC-Master, AZ Legal-A
Ana Chavez, BS, CHI
Karla Velazquez, CHI
Nancy Ramirez, CHI

OBJECTIVES

- Explain why language interpretation services are critical to support knowledge-transfer for effective patient-family education.

- Discuss how to use the different modalities of interpretation for patient-family education, including recognizing when to use which resource.

- Provide tips for implementing Over-the-Phone Interpretation (OPI) and Video Remote Interpretation (VRI), including tips for staff education.

- Review patient and family education strategies for Deaf and Hard of Hearing patients.

Introduction

This chapter will outline the multiple modes of interpretation and language service best practices needed to support patient and family education, regardless of the healthcare setting. Using language resources supports effective communication, which is needed to maximize knowledge-transfer. *Knowledge-transfer,* as discussed in Chapter 1, is an exchange of information that is a result of effective communication. For example, a nurse transfers knowledge to a patient and family on how to give medications, change a dressing, or care for a central line. Clear communication is an essential component of the knowledge-transfer process.

Victor's Story

It was June 2002; I was happily married to the love of my life, a Deaf woman named Naureen. One afternoon while at work, just a few hours after sharing a wonderful lunch with my wife, I received a Teletype (TTY) call from Naureen that just said "Hurry home."

After rushing back to our apartment, I found my wife semi-conscious and surrounded by police. I explained to the police that I was her husband and that she was Deaf, and they called for an ambulance.

When we arrived at the hospital, I requested a certified American Sign Language (ASL) interpreter. Although the hospital personnel did their best by calling local agencies, it was taking time to find one who was available immediately. I was not a certified interpreter at the time but very fluent in ASL, so I started to interpret for my wife—who gained consciousness once we arrived at the hospital—as the doctors and nurses ran tests. Before a certified interpreter could arrive, the doctor diagnosed her with a heart arrhythmia and said that they would need to sedate her and suction out fluid that was building in her lungs. Before they sedated her, I looked her in the eyes and promised that when she woke up, I would be the first person she would see.

Unfortunately, I couldn't keep that promise. Her conditioned worsened and I lost her.

I believe no one should have to experience the same situation that I went through—when a loved one is sick and in pain, the last thing anyone should worry about is accurately interpreting medical instructions. In a time-sensitive situation like the one I experienced, Video Remote Interpretation would have allowed me to be a husband to my wife, instead of her interpreter.

The Joint Commission (2010) defines effective communication as:

> *"the successful joint establishment of meaning wherein patients and healthcare providers exchange information, enabling patients to participate actively in their care from admission through discharge, and ensuring that the responsibilities of both patients and providers are understood. To be truly effective, communication requires a two-way process (expressive and receptive) in which messages are negotiated until the information is correctly understood by both parties. Successful communication takes place only when providers*

understand and integrate the information gleaned from patients, and when patients comprehend accurate, timely, complete, and unambiguous messages from providers in a way that enables them to participate responsibly in their care." (The Joint Commission, 2010, p. 1)

The standard communication process as shown in Figure 9.1 doesn't take into account the factors affecting the receiver's ability to understand the message. These factors can include the receiver not being able to hear the message, the receiver not understanding the language, or the sender using an approach that does not permit the receiver to take in the right kinds of information.

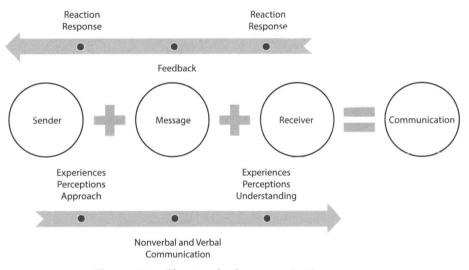

Figure 9.1   The standard communication process.

Consider an example of an exchange between a nurse who speaks only English and a patient who speaks Spanish and very limited English. The patient is being sent home from the hospital with a PICC line and home antibiotics. The nurse, who has three other patients, is busy, but this patient is going home tomorrow and needs to learn how to flush the PICC line.

Nurse (in English): You are going home from the hospital tomorrow.

Receiver (in English): [Shaking head] Yes.

Nurse (in English): I need to teach you how to flush your PICC line.

Receiver (in English): [Shaking head] I can do.

Nurse (in English): Great, so you are ready to go home.

Receiver (in English): [Shaking head] Yes.

There is communication taking place, but it is not leading to an accurate information exchange. The hurried nurse might take the nonverbal gestures as a sign of affirmation that the patient already knows what to do.

Using this example, let's explore the patient education process from the effective communication lens. In this view, the nurse accounts for her role in determining the "approach" to delivering the message. This means using a language resource as part of the process via an interpreter, who ensures the message is received and that the sender has the right feedback from which to carry out the education plan (see Figure 9.2).

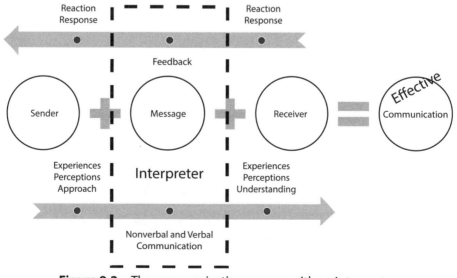

Figure 9.2 The communication process with an interpreter.

Using this example of a patient going home from the hospital:

Nurse (in English): I need to teach you how to flush your PICC line.

Interpreter (in Spanish): I need to teach you how to flush your PICC line.

Receiver (in Spanish): What is a PICC line?

Interpreter (in English): What is a PICC line?

Nurse (in English): A PICC line is a …

Receiver (in Spanish): My wife can do this if you show her how.

Interpreter (in English): My wife can do this if you show her how.

As you can see, using an interpreter becomes critical to the knowledge-transfer process, in which the exchange of information cannot take place without the two-way communication. This ensures that patients and families are engaged in their care. Significant quality and safety issues arise when there are miscommunications.

What Happens When Language Services Are Not Provided?

Many things can go wrong when the proper and full exchange of information doesn't take place. Here are just some of the issues you can run into:

- **Increased risks of medical malpractice and negligence:** Healthcare providers' failure to make effective language assistance available is inextricably linked to issues of standard of care, negligence, and medical malpractice. If a patient does not understand medical information conveyed by healthcare professionals because of a language barrier, there can be no informed consent to a specific medical procedure. Without informed consent, providers face significant liability for negligence and malpractice, plus monetary damages for national origin discrimination pursuant to Title VI of the Civil Rights Act of 1964.

- **Increased fines and rates of readmission:** Hospitals nationwide continue to face increased fines under a portion of the Affordable Care Act. If patients are readmitted unnecessarily—and LEP (Limited English Proficient) patients tend to have higher rates of readmission—hospitals receive penalties if the rate surpasses a given threshold. Medicare can cut its already low-margin reimbursements by as much as 3%. The greater the proportion of Medicare patients at a facility, the bigger the financial risk hospitals experience under the new system. In 2014, 2,610 facilities nationwide failed to meet the Act's criteria and will face stiff financial penalties (Rau, 2015). Hospitals can also receive fines for noncompliance with Title VI of the Civil Rights Act of 1964, and for noncompliance with the National Standards for Culturally and Linguistically Appropriate Services in Health and Health Care (the National CLAS Standards).

- **Lower HCAHPS scores:** The Hospital Consumer Assessment of Healthcare Providers and Systems (HCAHPS) Survey is the primary tool used to measure patient satisfaction in relation to ACA-based initiatives. Unfortunately, hospitals' efforts to improve overall HCAHPS Survey scores are often less successful with LEP patient populations and, conversely, service improvements for LEP patients often aren't reflected in improved HCAHPS scores due to low survey response rates.

- **Joint Commission non-compliance:** Hospitals with Joint Commission accreditation, and those seeking accreditation, will be scrutinized regarding their language services programs and processes for working with LEP patients throughout the provision of care.

- **Americans with Disabilities Act and Rehabilitation non-compliance:** Providing a qualified ASL interpreter to ensure effective communication with people who are Deaf or Hard of Hearing is required under the Americans with Disabilities Act and Rehabilitation Act of 1973. When a qualified interpreter is not used for medical interpreting, the patient as well as the hospital are at risk. Miscommunication can lead to mistakes in patient health and safety.

It is important to for you to understand an interpreter's role and performance expectations before the specific interpreting tools available for patient and family education are discussed.

> ## Case Example
>
> ### Using Qualified Interpreters Can Be a Matter of Life and Death
>
> "I was working over a period of time with a Guatemalan family. Once, when there was a long time to wait for the next available hospital interpreter, the clinician used an unqualified but bilingual hospital employee to interpret that a bone marrow transplant along with chemotherapy would increase the patient's chances of surviving. The family refused the bone marrow treatment, and when the patient's cancer relapsed, they came to the doctor to ask for the transplant. Unfortunately, the treatment could have only been done when the option was first presented to them. Based on the family's reaction, it appeared that there had been miscommunication, and I can't help but wonder if the patient would have survived if there had been a qualified medical interpreter there to interpret correctly for them the first time." –Certified Healthcare Interpreter

The Ethics and Standards of Interpretation

The role of the interpreter is to render a message from one language into another in a meaning-for-meaning manner without adding, omitting, or substituting information. A good interpreter will clarify, correct errors, and maintain transparency to ensure an accurate interpretation. To be effective, interpreters must refrain from advising or projecting their personal beliefs and biases through verbal or nonverbal communication and from becoming personally involved.

One of the main roles of an interpreter is to act as a cultural broker to facilitate communication across cultural differences. Whether it is cultural practices or beliefs, an interpreter should be culturally responsive. Finally, an interpreter must uphold HIPAA regulations and must not disclose information acquired in the course of interpreting. All notes taken during the interpretation session are to be destroyed as quickly as possible.

There are many modes of interpretation, but the most commonly used forms of interpretation are (Mikkelson, 1999):

- **Simultaneous**: The interpreter starts interpreting as soon as the speaker does so they are speaking at the same time.

- **Consecutive:** The interpreter waits until the speaker has finished before beginning the interpretation.

Simultaneous interpreting is more commonly used for conferences, and it is the preferred method for the United Nations and European Union.

Most medical interpreters use consecutive interpreting, which allows them to consistently and accurately convey the tone, meaning, and nuances of the original message. Using consecutive interpretation, medical interpreters are also able to look up terms, request repetitions, take notes, and verify critical information to ensure accuracy.

Best Tips for Working Effectively with an Interpreter

Consider these tips when working with an interpreter, for best results:

- **Allow the interpreter to greet you and provide an interpreter ID number.** All phone and video interpreters have a short script that they need to go through when they answer a call. Let them introduce themselves and state their ID number. Write the interpreter ID number in the patient's file or progress notes.

- **Provide the interpreter with a brief explanation.** Giving the interpreter a few sentences of background information about the patient interaction provides the context interpreters need to be more effective. It may be helpful to let the interpreter know if this will be a routine follow-up or a delicate situation, so that the interpreter can prepare to convey the appropriate tone. For example, "Hi, interpreter, I'm here with Mrs. Lin to follow up on the results of her appendix surgery."

- **Allow the interpreter to introduce herself to the patient.** The interpreter will quickly explain to your patient that they are a professional interpreter and will be interpreting everything that is said. Not only does this help clarify what is happening for the patient, especially in phone interpretation scenarios, it often is very reassuring to patients. This interpreter introduction may be a meaningful point in their healthcare experience in which they understand that the hospital cares about them and will communicate with them on any level. It can be a key step in the patient experience.

- **Speak directly to your patient and make eye contact. Speak in first person.** Using an interpreter doesn't mean that care has to be less personal. Speak to your patient as you would without an interpreter. If it is an in-person interpreter, pretend the interpreter isn't even there. If you are communicating via a phone interpreter, try not to look at the phone, but rather directly at your patient as normal. Speak in the first person, not the third. It is much easier and far more effective for an interpreter to interpret first-person interactions. Do not say, "Tell Mrs. Lin that her test results look very promising," but rather, "Mrs. Lin, your test results look very promising."

- **Use short but complete sentences.** This one is difficult to get used to at first, but using short sentences gives the interpreter a chance to relay what you are saying effectively. Interpreters may take notes to remember key things you say during a more "long-winded" sentence, but short and complete sentences ensure that no detail is left out.

- **Avoid slang, jargon, and metaphors.** Phrases like "it's raining cats and dogs" or "on the same page" may not translate very well into other languages. You could end up confusing a patient and affecting their understanding of treatment. Avoid these scenarios by choosing straightforward words and analogies.

- **Allow the interpreter to clarify linguistic and cultural issues.** Even if the interpreter is highly qualified, cultural issues may still arise. For example, the Spanish language has many dialects, with different words for the same subject. Bus is normally "autobus" in most Spanish dialects, but in Caribbean Spanish it is "guagua." If the interpreter notices that the patient does not understand something adequately, they may ask for a moment to clarify your message with the patient to ensure that the patient understands. Don't be concerned if this happens; it can be very helpful for all parties.

Different Ways to Deliver Language Interpretation

Your health system should utilize a diverse range of services to meet patient and family education needs. What you use will depend on the language and complexity of the learning need.

There are multiple modes of language interpreting:

- **Over-the-Phone Interpretation (OPI)**: One phone line with an English-speaking provider, an LEP (Limited English Proficient) patient, and an interpreter.
- **Video Remote Interpretation (VRI)**: Providers and patients use video chat with a qualified interpreter.
- **On-site Interpretation**: A physically present, qualified interpreter.

The most successful programs use technology interpreting and live interpreters in conjunction.

In-Person Interpreting

Many hospitals have designated Spanish interpreters, and some language services departments have a person onsite 24/7. Large health systems and organizations are encouraged to have an in-person interpreter available for medical staff who need to obtain consents, hold family conferences, discuss end-of-life issues, and support medical emergencies such as a code blue or trauma. Bedside nurses typically find that having an in-person interpreter has a positive impact on their relationship with the patient and her family.

Estimated length of the encounter: Best for 30 minutes or longer but determined by the type of encounter, simple vs. complex, when in person is an option.

Content of the encounter: You would use in-person interpreting for highly serious content, including new diagnoses, terminal diagnoses, end-of-life/palliative care, mental health, do-not-resuscitate (DNR) orders, complex instructions, and skill based-teaching.

Less serious content encounters that may be ideal for the use of OPI or VRI include admissions, registration, billing, insurance, and so on.

Teaching and educational encounters may also require the use of a face-to-face interpreter due to their hands-on nature; examples include respiratory therapy sessions, wound care, IV therapy, stoma care, etc.

Time-sensitive nature of the encounter: You would need to pre-schedule. Each health system has a process to request interpreters.

Language availability: Provided by your organization and health system.

Case Example

Staff Interpreters Support Continuity of Care

Interpreters often hold a dual role of both interpreting and translating. When the interpreter is constant during the patient's healthcare experience, he or she can help mitigate issues. For example, a patient was going home pending a transplant that required a special diet. A dietitian came on his last day to review his new diet and restrictions. An interpreter who was stationed in the unit was translating his discharge orders, to have a "regular for age diet." The interpreter immediately notified the nurse of the error, who communicated to the doctor on the floor that the patient was to have a new diet and teaching had taken place. Because of having a designated interpreter, they were able to help avoid an error in his care. If his orders were translated by another of the department language staff, they would have not known the medical background of this patient, and no one would have known to advocate on his behalf. Nurses can change from day to day, attending doctors change every couple of days/weeks, residents rotate, but the designated interpreter often remains the same, making continuity an essential part of the patient's healthcare journey.

Case Example

Choosing the Right Resource for the Situation

When a facility has a variety of language resources available, it is important to figure out what resource is the best fit to a given encounter. The interpreter walking around the inpatient units had the opportunity to observe a clinician utilize OPI to communicate very complex diagnostic information to a Spanish-speaking family with low literacy skills. The interpreter decided to interrupt the conversation, because the clinician was utilizing very high-registry vocabulary to explain the patient's complex condition. The OPI interpreter was doing a great job interpreting; however, there was no way for him to know that the family did not understand such a high registry. The staff interpreter politely interrupted the conversation and explained to the clinician that this particular family had low literacy skills and that maybe utilizing lay terms might be a better way to communicate with this family. This was an important step, because many families with low literacy skills traditionally follow doctor's orders and do not ask questions. This family just nodded to what was being said to them without having a full understanding. The interpreter took over the interpreting session from the OPI. During the rest of the encounter, the interpreter continued to remind the clinician about using less technical terms.

Telephonic Interpreting and Video Remote Interpreting

The choice of OPI and VRI can be the most efficient use of resources when interpreting encounters that are very short. For example, you would use this to complete a learning needs assessment or help a patient or family learn care routines by reviewing a plan for the day. This also includes preparing for self-care and reviewing discharge/home-care instructions.

Estimated length of the encounter: These encounters last 10 minutes on average.

Content of the encounter: The seriousness of the content of the encounter is an important factor to consider. Very serious cases may require the use of a face-to-face interpreter in order to provide more personal and intimate care for the patient.

Time-sensitive nature of the encounter: OPI and VRI interpreters can be secured in a matter of seconds. OPI and VRI can also be more efficient during night and weekend shifts, when the availability of face-to-face interpreters is reduced (CRICH, 2014).

Language availability: Legally, hospitals must provide interpretation services, no matter the variety of languages spoken by the patient population. One of the clear advantages of OPI is the large number of languages that are available. VRI usually has fewer languages available, but most companies have anywhere from 10 to over 20 languages.

Case Example

When a Language Is Rare, OPI and VRI Are Necessary for Communication

"One time we had a critically ill patient transferred to our hospital. The patient was admitted directly into our intensive care unit and was accompanied solely by a family member. When I was called to interpret to explain the patient's condition to the family member, I realized he had very limited Spanish comprehension and only spoke Mixteco Alto, an indigenous Mexican language for which we have no on-site interpreters available. Thankfully, our OPI vendor had a Mixteco Alto telephonic interpreter, and the doctor was able to explain how seriously ill the patient was. This patient ended up staying for a few months, and made a full recovery in our skilled nursing unit. Throughout his entire stay, the family was kept well-informed because of the use of telephonic interpreters." –Certified Healthcare Interpreter

Many times, depending on the geographic area where a hospital is located, face-to-face interpreters are only available for a very limited number of languages. It can also be difficult to provide face-to-face interpreters for Languages of Lesser Diffusion (LLDs)—those languages least requested.

Versatility of Telephonic Interpretation

The Toronto-based Center for Research on Inner City (CRICH) Health Survey Unit published a study in July 2014, detailing St. Michael's Hospital's year-long use of OPI in its language services program. The results showed that OPI added convenience and appropriateness in emergency situations when compared to on-site interpreters. Providers could treat patients without waiting for an interpreter to arrive, which, depending on the language, could take several hours (CRICH, 2014). The majority of providers for the Toronto study (2014) felt that OPI was appropriate in most cases. For a break down:

Type of Care	Percentage Who Said It Was Appropriate
Supportive Care	90%
Acute Care	88%
Chronic Care	86%
Mental Healthcare	73%

As for why OPI was reported to be less appropriate for mental healthcare, providers explained that for those patients who were experiencing paranoia, dementia, or delusions, a disembodied voice could be difficult for these patients to work with.

Taking into account these and other factors can help hospital staff to choose the appropriate mode of interpretation in a more conscious and deliberate way. This, in turn, can help to reduce the scheduling and budgetary pressures on hospital staff interpreters and contracted agency interpreters.

Review of Interpreting Methods

On-Site Interpretation

Estimated length of encounter: Long

Time-sensitive nature of encounter: Scheduled

Content of the encounter: Highly serious content, including terminal diagnoses, end-of-life/palliative care, mental health, and do-not-resuscitate (DNR) orders

Language availability: Common

Over-the-Phone Interpretation

Estimated length of encounter: Short, medium

Time-sensitive nature of encounter: Immediate, quick, routine

Content of the encounter: Average consultation, scheduling, admissions, quick check-up, billing insurance

Language availability: Various, including Languages of Lesser Diffusion

Video Remote Interpretation

Estimated length of encounter: Short, medium

Time-sensitive nature of encounter: Immediate, quick, routine

Content of the encounter: Average consultation, scheduling, physical therapy, American Sign Language

Language availability: Common

Best Practices and Tips for Implementing OPI and VRI

Of the two main language service technologies, OPI is by far the easier to use. Most companies that offer OPI provide access through a toll-free number or a smartphone app for easier access. In addition, there are a few things that you can do to use phone interpretation effectively in your hospital systems. See Figure 9.3.

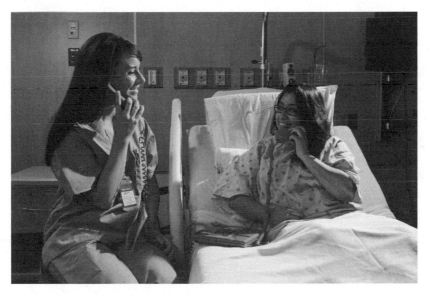

Figure 9.3   Over-the-phone interpretation.
Photo courtesy of CyraCom International, Inc.

Easy Access Checklist for Over-the-Phone Interpretation

Make phone interpretation easy for staff to access by:

- Placing cordless phones on every floor.
- Placing interpreter phones in areas of higher usage, such as the emergency department.
- Setting speed dials for both the hospital's internal telephone network and for interpreter-specific phones; when staff use these speed dials, they do not need account numbers or other information to gain access to an interpreter.

- Providing hospitalists with interpreter apps. Many OPI and VRI companies have smartphone and tablet apps; these are the perfect solution for staff who provide care in homes and in areas outside the hospital.

TIP

Some other great ideas include:

- Keep instructions and speed dial extensions on each provided interpreter phone.
- Provide all staff with ID badges on lanyards with the speed dial extensions and instructions posted on the backs so they always have the info with them and can use any phone available.

Make phone interpretation easy for patients to access by:

- Placing language service posters at all points of entry.
- *What*: These posters should display translated text announcing that language services are available.
- *Where*: In many hospitals, there are separate entrances apart from the main hospital entrance for women's centers, clinics, and emergency departments. It's a good idea to put posters at all points of entry so that all patients entering the hospital can see that language services are available.
- Placing stand-up posters at each admission station. These posters should be translated into the top languages for each hospital and say, "Please notify your caregiver if you speak [language]. Interpretation services are provided at this facility free of charge."

TIP

Try quick access cards. These cards can be provided to LEP patients with their name and language so if they visit the hospital regularly, they can just check in by showing the card with their personal ID.

Video Remote Interpretation Specifics

Video Remote Interpretation (VRI; see Figure 9.4) is a relatively new technology and may require more careful planning and configuring than OPI. Depending on your VRI vendor, your hospital may need to use the company's provided VRI equipment or invest in high-quality VRI equipment and accessories to use the service efficiently.

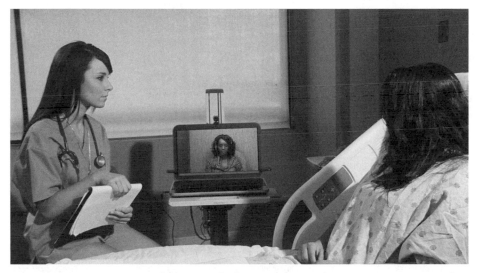

Figure 9.4   VRI equipment being used. Photo courtesy of CyraCom International, Inc.

VRI can be accessed through desktop computers, laptops, tablets, and smartphones, and there are many options to choose from. Keep the following considerations in mind when selecting your equipment:

- **Screen size**: Because a key component of VRI is the video, screen size will need to be large enough to be effective.
- **Integrated webcam and speakers**: Some devices have an integrated webcam and speakers, which can make for easier access.
- **Portability**: VRI units will need to be portable to be accessible to every patient.
- **Security**: VRI units will need to be secured in your facility.
- **Charging**: Portable VRI units will run off of battery and need charging.
- **VRI app**: Some devices will be able to access a vendor VRI app, which may make for easier access.

Equipment needed for VRI:

Equipment	Desktop Computer	Laptop	Tablet	Smartphone
Pros	Screen size	Screen size Portable	Portable webcam built in to VRI app	Very portable VRI app
Cons	Need webcam and speakers Not portable	Security Charging required	Screen size Security Charging required May need speakers	Screen size

Accessories needed for VRI:

Laptop Cart	iPad Cart	Webcam	Speakers
A laptop cart will provide a mobile platform for VRI laptops. It is adjustable to position the camera in front of the patient, and can lock the laptop in place to keep it secure.	An iPad card will provide a mobile platform to hold the VRI iPad or tablet. It is adjustable to position the iPad in front of the patient, and can lock the iPad in place to keep it secure.	Some computers will need a higher-quality external webcam to provide optimal video relay.	Some computers or tablets will need external speakers to allow everyone to hear the interpreter.

In 2015, most current users of VRI in hospitals access the service through laptops. This is a robust solution that allows for a large screen, high-quality webcam and speakers, and sometimes already existing infrastructure. If you've selected a vendor with a VRI app, this opens up your equipment options to include tablets and smartphones. Many hospitals have started using iPads for VRI, which is a very portable, battery-efficient, and high-quality option. In either case, the best practice here will be to get carts/stands to accompany your laptop or tablet devices. A cart will enable you to secure the VRI device and position the camera and screen right in front of your patient for optimal viewing.

Working with Your IT Department

By far the most critical area for video-interpreting success will be configuring the technology correctly.

Involve your IT department in VRI setup as soon as possible. Set up a conference call or meeting with your telecommunications staff so you can get them invested in configuring it to work reliably early on. Most language services vendors have documents or implementation staff that can help IT identify and work through typical areas of concern. The sooner these issues are solved, the smoother the VRI implementation will be. You'll need to address issues such as the following:

- **Firewall permissions**: Firewalls help restrict access to certain sites. IT can adjust the firewall lists to allow access to VRI clients.
- **Bandwidth limitations**: VRI requires a significant amount of Internet bandwidth. Make sure your hospital has enough bandwidth to support at least 1 Mbps download and upload speeds.
- **QoS regulations**: Quality of Service (QoS) regulations are set to allow certain users and actions to take up extra bandwidth on your network. Set your QoS to prioritize VRI calls to allow maximum bandwidth.
- **Wi-Fi reach**: Whether due to building design or equipment placement, sometimes hospitals have Wi-Fi dead zones. Find spots with problematic Wi-Fi signals so that your IT staff can fix them.

It may take a fair amount of investigating and problem-solving, but once your team resolves these common issues, VRI will run smoothly.

VRI best practices checklist for storage:

- Store VRI carts where they are available 24/7 but secure.
- Place one unit in ED.

- Place additional units in areas of higher usage.
- AoD or nurse manager will be in charge of VRI unit. Nurses check out VRI cart when needed.
- When not in use, check back into nurse station for charging.

Patient experience checklist:

- Position unit in front of patient so they can see screen.
- Nurse/doctor should stand behind or right next to screen and keep eye contact with patient. The nurse or doctor will not actually need to see the screen, because he or she will be listening to the audio from the interpreter and taking facial cues directly from the patient.
- Maximize video window to full screen.

Providing the Best Care for Deaf and Hard of Hearing Patients

"Since I lost Naureen, it has been my personal mission to provide services that allow Deaf and Hard of Hearing patients to obtain clear and precise instructions and information regarding their healthcare situation, through access to a professionally trained ASL interpreter in a timely manner. With improvements in technology making VRI a viable option, I believe it is our responsibility to provide it to those families who need it." –Victor Collazo

Understanding the Deaf and Hard of Hearing (HOH) Culture

Using one's voice is not the only way to communicate. Deaf and HOH people use sign language, vocalizations, lip reading, and so on to communicate (see Figure 9.5). Understanding the basic principle that ASL is a visual language and understanding how the Deaf and Hard of Hearing people identify themselves is key to understanding their culture. The Deaf and Hard of Hearing community is a diverse one with variations in the cause and degree of hearing loss. A term seen as all-inclusive by some is "people with a hearing loss," but some people who are born deaf or hard of hearing do not think of themselves as having lost their hearing. The three most common terms accepted by the Deaf and Hard of Hearing communities are deaf, Deaf, and Hard of Hearing (HOH).

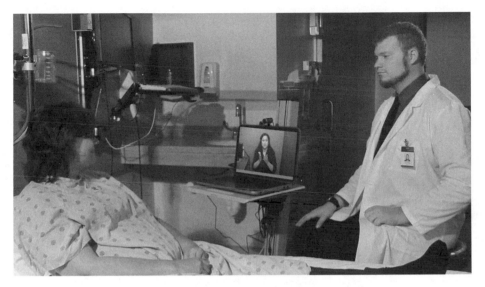

Figure 9.5   American Sign Language interpreting using VRI.
Photo courtesy of CyraCom International, Inc.

What is the difference between Deaf and deaf? According to Carol Padden and Tom Humphries, in *Deaf in America: Voices from a Culture* (1988):

> *"We use the lowercase deaf when referring to the audiological condition of not hearing, and the uppercase Deaf when referring to a particular group of deaf people who share a language—American Sign Language (ASL)—and a culture." (p. 2)*

In the Deaf community, "Deaf" is not a bad word. Hearing individuals grow up learning politically correct (PC) terms like hearing-impaired. In the Deaf community, the word "Deaf" refers to a community with a shared language, values, and traditions. Deaf individuals don't see themselves as impaired.

Hard of Hearing (HOH) can mean a person with a mild to moderate hearing loss. These people can sometimes find themselves walking that fine line between the hearing and the deaf world, while some can comfortably see themselves as a member of both.

Labels That Are Not Culturally Acceptable

Deaf and Dumb: This very offensive term was first used by Greek philosopher Aristotle because he thought that deaf people were incapable of being taught, of learning, and of reasoned thinking. This is untrue of course, as Deaf and HOH people have proven they have much to contribute to society.

Deaf-Mute: Another offensive term from the 18th to 19th century, "mute" is a term that is technically inaccurate and means silent and without voice. Deaf and HOH individuals use various methods of communication other than or in addition to using their voices, so they are not truly mute.

Hearing-Impaired: This term was once seen as acceptable and PC (politically correct). To call someone deaf or blind outright was considered rude and impolite. However, the term *hearing-impaired* is viewed as negative because the word focuses on what people can't do. It establishes the standard as "hearing" and anything different as "impaired" or substandard.

Important Tips for Communicating with the Deaf

Keep these important points in mind when communicating with the Deaf and Hard of Hearing:

- **Keep eye contact:** We "hearing" people often speak to each other without keeping constant eye contact.

- **Facial expression:** Be mindful of your facial expressions. In ASL, facial expression is a very important part of the language.

- **American Sign Language is not universal:** Each country has its own distinct form of sign language.

- **Be considerate to your Deaf patients**: Learn some basic ASL signs (see Figure 9.6).

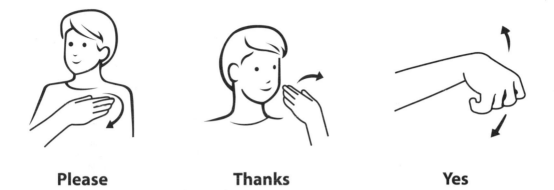

Please   **Thanks**   **Yes**

Figure 9.6   Be considerate to your deaf patients by learning some basic ASL signs. iStock photo licensed by CyraCom International, Inc. for use in this book.

Tips When Using an ASL Interpreter to Communicate with the Deaf

When interacting with a Deaf or Hard of Hearing individual who is using a certified ASL interpreter, keep these points in mind:

Do	*Don't*
Speak directly to the Deaf individual	Speak directly to interpreter
Use I and you: "What's your name?"	Use her or him: "What's her name?"
Speak in a normal tone	Speak loudly

Using Video Remote Interpretation to Communicate with ASL Users

With the improvements of technology, VRI is utilized more often as a good tool to provide ASL users with immediate access to an ASL interpreter. Both the National Association of the Deaf (NAD) and Registry of Interpreters for the Deaf (RID) have stated that VRI is an appropriate tool for communicating with the Deaf.

Excerpt from National Association of the Deaf (NAD) VRI position statement (2015, website):

> *"VRI is a means of providing qualified interpreter services to ensure effective communication with individuals who are deaf and who communicate using sign language. VRI uses videoconferencing technology, equipment, and a high-speed Internet connection with sufficient bandwidth to provide the services of an interpreter, usually located at a call center, to people at a different location. VRI is currently being used in a wide variety of settings including hospitals, physicians' offices, mental healthcare settings, police stations, schools, financial institutions, and workplaces. Entities may contract for VRI services to be provided by appointment or to be available 'on demand' 24 hours a day, seven days per week. As such, there are significant possibilities for the use of VRI technology and services."*

Excerpt from Registry of Interpreters for the Deaf (RID) VRI practice paper (2008, p. 1):

> *"When used appropriately, VRI has several benefits such as 'providing easier and faster access to communication, access to quality services, and effective use of fiscal resources.' VRI provides communication access for situations with an immediate need for interpreters; in addition, it meets interpreting demands when qualified on-site interpreters are not available, especially in rural areas where qualified interpreters are less accessible. VRI can reduce interpreting costs through fee structures and elimination of travel and mileage costs. While providing a viable option for interpreting services, VRI is not a comprehensive replacement for on-site interpreting. In order to assure that equal access is achieved, the decision to utilize VRI should be made with input from all participants."*

Training Your Staff in Your Language Service Program

Without properly training your staff, no system or program—no matter how thoughtful or prepared—will work. Your hospital must ensure that all staff knows how to access language services.

Find Your Champion

First, find a champion and expert for this program. Their passion and dedication will encourage adoption of the program among the staff. If there are any problems or questions, staff can find this person to get a resolution.

Most VRI and OPI companies have a variety of tools that hospitals can use to properly train their staff. For example, they offer videos, manuals, in-services, in-person demonstrations, etc. so that hospital staff understands exactly how to work the services. It's also important to pick a language service provider who has 24/7 customer support to help you and your staff if you encounter problems.

Training Ideas Checklist

- Take advantage of new-hires training and annual re-orientation days to provide training and a refresher course on how to use equipment and request interpreters.
- Have all staff sign that they've completed the training and understand how to request interpreters and use equipment.
- Hold a day-long training session with planned half-hour demonstrations and breaks for unplanned walk-ins for busy physicians.
- Hands-on demonstrations stick better than just explaining the service.
- Show how quickly you can connect to an interpreter.
- Tie in interpretation services with policies your hospital already has, and create an informational flyer that explains why using qualified medical interpreters fits into your hospital policies.
- Create informational flyers and quick access pages with information like:
  - How to access
  - How to use each modality

- HIPAA regulations
- Other laws and regulations regarding language services
- Make easy reminders of the process by placing log-in instructions on each phone and VRI cart.

Special Considerations When Caring for a Diverse Patient Population

When it comes to language support, you need to remember that translation is for written information and interpretation is for oral conversations (U.S. Department of Health and Human Services [USDHHS], 2014). A healthcare organization cannot translate everything, so there are guidelines on what must be translated. An organization is required to translate vital documents as mentioned in the Office of Civil Rights Title VI:

> *"Whether or not a document (or the information it contains or solicits) is 'vital' may depend upon the importance of the program, information, encounter, or service involved, and the consequence to the LEP person if the information in question is not provided accurately or in a timely manner. Where appropriate, recipients are encouraged to create a plan for consistently determining, over time and across their various activities, what documents are 'vital' to the meaningful access of the LEP populations they serve. Thus, vital documents could include, for instance, consent and complaint forms, intake forms with potential for important health consequences, written notices of eligibility criteria, rights, denial, loss, or decreases in benefits or services, actions affecting parental custody or child support, and other hearings, notices advising LEP persons of free language assistance, written tests that do not assess English language competency, but test competency for a particular license, job or skill for which knowing English is not required, or applications to participate in a recipient's program or activity or to receive recipient benefits or services." (USDHHS, 2015, website)*

Common vital content that is translated in the hospital and clinical setting includes documents that are directly related to patient care such as consent forms, education handouts, discharge instructions, and summary sheets for clinics. Additionally, a health system should translate vital documents for frequently encountered languages.

> *From the Health and Human Services Language Access Strategic Plan*
> *Element 3. Written Translations: "Each agency, program, and activity*
> *of HHS will produce vital documents in languages other than English*
> *where a significant number or percentage of the customers served or*
> *eligible to be served has limited English proficiency. These written*
> *materials may include paper and electronic documents such as*
> *publications, notices, correspondence, websites, and signs."*
> *(USDHHS, 2000, p. 3.)*

Your organization might have a policy in place specifying when to translate vital content, but a good rule of thumb is when the language represents 5% or greater of the total patient volume.

TIP

What do you do if the vital content cannot be translated? If a language need is required after business hours or for a language in which a translator is not available, you must use an interpreter to read and review the English document using the read-back method to verify comprehension and understanding. If in-house translation services are available for a specific language, your organization might recommend using OPI or VRI, then translate the content during business hours and mail to the patient's home. Please check with your organization's language services program and review policies for additional information.

Patient education materials are vital in the learning process of a patient's overall medical care (USDHHS, 2015). Any information that cannot be remembered at the time of the teaching can always be referenced back to the education materials given to the patient and his or her family. It helps patients and their families learn and understand about the different aspects of their care. It can include surgical procedures, nutrition, pain management, and medical conditions when diagnosed, to name a few. Handouts are one form of patient education materials. These handouts come primarily in English and are required to be translated into different languages to benefit your LEP (Limited English Proficient) patient population. There are a couple of resources that can help with translating the patient education material. One of them is a translator, someone who translates from one written language into another written language. The other resources are online translation tools, which are not recommended for use in healthcare settings.

> ### TIP
>
> A word of caution on the use of translation tools such as Google Translate for healthcare translation. Unfortunately, you cannot rely fully on such translation tools, because at times the translation can be too literal, and it will lose the meaning of the message that needs to be conveyed.

Assistive and Adaptive Technologies

It is important to support language needs for patients who are dependent on a mechanical ventilator or require adaptive technology communication. It is known that communication is critical to a patient's overall care, psychological functioning, and social interactions. For this particular patient population, things that can help with nonverbal communication are lip reading, communication boards, writing or typing, and computerized augmentative communication systems (Leder, 1990), which are discussed in greater detail in Chapter 10.

There are three important considerations for you to keep in mind. First, a patient may still need an interpreter to work between them and the team for words and choices not available on their devices. This means a patient may have to learn a new system in order to communicate. However, if a device is programed in a language other than English, the interpreter needs to make sure the healthcare providers fully understand what is being communicated. Simultaneously, you must utilize an interpreter to teach and guide the process.

> ### TIP
>
> A word of caution: A lot of these patients present with brain injuries and become cognitively flooded by the excessive verbal input and may shut down as a result.

Second, translation may be required for instructions and information that explains home-care routines or treatment plans. Low-tech communication systems are usually printed in the primary language and English to allow bilingual communication. Picture icons are available with premade layouts for these devices with a variety of ethnicities and gender specificities. Consider that a patient might need an augmentative and alternative communication (AAC) tool to communicate to the medical team but can read/understand information. This is key in self-determination when it comes to decision-making and engagement in their care.

Finally, even if the patient is able to communicate effectively with his or her AAC tools, if a family member or caregiver has limited English proficiency, it is critical to use an interpreter to ensure the most effective communication exchange takes place so that all knowledge and skills related to home care are fully understood and handed off to care-givers. Some AAC devices have multiple languages available; however, if a huge language barrier remains, you need to have an interpreter present for all exchanges with communicative partners who don't speak the primary language.

Conclusion and Key Points

As a nurse, you play an important role by supporting knowledge-transfer, which is based on effective communication. The key is to draw upon the patient and family's "story" to know their preferred language for speaking with medical providers and if they want to receive printed materials. Contact your department to learn more about the tools available to you. It is important for a language service department to provide you with a listing of available resources, including how to access them. Be sure to know your resources and how to use them.

Additionally, using language resources for patient and family education helps to re-duce healthcare disparities and address equity of care issues. This will be discussed more in Chapter 14. Healthcare disparities occur when different care is given to patients with the same diagnoses. A disparity based on language includes use of a language other than the patient's and family's preferred language for oral and written needs. An example you might be aware of is when a patient is Spanish-speaking but teaching is done in English.

Keep in mind that effective communication in a patient's language impacts care quality and safety. For example: medication errors such as taking too much or too little medication or the wrong medication (and the risk increases with multiple prescriptions); being comfortable in speaking up when safety issues are recognized, such as providers checking ID bands or washing their hands; participation in family-centered rounds; and involvement in decision-making, which affects adherence to treatment plans.

Remember that words do not have the same meaning across languages and cultures. If you have been exposed to Western medicine, it may seem very simple and straightforward to comprehend the language used when describing a medical history, requirements for monitoring such as multiple blood draws, and consent and the legality behind the many forms you ask the families to sign. However, in other languages, these concepts may not be as straightforward or common as they initially seem.

By being mindful of the words and language used when teaching, you can better help patients and their families understand their care and avoid all hindrances that may complicate a successful outcome in their medical care.

References

CRICH Survey Research Unit, St. Michael's Hospital. (2014). *Reducing the language accessibility gap: Language Services Toronto program evaluation report.* Retrieved from http://www.stmichaelshospital. com/crich/wp-content/uploads/LST_Program_Evaluation_Report_July31_one-up.pdf

Harris, Sydney. "The two words information and communication are often used interchangeably, but they signify quite different things. Information is giving out; communication is getting through." http://www. wordsmith-communication.co.uk/how-often-do-your-audiences-want-to-hear-from-you/

Leder, S. B. (1990). *Importance of verbal communication for the ventilator-dependent patient. Chest. 98*(4), 792–793. doi:10.1378/chest.98.4.792 Retrieved from http://journal.publications.chestnet.org/article. aspx?articleID=1063282

Mikkelson, H. (1999, January). *Interpreting is interpreting—Or is it?* Paper presented at the GSTI 30th Anniversary Conference. Monterey, CA. Retrieved from http://www.acebo.com/pages/interpreting-is-interpreting-or-is-it

National Association of the Deaf (NAD). (2015). *VRI services in hospitals* (Position statement 2008). Accessed from http://nad.org/issues/technology/vri/position-statement-hospitals

Padden, C., & Humphries, T. (1988). *Deaf in America: Voices from a culture.* Cambridge, MA: Harvard University Press.

Rau, J. (2015, October 2). Medicare fines 2,610 hospitals in third round of readmission penalties. *Kaiser Health News.* Retrieved from http://kaiserhealthnews.org/news/medicare-readmissions-penalties-2015/

Registry of Interpreters for the Deaf (RID). (2010). *VRI practice paper.* Retrieved from https://drive.google. com/file/d/0B3DKvZMflFLdTkk4QnM3T1JRR1U/view?pli=1

The Joint Commission (TJC). (2010). *Advancing effective communication, cultural competence, and patient- and family-centered care: A roadmap for hospitals.* Oakbrook Terrace, IL: The Joint Commission. Retrieved from http://www.jointcommission.org/roadmap_for_hospitals/

U.S. Department of Health and Human Services, Office for Civil Rights (USDHHS). (2015). *Questions and answers regarding the Department of Health and Human Services guidance to Federal financial assistance recipients regarding Title VI and the prohibition against national origin discrimination affecting Limited English Proficient persons.* Retrieved from http://www.hhs.gov/ocr/civilrights/resources/specialtopics/lep/finalproposed.html

U.S. Department of Health and Human Services, Office for Civil Rights (USDHHS). (2000). *Strategic plan to improve access to HHS programs and activities by limited English proficient (LEP) persons* (Report submitted to the U.S. Department of Justice December 12, 2000). Retrieved from http://www.hhs.gov/ocr/civilrights/resources/specialtopics/lep/lepstrategicplan2000.pdf

U.S. Department of Health and Human Services, Office for Civil Rights (USDHHS). (2014). *Compliance review initiative: Advancing effective communication in critical access hospitals.* Retrieved from http://www.hhs.gov/ocr/civilrights/activities/agreements/compliancereview_initiative.pdf

"No man has the right to dictate what other men should perceive, create or produce, but all should be encouraged to reveal themselves, their perceptions and emotions, and to build confidence in the creative spirit."
–Ansel Adams (n.d.)

Augmentative and Alternative Communication Needs and Patient-Family Education

Katy Peck, MA, CCC-SLP, CBIS, CLE, BCS-S
Kimberly Loffredo, OTR/L

OBJECTIVES

- Identify key elements to equipment selection and access considerations when using AAC (augmentative and alternative communication).

- Articulate key early identifiers for patients with communication needs requiring AAC.

- Determine strategies to incorporate AAC into the patient and family education plan.

- Define the role of the medical team in implementation of AAC used to empower patient and facilitate patient-family education.

Introduction

In its simplest form, communication is a rudimentary human behavior that establishes interpersonal connections and builds relationships through which we learn and thrive. The ability to request, share, question, and comment during information exchange is typically anything but simple. According to Beukelman & Mirenda (2013), communication involves expression using verbal and nonverbal language to send an intended message. This concept transcends all cultures, ethnicities, genders, and ages. Verbal communication begins with a concept or belief that is then synthesized into an intact sentence through which speech production ensues. There are some aspects of verbal language, aside from word choice and thought organization, that may additionally change meaning or the message during delivery. For example, use of inflection or changes in intonation (pitch) may be used to convey a question versus a statement. Overt changes in intonation during speech production may also indicate that the speaker is emotionally charged about the topic of conversation during delivery. Speakers place stress on specific words or phrases to intensify communication. Nonverbal components of communication additionally contribute to the meaning during the communicative exchange. Facial expression, eye contact, gestures, proximity, and body posture may alter the meaning of the actual message.

The verbal messages and nonverbal components of communication described are received by your communicative partner through auditory, visual, and cortical channels. The listener has to perceive the sounds and attach meaning to the message constructed based on the content and delivery of the message received. This involves vision, hearing, and cognitive functioning. The listener must be able to accurately hear what has been delivered, which may be difficult depending on competing acoustics in the immediate environment, attention, and auditory acuity of that individual. The listener attaches meaning to what she hears based on her own personal interpretation. We have lenses through which we perceive language, which we may alter based on the situation. For example, a patient who underwent surgery and was intubated for 2 weeks, now presents with weak vocal quality and poor breath support for speech due to general deconditioning. This patient may state, "want water." A healthcare worker might assume that the patient is thirsty. Upon further questioning, it may be revealed that the patient has significant fear related to drinking and swallowing. The patient was actually requesting a wet swab, similar to those used in standard oral care, to reduce the discomfort of his dry mouth.

According to the American Speech-Language-Hearing Association (ASHA):

> *"A communication disorder is an impairment in the ability to receive, send, process, and comprehend concepts or verbal, nonverbal and graphic symbol systems." (ASHA, 1993, p. 1.)*

Throughout this chapter, we will think over what happens when this complex chain of exchange becomes disrupted, rendering a child or adult limited and at times helpless in attempts to communicate successfully. We will also discuss how you may be able to empower your patient through communication despite identifiable limitations.

Healthcare workers in all settings will encounter patients with communication deficits. You should view barriers to successful communication as a disability requiring support, similar to a patient who requires crutches in order to walk. It is important to avoid situations in which you are forced to "guess" or assume the content during an exchange. You may unconsciously do this in an effort to decrease the duration of the exchange, avoid uncomfortable periods of silence during a social exchange, or reduce patient frustration. The aforementioned reasons described fall under the pretense of good intentions; however, the resulting miscommunications may be more devastating and potentially harmful than those variables suggest. This chapter will assist you in recognizing barriers to communication in any medical setting.

This chapter will provide you with tools to facilitate the highest possible level of communication for all diagnostic groups, ages, and cultures. You will learn to recognize barriers to successful communication in various medical settings, including hospital, rehabilitation, home health, or school-based settings. You will learn strategies to enable patients to access communication supports and function independently within their environment.

Understanding Augmentative and Alternative Communication (AAC)

As a medical caregiver, it is imperative that you are able to clearly communicate with your patient. However, what happens when your patient is rendered unable to speak? In order to be an effective caregiver, you must employ alternate methods of communication (Beukelman & Mirenda, 2013). This is where augmentative and alternative communication techniques come into play.

> *"Augmentative and alternative communication (AAC) includes all forms of communication (other than oral speech) that are used to express thoughts, needs, wants, and ideas. We all use AAC when we make facial expressions or gestures, use symbols or pictures, or write." (ASHA, 2015, p 1.)*

Typical and simple forms of AAC include use of communication aids such as a communication book, board, or chart. More sophisticated forms of AAC also exist. These include the use of computers and mechanical or electronic devices. A person is also using AAC when he/she employs a specific strategy or technique to convey a message.

It is typically time- and cost-effective to employ a simple form of AAC such as those listed above. However, what if your patient's disability precludes them from using a simple communication method? What if they are unable to use simple movements in order to use the aforementioned techniques? Perhaps there is a more efficient method available which requires less energy expenditure. This will afford access with greater ease, resulting in an upward trend of frequency of use throughout the day. In such a situation, your patient may benefit from an assistive technology evaluation.

The term *assistive technology device* is defined as:

> *"Any item, piece of equipment, or product system, whether acquired commercially off the shelf, modified, or customized, that is used to increase, maintain, or improve functional capabilities of a child [person] with a disability." (Individuals with Disabilities Education Act [IDEA], 1997, amended 2004.)*

The passage of the Technology-Related Assistance for Individuals with Disabilities Act (Tech Act) of 1988 has contributed to increased attention on the role that assistive technology (AT) can have in improving the functional needs of individuals with disabilities (Alper & Raharinirina, 2006). See Figure 10.1.

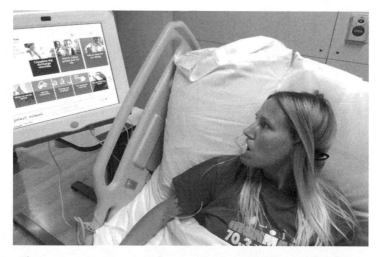

Figure 10.1 The patient is accessing the computer-based hospital interface and Internet through the act of producing a "sip" and "puff" to visually scan the available options. Photo courtesy of Kimberly Loffredo.

Roles of Professionals During AAC Implementation

Referring your patient to a speech-language pathologist (SLP) and an occupational therapist (OT) is crucial to help her develop an effective communication system. The SLP, OT, and bedside nurse will all work in unison so that effective communication can be implemented.

Speech and language pathologists are trained to determine the most efficient communication system, given a patient's level of function. The SLP will consider elemental components of communication delivery, including:

- Motivation of the patient and caregivers
- Premorbid level of functioning
- Communication supports previously in use
- Psycho-social issues
- Cultural issues

This chapter will guide you through further examination of these quintessential aspects in greater detail as you learn about AAC and environmental access in healthcare.

An occupational therapist (OT) also plays an essential role in AAC system selection, development, and implementation of use. Occupational therapists receive training in how to optimize access to the device. The OT may help the SLP orient the symbols on a communication board based on visuospatial assessment. If a client is having difficulty holding a stylus in order to access a communication board or write on a tablet, the OT is skilled in adapting the tool's weight or circumference in order to allow for improved grip and control of the tool. This will result in better hand control of the stylus and ultimately increases independence with the communication system.

An assistive technology evaluation is all-encompassing. Leading the evaluation process is patient and family preference and their cultural practices. When assessing a client's potential for use of a piece of assistive technology, the focus must remain on the patient and not the tool itself. A patient cannot be made to fit a tool such as a tablet or speech-generating device. Instead, the right tool will surface with careful evaluation of the client's abilities, goals, and cultural practices.

Familiar caregivers, including the nurse, play an additional vital role on the journey to establish a communication system for the patient. Due to your familiarity with the patient and his preferences, bedside caregivers become the voice for the patient. You and the patient's family provide essential input from the very beginning of system development. Staff and caregiver perceptions on the need for this assessment may vary (see Table 10.1). Although the medical model consists of healthcare workers with the best intentions, we may forget to employ specialty services due to the following factors:

- Pressing medical necessity (e.g., focus of care on life-saving measures)
- Lack of awareness of the services available
- Lack of awareness about how a communication-needs assessment will positively impact interactions, empower patient, and help the family coping with recent changes in the patient's level of functioning

Table 10.1   Common Misconceptions of the Healthcare Team

MD/RN	SLP	OT	Caregiver
"I don't think an AAC assessment is needed because we can communicate with the patient just by asking yes/no questions." "The patient gets my attention by tapping on the bedrail or gesturing."	"Instead of using only yes/no questions, which limits the patient's ability to communicate fully, we can use a communication board. Present pictures on the left side of the board. Start with 'category cards' to narrow down what he is trying to say (pain, change in position, etc.)."	"Since the patient is unable to press the nurse call button, use this adaptive switch to make sure he can get your attention at any time."	"I really appreciate the pictures you provided. Now I am able to figure out what Johnny is trying to say quicker." "It makes me feel better to know that Johnny can call the nurse with his special button if I am not in the room to do it for him."

Barriers to Successful Patient-Family Education

You will encounter many hurdles alongside the SLP and OT when implementing use of communication supports. Such barriers may be due to caregiver training needs or difficulty with carryover across medical professionals during encounters with the patient. The family's and associated caregivers' literacy level may affect selection of a communication system. Patients with a low level of cognitive functioning may have to rely on the caregivers' presentation of a system in order to succeed. For example, a patient may be able to communicate through shaking one finger to respond affirmatively and two fingers to communicate negation in response to binary questions (i.e., yes/no questions). The SLP may provide training for the family to only present short sentences of four to six words at a slow rate of presentation using a question-and-answer format to allow optimal comprehension of question content.

Medical literacy additionally becomes an issue during training, because the caregiver may be asking questions related to pain and medication. The caregiver must understand instructions regarding how to question the patient about their pain level or need for intervention. If there is a breakdown in communication, it could lead to unnecessary use of pharmaceutical intervention such as pain medication. All caregivers, including you as the nurse, are responsible for assessing literacy levels and screening for comprehension of information presented. When introducing AAC, specific support can be used to supplement education. This includes use of pictures for visual learners, demonstration and modeling for kinesthetic learners, and frequent rephrasing for auditory learners. You should provide all written education at a level commensurate with the 4th-grade reading level and monitor materials provided by other medical professionals to ensure compliance. The SLP may assist you throughout implementation of AAC to help you gauge the patient's and family's literacy levels through ongoing assessment. You will help facilitate carryover of use of communication systems by presenting discrete trials under the supervision of the SLP, including direct observation, guided practice, and independent use of communication systems with patients.

Cultural and Social Sensitivities in Patient-Family Education

Communication by its very nature is culturally dependent. ASHA defines a *communication difference/dialect* as:

> "*A variation of a symbol system used by a group of individuals that reflects and is determined by shared regional, social, or cultural/ethnic factors. A regional, social, or cultural/ethnic variation of a symbol system should not be considered a disorder of speech or language.*" (*ASHA, 1993, Section II. Communication Variations. A.*)

Caregivers need to be ready to interact in a patient's native language via use of translation and interpretation. A caregiver also needs to accommodate for cultural practices and preferences as they relate to communication. For example, it may be difficult for some cultures to slow their rate of speech or reduce the length of utterances. Quiet pauses after presentation of a phrase may not be a comfortable practice for certain cultures. Individuals may produce frequent repetitions and increase the intensity of their voice as a result of discomfort with impending silence during each exchange. Silence during a communicative exchange allows an individual to perform the following:

- Process the message on a cognitive level
- Elicit a motor response
- Achieve the target motor movement to respond

These culturally-based communication habits may override the specific accommodations needed to succeed during a conversation.

You must also be mindful of cultural sensitivities, specifically individual and familial preferences. For example, a family from certain cultures may insist that their nonverbal child talk to communicate wants and needs, even when physically not possible. Their belief system may incorporate standards for development unrealistic in comparison to their child's current level of functioning. Given these expectations and cultural beliefs, bedside caregivers on the AAC team must be creative and gently suggest alternatives to talking and patiently wait until the family is ready for AAC intervention. When using communication boards, icons and pictures must reflect the culture of the patient. For example, after the earthquake in Haiti, several children were hospitalized in the United States and required AAC interventions to communicate basic needs with nurses and doctors. However, according to representatives of that culture, picture icons used as symbols to represent healthcare needs did not represent the intended message. Age and gender variables may also be applicable. Men and women tend to speak about dissimilar topics and even prefer different core vocabulary than that of the opposite sex (Blackstone, Garret, & Hasselkus, 2011). Children and adults also vary in topics of conversation and word choice. A teenager may prefer slang and sarcasm, while an elderly patient may choose more formal language to communicate the same message.

Communication Vulnerability

Any individual who faces communication breakdowns or barriers has communication vulnerability.

Communication vulnerability includes:

> *"…those who have no voice or severe voice disturbance; have hearing, vision, or cognitive impairment; speak a language other than English; have limited literacy or knowledge about health care; or have sexual identity, cultural, or religious differences." (Blackstone et al., 2011, paragraph 2)*

Since January 2011, compliance with the Provider Communication Standards has been reinforced by the Joint Commission. The standard is set to ensure that patients who have communication impairments have access to all supports—including glasses, hearing aids, AAC systems, and interpreters when applicable—in any accredited institution. *Communication vulnerability* is a term used to describe a significant change in a person's functional status resulting in reduced ability to interact with individuals in their environment. In the medical setting, your patients are specifically vulnerable as a variety of tasks are done to them (for example, blood draws, catheterization, and dressing changes). The initiative and regulatory measures urge healthcare workers to foresee the necessary steps to identify vulnerable individuals and empower them to communicate in whatever capacity possible. This includes communication supports already in place prior to admission as well as implementing any newly required supports. Healthcare workers should be aware of devices and/or supports already in use prior to admission and encourage family members to have them readily available for use.

You may interact with patients as they wake from sedation, confused. Given limited responsiveness and only brief periods of arousal, you may perceive that the patient is not able to understand what is happening around them. Research has shown that one's perception regarding a patient's arousal level may be inaccurate. In fact, the patient often has transient periods of arousal as the physicians wean medications often known to alter mental status. Empirical evidence suggests that providers give unnecessary additional sedation due to patients' anxious behaviors that manifest as a result of not being able to readily communicate with caregivers or family. For patients on ventilators, Bergbom-Engberg and Haljamae (1989) found that the primary reason for feeling fear, anxiety, insecurity, and panic was being unable to talk.

Assessing the Patient

Your diagnostic journey begins with analysis of the patient's abilities. The PPFEM "story" discussed in Chapter 1 serves as a foundation to comprehensively assess the patient and their caregivers. The devices and systems you select to best meet the communicative needs of your patient are an adjunct to their story. The diagnostic assessment begins with multiple areas of consideration.

Let's look at common patient classifications in order to understand how to select the appropriate diagnostic pathway. We will arrange groups by arousal level and then consider their current level of cognitive functioning, sensory and motor skills, and language.

Low Arousal Level

This is the patient who is emerging from a comatose state and may currently remain in a semi-comatose level of arousal. The nurse will be asked by the SLP how the patient typically communicates. Healthcare workers do not typically receive training on how to communicate with this patient population, because you are typically attending to the potential life-threatening, immediate medical needs of the patient.

The SLP will explain how all patients should be empowered to interact with their environment through bi-directional communication. This includes the ability to alter what is done to them, when it is done, and provide feedback to the healthcare team on how interventions are being perceived. Does this patient want to know before you do a blood draw? Is this patient uncomfortable when you move them a particular way? This may seem insignificant in comparison to providing life-sustaining medical care; however, when you ask patients who are able to recall their experience, you will find that this aspect of their care is comparable to the need for life-saving measures taken by the medical team to sustain life.

Researchers have found that inefficient communication between patients and providers has been a significant factor contributing to adverse outcomes in healthcare.

> *"Being unable to communicate is emotionally frightening for children and can lead to an increase in sentinel events, medical errors and extended lengths of stay." (Costello, Patak, & Pritchard, 2010, p. 289)*

Costello, Patak, and Pritchard (2010, p. 289) additionally noted the following:

> *"When patient-provider communication improves, treatment success goes up, hospital-caused errors decrease and patient and family satisfaction improve."*

To further highlight this disparity in health care provision, according to Barlett, Bliis, Tamblyn, Clermont, and MacGibbon (2008, p. 1559):

> *"...patients with communication problems were 3 times more likely to experience a preventable adverse event than patients without such problems."*

Figure 10.2 shows an action plan to assist you when providing care to this cohort of patients presenting with a low level of arousal in any setting.

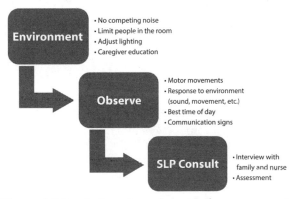

Figure 10.2   Action plan schematic for assessment.

Environment

The nurse is an integral member of a comfort team. You play a key role in making sure the environment is promoting patient success. The nurse, for instance, has the ability to minimize competing acoustics. If multiple family members are talking and the television is on in the background, the patient may feel sensory overload, unnecessarily. If the shades are open or a light is on over the patient after a procedure that took place hours prior, the patient may be uncomfortable. If you move a patient quickly without warning them, their sensory system may not be able to process and balance the unexpected bombardment of input. Overwhelming the patient is preventable when an effective communication system is in place (see Figures 10.3 and 10.4). Caregivers may not be aware of these factors related to sensory processing; therefore, education is necessary at this point of patient care.

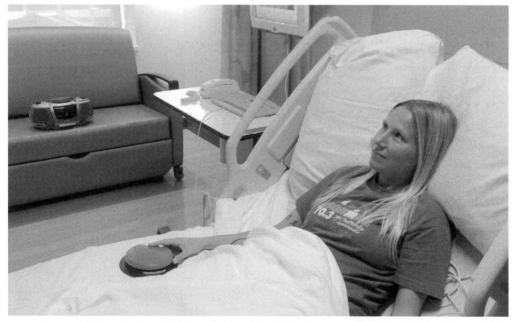

Figure 10.3   Optimal environment with minimal competing acoustics or visual distractions present. The patient is listening to music and has a switch to remotely turn it off when not desired. Photo courtesy of Kimberly Loffredo.

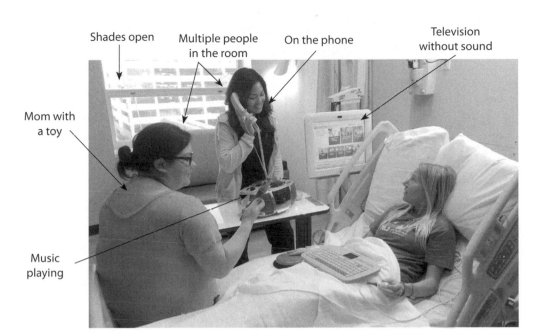

Shades open   Multiple people   On the phone   Television
in the room   without sound

Mom with
a toy

Music
playing

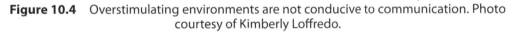

Figure 10.4   Overstimulating environments are not conducive to communication. Photo
courtesy of Kimberly Loffredo.

Observation

At the start of your shift, you can begin your surveillance of patient abilities. Ask yourself, "Is the patient moving volitionally, and if so, what is the quality of the movement?" You need to identify conditions within the environment that optimize patient comfort as well as any breakdown in the environment that may induce stress. Share your observational analysis with other caregivers so that they too can benefit from strategies that you use. For example, do you ask questions of the patient? Do you wait for the patient to demonstrate signs of discomfort? Do you look for indications that the patient is attempting to communicate?

As a healthcare worker, you are able to pinpoint certain times of the day and/or conditions in which the patient performs better. For example, a pediatric patient may perform more consistently with a familiar caregiver. A patient may present with passive participation for a maximum of 1 to 2 minutes in the early morning. However, the same patient may sustain attention for 5 to 10 minutes in the early afternoon due to changes in sleep patterns or pharmaceutical side effects.

You are the detective monitoring movements that are automatic and purposeful, and trying to differentiate between the two. You will have to decide whether the movements you observe are deliberate, purposeful motor acts. The following list explains some examples; however, note that any intentional movement that is not a reflex (e.g., repetitive eye blinking) or an involuntary motor response (e.g., hand clinching during hand holding) applies.

Identifiable motor movements for early communication:

- Eye blinking
- Eye scanning
- Gesturing
- Opening the mouth
- Wiggling the toes
- Tilting the head
- Hand squeezing
- Mouthing words

Questions

The healthcare worker has determined that this patient with a low level of arousal may benefit from an assessment with an SLP. Remember, even patients who are sedated for the majority of the day may be appropriate to participate in an AAC evaluation. No matter the level of alertness or arousal, each patient has the potential and the personal right to communicate. We, as caregivers, would never think of preventing an able-bodied person from speaking. Yet, we are actually preventing a person who has a low level of arousal from communicating if we do not empower them with the appropriate alternative methods for communication. In a sense, without alternative and augmentative communication systems in place, it is as if we have removed their figurative voice box.

The SLP will interview the caregivers and healthcare workers to learn from you, given your history with the patient. They complete a more comprehensive assessment of sensory, motor, cognitive, and language abilities, which we will hash out during a broad-spectrum overview of assessment. The SLP, in collaboration with an OT, may ascertain a more efficient method for communication that requires less energy expenditure during their assessment.

Moderate to High Arousal Level

This category includes the remaining population with which you may interface. These patients maintain an alert state of arousal for a sustained duration of time. They are more participatory and therefore will be able to tolerate comprehensive testing with SLP and OT. We will provide a gestalt of the areas we consider so that you are more aware with the process. See Table 10.2.

Table 10.2 Components of a Comprehensive AAC Assessment

Area Evaluated	Specialty Service	Clinical Presentation Neurological Change or Disease Resulting In	Remediation
Motor Skills			
Trunk Stability	OT and PT	• Poor endurance • Weakness • Spasticity • Dystonia	• Moving the patient out of bed into a supportive chair • Adapting bed or wheelchair with specialty cushions
Range of Motion	OT	• Weakness • Orthopedic fractures	• Modification of placement of communication aid to an accessible location • Use of adaptive equipment to mount communication device in optimal positions

continues

Table 10.2   Components of a Comprehensive AAC Assessment (continued)

Area Evaluated	Specialty Service	Clinical Presentation Neurological Change or Disease Resulting In	Remediation
Motor Skills			
Visual and Auditory Perception and Acuity	OT and SLP	• Blindness • Low visual acuity • Visual perceptual • Lack of attention to certain quadrants in the visual field • Neglect to perceive one side of the visual field • Color and light sensitivity • Hearing impairment	• Large, bright font • Use of magnified glass • Modification of room lighting • Use of Braille • Placement of words or picture in areas of visual attention • Use of marker lines (red tape) to cue patient to scan the entire visual field • Use of key guards to facilitate tactile scanning of all items in the visual field • Use of tactile sensation to identify objects • Use of hearing aids
Cognition	SLP	Acquired brain injury or disease progression with or without pre-existing congenital anomalies resulting in:	

Endurance	• Reduced attention • Poor stamina or endurance	• Offer structured opportunities to practice using the system during optimal periods of arousal • Provide short increments of practice multiple times throughout the day with multiple different communicative partners
Attention	• Inability to focus, sustain, or alternate attention • Poor awareness of deficits or ability to monitor performance • Pharmaceutical side effects	• Simplify the system based on the level of attention to task present • You want to make the system functional for use. The SLP may choose a system that will not overwhelm the patient. This may not be consistent with their potential, but offer more success
Initiation Time	• Delay in initiation of motor movements may be present and take up to 4–5 minutes at times	• Teach communicative partners to provide time for the patient to respond during an exchange
Memory	• Working and short-term memory deficits • Inability to recall device layout and how to efficiently select picture/words from one day to the next	• Structured practice throughout the day • Use of pictures of family members and familiar items instead of pictures available on computer software

continues

Table 10.2 Components of a Comprehensive AAC Assessment (continued)

Area Evaluated	Specialty Service	Clinical Presentation Neurological Change or Disease Resulting In	Remediation
Organization		• Fragmented thinking • Inability to functionally use systems with multiple screens or hyperlinks	• Organize the system by colors, categories, or most frequently used phrases/words
Motivation		Patients may not be willing to use a device, they prefer to not communicate	Address reasons behind lack of motivation

Literacy		• Literacy level not commensurate with how patient was able to function previously in areas of:
		  • Reading
		  • Spelling
		  • Writing
			• System should reflect current level of functioning
			• Consider if change in status is possible: Decline due to disease progression (tumor growth, demyelinating condition, etc.)
			  • Improvement due to recovery (from acquired brain injury, seizure exasperation, infections, etc.)

Receptive Language	SLP	Acquired brain injury or disease progression resulting in:	

Understanding Words, Phrases, and Conversation		• Difficulty understanding words, phrases, or conversation • Inability to identify words or pictures • Poor comprehension • Difficulty understanding verbal or written instructions	• Utilization of pre-existing communication supports • Selection of a device based on current level • Simplified systems to achieve functional use and success
Expressive Language, Speech, and Voice	SLP	Acquired brain injury or disease progression resulting in:	
Language Use		• Limited ability to combine words or pictures into phrases • Not able to generate and organize thoughts • Concerns related to socialization	• Simple AAC devices with few words or pictures • Complex dynamic display, voice output devices • Speech therapy to address deficits
Speech Production		• Able to speak, but not to be understood due to weakness of the oral musculature	• Short-term use of communication systems • Speech therapy to increase intelligibility
Voice		• Reduced respiratory stamina/volume to support speech resulting in voice low in intensity • Swelling in the glottis or vocal fold paresis (incomplete closure) as a result of prolonged intubation	• Voice amplification (microphone pinned on patient's gown or shirt) • Speech therapy, respiratory therapy, and physical therapy to restore respiratory stamina and volume during speech production

continues

Table 10.2	Components of a Comprehensive AAC Assessment (continued)		
Area Evaluated	Specialty Service	Clinical Presentation Neurological Change or Disease Resulting In	Remediation
*Physical Therapist (PT)			
*Occupational Therapist (OT)			
*Speech-Language Pathologist (SLP)			

Communication Devices

A communication system may be classified as "low technology" or "high technology." Examples of low-technology communication devices include communication boards, simple switches with voice-output capability, and basic gestural systems. For an individual to benefit from this level of technology, he would need to have a functional understanding of symbolic representations as a baseline skillset. In other words, he demonstrates the ability to grasp the relationship between symbols (e.g., pictures, line drawings, photographs) and their referents (Blackstone et al., 2011). Examples of high technology include computerized systems with pre-stored messages and voice-output capabilities. The sophistication of voice software available currently on the market allows patients to select a voice using qualifiers, such as age, gender, and ethnicity. These systems have word prediction, similar to when you text on a cell phone. This affords rate enhancement and reduces fatigue. The SLP will consider the following factors when trying to decipher between low-tech and high-tech options:

- Knowledge and skill barriers: Reference Table 10.2.

- Access barriers: Reference Table 10.2.

- Message acceleration and rate enhancement: Identify words or phrases used frequently, and adapt encoding strategy to minimize effort through diminished keystroke or frequency of selection (Blackstone et al., 2011; Patak et al., 2009).

- Patient's motivation with appropriate options: Often, a family may prefer to use a tablet due to social stigmas they perceive as undesirable, despite the fact that this system does not best suit the patient.

- Funding resources and policy barriers.

- Systems that reduce the workload of AAC facilitators.

Low-Tech Communication Options

Your patient may only be able to wiggle a toe in her efforts to communicate. This represents the foundation of a communication system enabling the patient to binary and/or conditional questions. For example, "wiggle your toe if you are in pain." When utilizing these types of individualized communication systems, it's important to perform intermittent comprehension checks to confirm the accuracy of the patient response. You may clarify and confirm the reliability of the response mode and determine the accuracy of response through reversal of questions. Using the example above, you may follow up through stating "wiggle your toe if you are comfortable." Using an antonym of the same question minimizes presentation of new words or altered sentence structure while confirming response intent. This may result in determining that your communication system needs modification. You may notice that a patient shakes their head in response to yes/no questions and assume this is the patient indicating "no." However, it is common for patients to move reflexively in this manner due to automaticity of the movement with no correlation to the actual communicative exchange. This represents another example of how simple movements may be misconstrued by medical professionals and caregivers when using low-tech communication options.

To avoid communication breakdown, empower the patient, and reduce unnecessary energy expenditure, communication systems should be documented and posted once developed. Nurses and therapists work together to write the communication strategies using simple terms and pictures. This may be posted in the medical record, interdisciplinary notes, or handoff communication, and most importantly at the bedside for all caregivers to reference. In the home environment, this may be posted in multiple areas of the home and available on a portable, laminated sheet for community outings. Refer to Figures 10.5 through 10.7 for sample communication systems.

Let's role play a conversation between the nurse and patient. In this model, the motor effort in response to verbal requests is movement of the index finger. You ask the patient to cease movement of this extremity if the response to the question or statement is "no." Please note that the SLP will further evaluate these movements; however, it is helpful for you to begin an early inventory to meet the immediate needs of the patient if early communicative efforts are existent.

You begin to make use of the purposeful movement through asking conditional questions with a mutually known response:

Nurse: "John, wiggle your finger if you are lying down."

(The nurse allows the patient time to respond, which may be seconds to minutes.)

John: Wiggles his index finger.

(The nurse then asks the question in reverse.)

Nurse: "Wiggle your finger if you are standing up."

John: No movement.

Nurse: "Wiggle your finger if your name is Mark."

John: No movement.

Nurse: "Wiggle your finger if your name is Sam."

John: No movement.

Nurse: "Wiggle your finger if your name is John."

John: Wiggles his index finger.

This confirms the patient's understanding of the question and the effectiveness of the communication system. You may observe signs of frustration as you ask questions in reverse. You can remind the patient that you are aware you are repeating the same question, but that it is necessary to make sure miscommunications do not happen. You may want to mention that this helps you to know how much the patient is able to comprehend given the current circumstances.

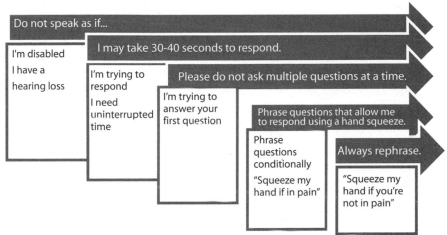

Figure 10.5   Single motor response communication system (hand squeeze).

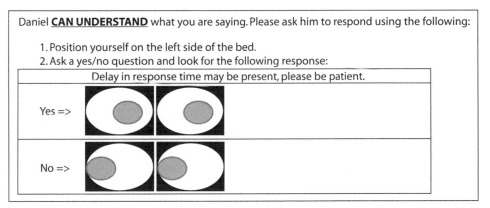

Figure 10.6   Eye gaze communication system.

Category				Yes/No Questions				
Pain				Sharp	Aching	Nausea	Dizziness	Need Medicine
Family				Mom	Dad	Johnny	Jacob	Hilary
Position				Up	Down	Legs	Back	Side
Environment				Cold	Hot	Loud	Quiet	Too Many People
Greetings/Questions	Hi	Who are you?	Will you come back later?	Will you please leave?		Bye		

Figure 10.7   This system utilizes visual scanning with organization of common
categories of communicative content available.

When your patient is unable to speak, a simple way of facilitating communication may be building a high-frequency word list (see Table 10.3). This is a basic list of words/phrases that are commonly used in a certain setting or situation, specific to that patient. It is optimal for the patient to participate in formulating the list herself. In some cases, the patient may be undergoing an elective surgery in which she is aware that she will be unable to communicate immediately following the surgery. Therefore, the patient will create a high-frequency word list with the help of the SLP to be used during the recovery phase when she is rendered unable to speak.

Furthermore, it is common for implementation of a communication system to begin after the barriers to communication are already present. This may be a result of trauma, post-surgical complications, intubation, acquired brain injury, orofacial procedures, or other medical implications. The nurse and the family engage with the patient throughout the day and have a unique grasp on concepts the patient may need to communicate given their current status and environment.

Table 10.3   A Typical High-Frequency, Core Vocabulary Inventory

Communication Inventory

Environment	People	Comfort	Frequent Requests
I'm hot	Mom	Head up/down	Please don't talk about me; talk with me.
I'm cold	Dad	I need my glasses	
It's too loud	Brother	I want a pillow	Please wait. I have something to say.
Lights out	Sister	I want to go to bed	
Lights on	Doctor	I want to sit on a chair	That's not what I meant.
Too many visitors	Nurse		
	Therapist	I am uncomfortable	I want to talk about _____.
		Please reposition me	

Feelings	Activities	Healthcare Needs	Responses
Happy	Computer	I cannot breathe.	Yes
Sad	Read	Leave me alone.	No
Scared	Television	I am in pain.	Maybe
Frustrated	Movie	Give me a tissue.	
Confused	Music	Clean my mouth.	
Anxious		Wipe my face.	
		I would like a blanket.	

The SLP will organize the vocabulary words to facilitate access and time enhancement. This may be categorical or color-coded, pictures or words. The list is presented in preferred languages, taking into account the patient's cultural considerations. All pictures and gestures are not universally understood; therefore, a picture of a person making the "ok" gesture may be meaningless to some cultures. Icons are pictures symbols that represent words or concepts. Positioning of the icons on the page or screen is important. Your patient may present with blind spots or visual neglect of a certain side or area. The icons may be deliberately presented on one side of a patient's visual field to accommodate for any visual neglect. Icons will also be personalized in the areas of font size and color to ensure successful viewing. The caregivers may provide input as to whether a patient would prefer to use a low-tech system (e.g., communication board) vs. a high-tech system (e.g., speech-generating device). See Figures 10.8 and 10.9.

You, as the bedside nurse, may find that through discrete trials throughout the day that the patient actually prefers a different method. Feedback from all familiar caregivers then allows the SLP and OT to adjust the plan accordingly to accommodate for such preferences. You are critical in monitoring the patient's success when using the communication system. Ongoing modifications in communication systems can only happen if the AAC team and healthcare workers maintain bi-directional communication throughout the process.

A communication board may be developed specifically for individual patients to meet immediate communication needs. The board will display printed words or picture icons to represent single symbols. Depending on a patient's cognitive and visual status, the therapist may limit the number of words or pictures per page. The therapist may alter the size of each icon (picture symbol) or change the orientation. For example, a patient with severe cognitive deficits may only be able to process two pictures presented at opposite ends of the visual field due to limited attention. In this case, the therapist alters the orientation to compensate for visual perception and attention. An individual functioning at a higher cognitive level (with intact fine-motor coordination) may be successful with up to 64 icons per page. Although this presentation may appear visually overwhelming initially, it allows the patient to readily combine icons to formulate sentences and elaborate thoughts.

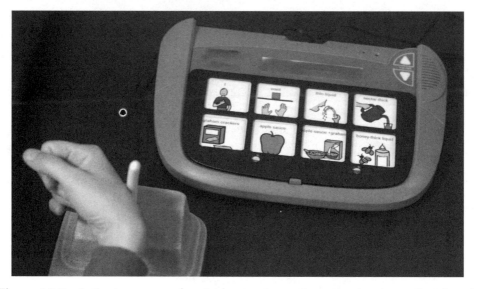

Figure 10.8   Patient accesses a low-tech scanning, voice-output system using dorsal aspect of hand. Photo courtesy of Christopher Stevens.

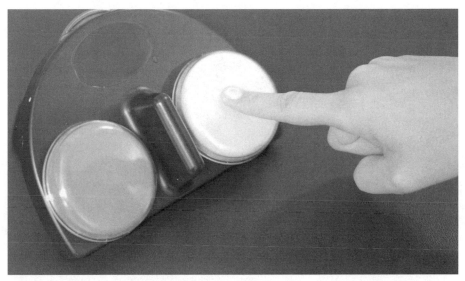

Figure 10.9   Patient uses pointer finger as a method of direct selection using this binary voice output switch. Photo courtesy of Christopher Stevens.

Communication Boards

A communication board (see Figure 10.10) may be mounted to improve accessibility and use. Communication boards are lightweight, inexpensive, and may be easily adjusted to meet the needs of your patient's changes in status (Berg, Doering, Fung, Gawlinski, Henneman, & Patak, 2006). You may want to use this tool on your unit for short-term communication support. These systems are typically replaced by more efficient methods of communication if long-term use is anticipated. Patients may only require use during a short-term hospitalization to meet their needs temporarily until their ability to communicate returns.

The SLP may supply nurses with low-tech options and provided training for immediate implementation. The teamwork lends an open exchange between the nurse and SLP as ongoing assessment of the system continues. Systems should not be recycled between patients or used without input from an SLP to ensure that this dyad is successful.

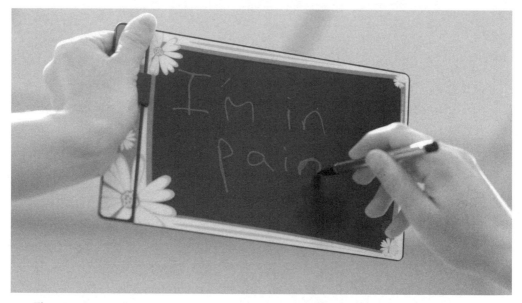

Figure 10.10   Patient uses a stylus to write a message while supine in bed. Photo courtesy of Christopher Stevens.

Voice Output Devices

These devices are simple switches that, when activated, will play a recording. The device may be prerecorded with the patient's or caregiver's voice. You may use switches with binary message capabilities through implementation of prerecorded messages such as "I'm ready" and "stop please" during daily care or medical procedures. This will allow the patient to guide your actions similar to how an oral-speaking individual does, as you have now provided a voice for this nonverbal patient. Switches may also function to gain the attention of friends, family, and caregiver in the immediate environment through simply recording a message, such as, "I need you." In the hospital, your patient may use a switch with voice-recording capabilities in connection with the nurse call light (in lieu of using a traditional nurse call system).

If further environmental adaptations are necessary, a referral to occupational therapy is appropriate. The occupational therapist (OT) on your AAC team is equipped with a variety of adaptive buttons and switches so that the environment may be adapted for greater independence. If the voice output device with prerecorded phrases is not loud enough for the nurses to hear the call for help, and the patient is unable to physically depress the nurse call button, the OT may adapt the nurse call system. An adaptive button can be placed in line with the hospital call light system so the patient may activate this universal system in an alternative way. For example, a large flat button requires only a gentle tap from a patient to activate the nurse call light. The button may be mounted at the leg, head, chin, or wherever the patient finds it the most convenient.

If the patient is completely unable to move, as in the case of quadriplegia, many high-tech options exist. One of the most common is a pneumatic switch. This dual switch is designed to be activated by breathing through a tube for individuals with severe physical disabilities. Sipping on the switch activates one switch; puffing activates the other. Pneumatic switches can be used to activate a variety of devices including the nurse call light, an augmentative communication device, or a wheelchair.

A variety of other adaptations are available to permit access to assistive technology. These include devices controlled by eye gaze, tongue movements, or mouth sticks, just to name a few. The occupational therapist will work with you, the patient, and the family to determine the most efficient adaptive switch to not only control the communication device, but to control as much of the immediate environment as possible. Please refer to Figure 10.9 for details. As you can see, switches are simple supports that can reconnect patients with their surroundings and empower them to be an active part of their surroundings and overall healthcare (Chlan, Grossbach, & Stranberg, 2011).

Conclusion and Key Points

When a low-tech option does not seem to meet the needs of your patient and/or caregiver, a high-tech option may be considered. Today, technology continues to evolve, allowing caregivers better communication with their patients. Speech-generating devices (SGDs) are a common option employed by the AAC team. SGDs are most appropriate for patients with higher-level cognitive functioning. As noted previously, there is a wide variety of tools available to access these systems. These include large or adaptive buttons used when a patient is unable to press the keys of the device in a traditional manner, as well as access systems that do not involve traditional motor movements, such as eye gaze, pneumatic controls, and tongue and mouth controls. Given the rise in technology, lighter-weight options similar to tablets are available with similar capabilities. Devices may allow a person to type with voice output, allowing others to hear the message. A variety of voices with consideration to age, gender identity, and ethnicity are available for selection on the majority of these devices.

Because technology continues to advance these complex systems, we have not discussed every option available to enhance communication in depth. This chapter has identified how you, as a nurse, can facilitate communication in collaboration with specialty services involved in a patient's care, and you can apply those same techniques to equipment selection, incorporating AAC into the patient and family education plan and facilitating patient-family education.

References

Ansel Adams. (n.d.). BrainyQuote.com. Retrieved June 1, 2015, from the BrainyQuote.com website at http://www.brainyquote.com/quotes/quotes/a/anseladams408598.html

Alper, S., & Raharinirina, S. (2006). Assistive technology for individuals with disabilities: A review and synthesis of the literature. *The Journal of Special Education and Technology, 21*(2), 47.

American Speech-Language-Hearing Association (ASHA). (1993). Definitions of communication disorders and variations. Retrieved from http://www.asha.org/policy/RP1993-00208/

American Speech-Language-Hearing Association (ASHA). (2015). Augmentative and Alternative Communication (AAC). Accessed at: http://www.asha.org/public/speech/disorders/AAC/

Barlett, G. R., Blais, R., & Tamblyn, R. (2008). Impact of patient communication problems on the risk of preventable adverse events in the acute care settings. *Canadian Medical Association Journal,* 178, 1555–1562.

Berg, J., Doering, L., Fung, N., Gawlinski, A., Henneman, E., & Patak, L. (2006). Communication boards in critical care: Patients' views. *Applied Nursing Research,* 19, 182–190.

Bergbom-Engberg, I., & Haljamae, H. (1989). Assessment of patients' experience of discomforts during respirator therapy. *Critical Care Medicine,* 17, 1068–1072.

Beukelman, D., & Mirenda, P. (2013). *Augmentative and Alternative Communication* (4th ed.), Baltimore, MA: Paul. H Brookes Publishing Co.

Blackstone, S., Garret, K., & Hasselkus, A. (2011). New hospital standards will improve communication: Accreditation guidelines address language, culture, vulnerability, health literacy. The ASHA Leader, January 2011, Vol. 16, 24–25. doi:10.1044/leader.OTP.16012011.24 Accessed at http://leader.pubs.asha.org/article.aspx?articleid=2278968

Chlan, L., Grossbach, I., & Stranberg, S. (2011). Promoting effective communication for patients receiving mechanical ventilation. *Critical Care Nurse, 31*(3), 46–62.

Costello, J., Patak, L., & Pritchard, J. (2010). Communication vulnerable patients in the pediatric ICU: Enhancing care through augmentative and alternative communication. *Journal of Pediatric Rehabilitation Medicine: An Interdisciplinary Approach,* 3, 289–301.

Individuals with Disabilities Education Act (IDEA), Assistive Technology Act. (1997, amended 2004)-;Authority: 20 U.S.C 1401 PUBLIC LAW 108–364—OCT. 25, 2004. Accessed at: http://idea.ed.gov/

Patak, L., Wilson-Stronks, A., Costello, J., Kleinpell, R. M., Henneman, E. A., Person, C., & Happ, M. B. (2009). Improving patient-provider communication: A call to action. *JONA, 39*(9), 372–376.

Vanderheiden, G., & Kelso, D. (1987). Comparative analysis of fixed-vocabulary communication acceleration techniques. *Augmentative and Alternative Communication, 3,* 196–206.

Establishing a Health System Approach for Patient and Family Education

"Begin with the end in mind."
–Stephen Covey (2000)

Patient-Family Education Documentation Processes and Systems

Christina L. Cordero, PhD, MPH
Lori C. Marshall, PhD, MSN, RN

Introduction

Patient and family education is an integral part of quality patient care. In order for patients and families to actively participate in care and make informed decisions, it is imperative that all involved understand the diagnosis and treatment information provided by the myriad of healthcare professionals they encounter. The documentation of patient and family education is a key component of your patient and family education process.

Documenting patient and family education allows the providers across your organization to capture information about the patient's and family's learning needs, the educational resources used by staff, their overall response to learning, and any future education needs the patient/family may have. Comprehensive documentation of patient and family education creates a roadmap of where the patient has been and where he or she is headed next.

This chapter discusses how to develop a process to consistently document patient and family education information, including the data elements to include in your documentation system, and options for aligning all of the important documentation components across the continuum of care. While we acknowledge that institutions may have a predominantly electronic, paper, or a hybrid paper-and-electronic documentation system, this chapter focuses on the development of an electronic documentation system for patient and family education.

Documenting Patient and Family Education Is Critical

Research has shown that strategies to improve patient education can reduce hospital readmission rates (Peter et al., 2015; Robert Wood Johnson Foundation [RWJF], 2010). When patients understand how to take medications or make follow-up appointments, the risk of being readmitted or visiting the emergency department decreases by 30%, as compared to patients who do not show a similar level of understanding (Jack et al., 2009). There is also evidence demonstrating that patients with limited English proficiency are more likely to experience an adverse event than English-speaking patients (Divi, Koss, Schmaltz, & Loeb, 2007). Identifying and addressing patient communication needs (such as preferred language or health literacy level) during the provision of care can improve patient safety (DeWalt et al., 2006; Flores, Abreu, Pizzo Barone, Bachur, & Lin, 2012).

Confusion about which educational content to use, storing resources in multiple locations, and lack of access to the area of the medical record used to document education have all been cited as challenges to routine documentation of patient and family education information (Buchko, Gutshall, & Jordan, 2012; Cook et al., 2008; Portz & Johnston, 2014).

> *"Developing a consistent approach to documenting patient and family learning needs, as well as the education provided, can greatly support your organization's efforts to deliver high-quality care."*

When you take a consistent approach to documentation, your staff will be able to access vital information about who should receive education, how they should receive it, and what education has already been received. A better understanding of where patients and families are in the learning process will enable your staff to work collaboratively to address any existing or pending educational needs. Appropriate documentation also decreases the likelihood of losing an opportunity to provide or reinforce educational material when necessary.

Common Challenges with Documentation

With so many healthcare professionals involved in educating patients and families during different encounters, it is important to design and implement a documentation system that addresses the challenges of managing multiple entries into the medical record (including fragmented, duplicate, and incomplete information) and relying on free text or narrative content to capture key data elements. Unfortunately, most healthcare organizations structure their documentation systems to meet regulatory or accreditation requirements, and the systems are not always developed to support a broader vision. Insufficient time and effort invested into identifying the necessary components for a patient and family educational documentation system can lead to several issues that may negatively affect the patient-family education process.

Dealing with Multiple Entries

Documentation of patient and family education (PFE) can occur at various points throughout the provision of care. An assessment of patient and family learning needs should take place early in the process, before any education is provided. However, after the initial assessment is completed, multiple providers will access the medical record to enter and update PFE information. If the documentation system is not designed to store the information in a single location or in a standardized format, it will be difficult for your staff to identify what was taught to whom, and by whom.

Fragmented Information

Often, patient and family education is documented based on an episode of care or a specific care setting. In some organizations, each department or setting may have its own process for documenting patient and family education. Some disciplines may have a specific area in the medical record to document education, while others may chart education as part of their progress notes. Entering information in multiple locations within the medical record makes it difficult for the nurse or other providers to identify the education already given and to follow through or reinforce the learning. A fragmented view of the education provided also prohibits your staff from getting a complete picture of the education process.

Duplicate Information

Another concern regarding multiple entries into the medical record is duplicated information. If there is no standardized format or location for entering information about patient and family education, different providers may unknowingly document the same learning needs or duplicate education efforts. Additionally, if the information entered is not linked to other entries about patient and family education, the healthcare team cannot easily see the progression of the learning process. Staff will need to spend extra time trying to piece the information together to understand what education was provided and whether reinforcement is necessary. For example, if a patient has five separate entries in the medical record pertaining to education about asthma, a nurse would need to review each teaching note to get a sense of what information the patient has already received and to identify if additional education or follow-up is required.

Incomplete Information

Documentation systems can be built to include data fields that capture the patient and family's learning needs, the individuals who received education, the date education was provided, and the staff member that did the teaching. However, even when a standardized process for documenting patient and family education is in place, the information collected may still be incomplete or documented inconsistently. The quality of the data collected depends on the provider being familiar enough with the patient and family educational process to ensure that all of the relevant information is recorded in the system.

One area of your documentation system that may require extra attention is the learning needs assessment. The learning needs assessment is used to identify crucial information about any barriers, limitations, or specific needs that should be addressed in the education plan. Typically, information such as the patient's preferred language for discussing healthcare, information regarding cultural or religious beliefs, health literacy needs, or physical or cognitive limitations are documented. It is also common to identify the patient's primary caregiver or other individuals that the patient would like to be involved in the education process. While it is helpful for the documentation system to provide areas to capture these data elements through drop-down menus or checklists, the provider must first acknowledge the importance of completing the entire assessment and incorporating additional detail when necessary. If the learning needs assessment is incomplete or the learning needs are defined inconsistently across departments, key pieces of information may be omitted from the medical record that can have a significant impact on the success of the education plan.

Relying on Free Text

Documenting patient and family education information using free text to capture narrative content, instead of incorporating drop-down menus or specific data fields, introduces variation in how staff record the components of the education process. As mentioned, inconsistent documentation of the learning needs assessment has the potential to negatively affect the education plan, because information can be inaccurate or omitted. Free text can also be problematic for documenting the evaluation of learning outcomes, because the information is left open to interpretation by other members of the care team.

The use of communication tools—such as Data-Action-Response-Plan (DARP), Situation-Background-Assessment-Recommendation-Question (SBARQ), or progress-style notes that have a header but include the pertinent information in the narrative section—can also lead to differences in the way staff document education activities. Some staff will write too much or include irrelevant details, while others may not provide enough information. Relying on free text is not only inefficient for the person entering the information, but it also creates challenges for future analysis of specific data elements identified during the education process. When details are embedded in narrative paragraphs, it can be difficult to extract, sort, and link data that may otherwise be available if collected in a structured format.

Designing a System to Document Patient and Family Education

It is not uncommon for disciplines and settings within the same organization to use completely different methods to document PFE information. While collecting the information through a variety of forms or notes may meet the overall requirement to capture the teaching and education provided, it can create several challenges with respect to the usability of the data at the individual and aggregate level. Designing a system to consistently document PFE information can improve your organization's ability to evaluate learning and identify opportunities to enhance your PFE process to increase care quality and patient safety.

Assessing the Current Process

The first step in designing a system to document patient and family education is to conduct an assessment of your current documentation process. Before developing new process steps or incorporating additional data elements, you need to understand the following:

- What PFE information is currently being documented?
- What are the common challenges or barriers to consistently documenting the information?
- What problems occur as a result of inconsistent documentation?
- Where in the medical record are staff documenting PFE information?
- How does each discipline or setting document the information (e.g., in progress or visit notes, or is there a specific area for education information)?
- Which staff members are responsible for documenting PFE information?
- How does each discipline or setting define patient and family education?
- What are the differences between how education is defined across disciplines or settings?
- How is PFE information incorporated into the education plan?
- Which staff have access to the information?
- What are the barriers to accessing the information?
- What are the challenges to incorporating the information into the education plan?
- What educational content and resources are being used in the different disciplines and settings at your facility?
- What content and resources are shared across disciplines and settings? What content and resources are unique?
- What is the process to catalog the different forms, notes, or resources being used across disciplines and settings?
- Where are the educational content and resources located within each discipline or setting?

Creating a Vision for a New Documentation Process

After identifying the benefits and challenges of your existing process for documenting PFE, you also need to consider how a new documentation system will be used during the different encounters and settings throughout your organization. In addition to addressing the documentation barriers in your current system, the new system should be designed with future data use in mind, including standardized terminology and specific data elements that can be analyzed at the individual, aggregate, or system level. Understanding how the data is intended to be used can influence the way you design the documentation system.

Another important component in the development of a new documentation system is the inclusion of key stakeholder input. It is beneficial to work collaboratively with an interprofessional team on the design and format of the documentation system, because the end users bring a valuable perspective on how the system fits into the current workflow and whether the system is intuitive and easy to use. Gathering staff feedback will help identify the documentation needs of the disciplines or settings that use the system and ensure that essential information is captured during the different types of encounters that occur across your organization.

Determining Crucial Data Elements

Determining the critical data elements to collect in your documentation system depends on the way the data is currently being used and how the data may be used in the future. Designing the system to collect information that can be extracted, sorted, and linked will allow you to analyze data at the individual and aggregate levels, which provides an opportunity to learn about the education provided to each patient and to the patient population as a whole. Collecting data through an institution's interactive patient care system (including utilization of video education, medication teaching, safety education content, and discharge preparation assessments) can add another layer of information. This will be addressed in more detail in Chapter 14.

Using Data at the Individual Level

Documenting PFE information at the individual level includes all relevant data about the patient, family, or caregiver's education experience at one moment in time. The learning needs assessment identifies critical data pertaining to barriers, limitations, or specific needs that should be addressed in the patient and family's education plan. It is also important to include standardized definitions for each of the learning needs, so that consistent information is documented, regardless of the discipline or setting in which the data is collected.

The data collected during the learning needs assessment should include any communication needs that can affect the patient and family's ability to understand the information provided and to communicate effectively with the healthcare team. The learning needs assessment also serves as a foundation for choosing the most appropriate method or format to use to present educational content. Recommended data elements related to communication needs include, but are not limited to:

- Preferred language for discussing healthcare—does the patient/family need a language interpreter and/or translated written materials?

- Race, ethnicity, or cultural information—are there any cultural considerations (e.g., customs and practices) that might influence the education provided?

- Religious or spiritual beliefs—are there any religious or spiritual considerations (e.g., customs and practices) that may have an impact on the education provided?

- Health literacy needs—does the patient/family need plain language material or supplemental information in alternate formats (i.e., written, audio, or video)?

- Augmentative and assistive communication resources—does the patient need augmentative and assistive communication resources, aids, or devices (see Chapter 10)?

Family members and caregivers are integral to the education process, and your documentation system should identify the patient's primary caregiver or any other individuals whom the patient requests to be included in the education. Patients may prefer to have extended family members participate or may only select a few individuals to involve in the process. The documentation system should be flexible enough to capture information regarding any relevant cultural considerations, family structure information, and overall patient preferences.

Using Data at the Aggregate Level

A well-designed PFE documentation system can provide valuable data for the analysis of quality measures and patient outcomes, and for other research purposes. If the documentation system incorporates standardized definitions for potential learning needs, and data elements are systematically collected through drop-down menus or checklists, individual-level data can be extracted from the system and aggregated for further analysis.

Using data at the aggregate level allows you to learn about the educational needs of the patient population your organization serves. Reviewing aggregate data about patient and family communication needs identified during the learning needs assessment may indicate an increase in the resources required for a specific population. For example, if there is an influx of patients and families that list Spanish as their preferred language for discussing healthcare, it may be necessary to expand your organization's resources for the Spanish-speaking population. This may include additional interpreters, translated materials, or staff training on the use of language services as it relates to interpreting requirements and vital documents. These issues are outlined in Chapter 9.

As discussed earlier in this chapter, a documentation system that relies heavily on free text to capture patient and family education information can create challenges for future data analysis. If learning needs assessment data is embedded in progress notes and narrative content, identifying and extracting specific pieces of information can be problematic. Although the learning needs data collected in this manner may still be useful at the individual level, it can be difficult to analyze and manipulate at the aggregate level.

Understanding the Electronic Health Record (EHR)

One of the most important components to designing a good documentation process is to start with an understanding of how your organization's EHR works. You may need to reach out to members of your Health Information Technology department to gain this knowledge, and typically, the individuals who are the most involved in the EHR's design are the clinical analysts who support the development process and build the tools. These individuals are knowledgeable about how a specific piece of data will behave based on which entry method is used. The EHR functionality has a language all its own, so be sure to learn the correct terminology and definitions to improve communication about future design options.

Using the Note

What are the differences between a *note* and a *form*? Both are documentation tools that can have unique properties and characteristics depending on how data is entered and what information needs to be available at a later time. In theory, both tools might accommodate multiple contributors and modifications and may cross the care continuum. In practice, however, if a *note* displays modifications in entries similar to track changes in a Microsoft Word document, it may be a poor design option for your EHR if you want to visualize information that may have been modified across multiple entries.

As shown in Figure 11.1, if revisions to the note are displayed in a track changes view, you can imagine that by the time three or four entries are made, the note will be difficult to follow. You can also identify multiple typographical errors over time. Another downside of this design option relates to future data needs. Easily leveraged data needs a discrete data field, and Figure 11.1 is an example of a setting-specific note with a topic heading, but it relies on free text entries that may be difficult to analyze at the aggregate level.

Date : ~~March 22, 2015 1708~~ March 23, 2015 1050
Name of person: ~~Lori Marshall RN~~ Christina Cordero, RN

In patient Learning Need: CPR Infant *(March 22, 2015 1708 Lori Marshall RN)*

Who was taught:
Mom *(March 22, 2015 1708 Lori Marshall RN)*
~~Uncle~~ Aunt *(March 22, 2015 1708 Lori Marshall RN)* (deleted in error) ~~Aunt~~ *(March 23, 2015 1050 Christina Cordero, RN)*
Dad *(March 22, 2015 1708 Lori Marshall RN)*
Uncle *(March 23, 2015 1050 Christina Cordero, RN)*

Information Giver to the learner:
Infant Choking and CPR *(March 22, 2015 1708 Lori Marshall RN)*
Infant CPR and Choking to Uncle *(March 23, 2015 1050 Christina Cordero, RN)*
Activating 911 *(March 22, 2015 1708 Lori Marshall RN)*
Calling for help and activating EMS *(March 23, 2015 1050 Christina Cordero, RN)*

Watched CPR video *(March 22, 2015 1708 Lori Marshall RN)*
Infant AHA CPR *(March 23, 2015 1050 Christina Cordero, RN)*

Response to learning:
Mom, Dad can do choking and CPR without help *(March 22, 2015 1708 Lori Marshall RN)*
Aunt needs more practice. Requires another class *(March 22, 2015 1708 Lori Marshall RN)*
Uncle did great. Auntie not going to be caring for the infant. *(March 23, 2015 1050 Christina Cordero, RN)*

Plan:
Have parents practice at bedside. Find alternate care giver instead of aunt. *(March 22, 2015 1708 Lori Marshall RN)*

Figure 11.1   Example of setting-specific PFE note with headings.

When a note is viewed in a standard mode that does not display each modification, as shown in Figure 11.2, it is difficult to identify which staff members entered information in the EHR when there are multiple contributors and multiple learners involved in the education process.

Date : March 23, 2015 1050
Name of person: Christina Cordero, RN

In patient Learning Need: CPR Infant

Who was taught:
Mom
Aunt
Dad
Uncle

Information Giver to the learner:
Infant Choking and CPR
Infant CPR and Choking to Uncle
Activating 911
Calling for help and activating EMS
Watched CPR video
Infant AHA CPR

Response to learning:
Mom, Dad can do choking and CPR without help
Aunt needs more practice. Requires another class
Uncle did great. Auntie not going to be caring for the infant.

Plan:
Have parents practice at bedside. Find alternate care giver instead of aunt.

Figure 11.2   Same note from Figure 11.1, this time in standard view.

TIP

One of the biggest mistakes people make when designing patient education documentation systems is to approach the design with only current needs in mind or with only a minimalist approach to satisfy regulatory needs. You will serve your patients and families better by thinking out 5 years in the future to what information will be important to collect and apply to the measurement of care outcomes. These are important design considerations. They can also help you determine which document type to use.

A form is the next most commonly used document type found in the EHR.

Using the Form Format

A *form* has many design possibilities, starting with the discrete data elements that can be pre-populated from another form or repurposed for future use. Designing a form with this functionality in mind saves time by leveraging one entry event that can populate a field required by another form, and it creates important connections between data elements. Forms provide the best platform for future data analysis, and Figure 11.3 is an example of a simple design for a form with standardized choices.

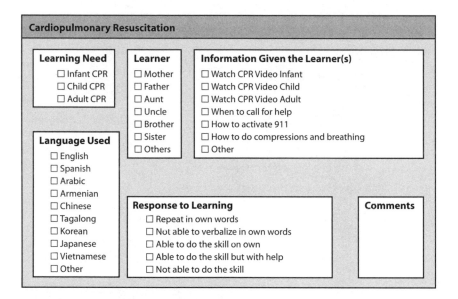

Figure 11.3   Example of a single-topic PFE form with standardized choices—simple design.

The form shown in Figure 11.4 is an example of a multi-contributor tool that accommodates a historical view of a specific learning need, showing a progression.

Generic Patient Education Form

Learning Need (s)	Who Was Taught	What Was Taught	How It Was Taught	Practice	Mastery of Knowledge and Skills	Comments

Figure 11.4   Example of simple generic PFE form using a row design.

Leveraging the row style, a form can be designed to go across the care continuum so staff and providers in all settings such as inpatient, outpatient, and emergency departments can easily view the content and add to it as part of an interprofessional education process (see Figure 11.5).

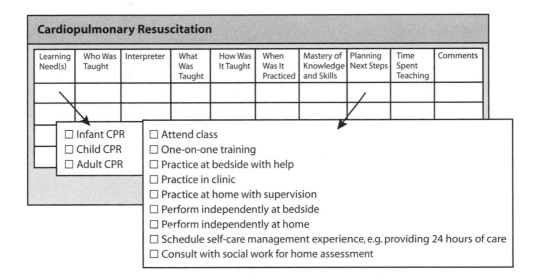

Figure 11.5   Example of single-topic cross-continuum PFE form using a row design.

The column names are simplified in the example shown in Figure 11.5, but the intent of each column is to capture key aspects of documentation so it is clear what was done, by whom, and the results of the education exchange. This expanded view links other data elements such as use of language services and time spent teaching that can be used when the form is interfaced with acuity systems. One of the objectives of the form is to use standardized terminology and provide choices that are available when you are charting rather than presenting a set of static choices for one person. This not only create efficiencies, but it allows for the collection and analysis of data for quality, outcomes, research, and disparity analysis.

Designing PFE Documentation

Once you understand what your EHR can do and what aspects to consider when weighing in on the design options, it is time to start the process. Refer to Table 11.1 for design considerations.

Table 11.1	Documentation Design Properties to Consider	
Properties	**Note**	**Form**
Multi-contributor	✓	✓
Crosses encounters	✓	✓
If modified, additional entries remain part of main documentation tool	In some systems it becomes an addendum below the original entry	✓
Keeps all entries in sequence		✓
Discrete data fields		✓
Easy for queries		✓
Converts to a note for summative viewing		✓
Easy to visualize progression and next steps		✓

Document Design Phases

There are five key phases when creating new PFE documentation. Each phase has its unique challenges, and it is important to dedicate sufficient time to each phase in the full project-planning process. A complete redesign can take up to 2 years depending on your organization's current design and culture.

- Phase 1: Create the concept framework with the end in mind.
- Phase 2: Design and build a prototype.
- Phase 3: Test and fix it.
- Phase 4: Implement and roll out new PFE documentation.
- Phase 5: Monitor and refine the redesign.

Phase 1: Conceptual Framework

During the conceptual framework stage, begin with the end in mind. This phase answers the question: What are the future desired outcomes of the new documentation process and what data needs to be entered?

The key steps in this phase include:

- Gather the key stakeholders.
- Review the current state from a change-management lens for a culture/practice change. What are your organization's practices?
- Review policies for timeframes specifying when staff must complete a tool (e.g., upon admission, within 24 hours, initiate in 24 hours, each clinic visit, annual at clinic visit) and how often (e.g., every admission, or review update if readmission is 30 days or less).
- It is important to separate the time parameters that are imposed by an outside agency or regulatory body from those the organization imposes on itself. This is particularly true when it comes to doing something because it has always been that way. Ask the question, "Does this need to be done this way?"
- Consider how a desired redesign matches current practice and capacity for a new process.

Have Realistic Expectations of What Is Possible

It is important to carefully assess your organization's readiness for advancing a specific note design. While the ultimate goal should be to move toward a health system design, the culture has to support this new way of thinking, so it may be necessary to consider it as a progressive, multiyear plan.

We recommend using a strategy where your concept development is part of a progressive, planned change process. For example, you might start by going from 100% free text as a note to a note with a framework as shown in the following figure. This approach works well to guide staff on the process of patient-family education and to think about key components related to that work. Consider headings such as:

- What is being taught
- Who was taught
- Language
- Response to learning
- Plan

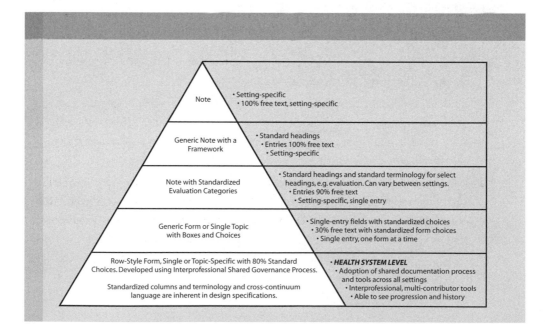

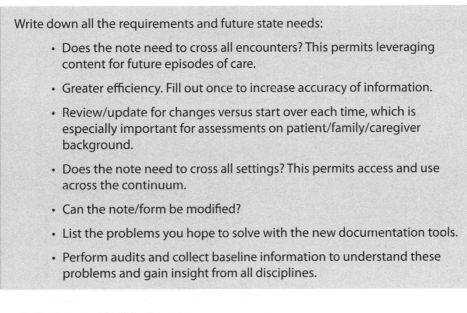

Write down all the requirements and future state needs:

- Does the note need to cross all encounters? This permits leveraging content for future episodes of care.

- Greater efficiency. Fill out once to increase accuracy of information.

- Review/update for changes versus start over each time, which is especially important for assessments on patient/family/caregiver background.

- Does the note need to cross all settings? This permits access and use across the continuum.

- Can the note/form be modified?

- List the problems you hope to solve with the new documentation tools.

- Perform audits and collect baseline information to understand these problems and gain insight from all disciplines.

Phase 2: Design and Build a Prototype

Phase 2 is the design phase and is done by your clinical analyst, who will take the requirements and build a prototype. In this phase, the clinical analyst recommends a documentation form/note design that matches your new vision with the functionality and features available within your hospital/health systems EHR.

Learning assessment documentation development tips:

- Use a tool that has distinct data fields.

- Use a self-rating approach for questions.

- Standardized questions with an 80/20 rule (less than 20% free text).

- Create a comprehensive assessment to include a wide range of items about background, family, available caregivers, learning preference, health literacy, and self-care management skills. Recommend using a "form style" as shown in Figure 11.6.

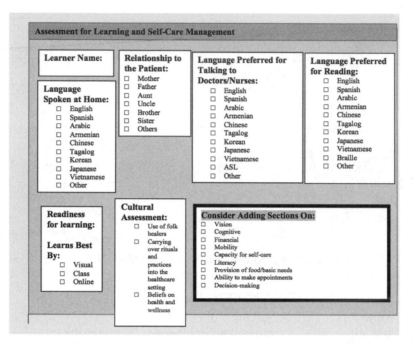

Figure 11.6 Assessment designed using form.

- Include a technology assessment of what they own and know how to use.
- Organize by priorities with regard to data that must be completed at a specific time in the first part of the document.

Learning needs can be documented in various ways based on care setting in line with state and other requirements, for example, in a separate tool identified as the multidisciplinary plan of care in the inpatient setting or rehabilitation setting, or a problem list in the clinical setting. EHRs can leverage features that permit organizing documentation notes, forms, and tools into a single source, making it easier to mimic the "lists" found in a care plan. Ensure that the processes are a good fit.

Documentation form—development tips:

- Include evaluating response to learning to documentation education-exchange process.

- Organize by system that guides "process," such as "tell-show-do-practice-review."

- Include date, time, learners taught, what was taught, and by whom.

For a health system approach, it's best to use a form following the 80/20 rule that is comprehensive and standardizes columns with responses, as you can see in the columns in Figure 11.7.

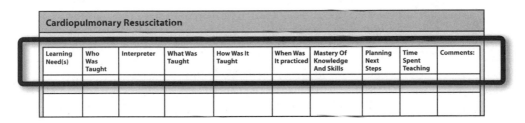

Cardiopulmonary Resuscitation

Learning Need(s)	Who Was Taught	Interpreter	What Was Taught	How Was It Taught	When Was It practiced	Mastery Of Knowledge And Skills	Planning Next Steps	Time Spent Teaching	Comments:	

Figure 11.7   Columns for row-style form.

TIP

If your institution/health system is transitioning from a paper to electronic system, keep in mind that not all forms are effective as recreations of current paper forms. Not taking advantage of the opportunity to redesign the form for an electronic environment may perpetuate poor processes.

A critical component to success is partnering with workgroups, shared governance councils, and other disciplines to develop note content (Leisner & Wonch, 2006).

- Start with problematic areas where issues exist and quality/safety concerns need to be addressed.

- Create interprofessional notes. A majority of learning needs are not exclusive to one discipline. As mentioned in Chapters 2 and 4, the nurse's role is to recognize how and when to facilitate learning, leveraging other disciplines and (when possible) planned partnerships in the form of a learning-need specific, interprofessional curriculum.

- Use related topic notes to guide best education practices. A well-designed documentation system will cover a majority of learning needs within a core set of notes. A generic note will capture the rest. As part of periodic review, analyze topics in generic notes to identify any potential standardized notes.
- Begin by brainstorming topics of commonly taught learning needs.
- Group by related areas of focus.
- Create a curriculum.
- List all the handouts given.
- List all the videos used.
- List all information that is given (verbal or demonstrated) to a learner.
- Specify learning objectives for a specific topic. What do you want the learner to be able to do or know as a result.?

List what constitutes mastery of the task and ensure the documentation form includes these choices. Janousek, Heermann, and Eilers (2005) identified a challenge for EHR PFE documentation: seeing mastery when there are multiple learners. The documentation tool design sample shown in Figure 11.8 provides a way to capture everything that was done or given to the patient and family. It sets the stage for others who must reinforce or continue supporting the learning need.

Phase 3: Test and Fix

In this phase, all key stakeholders go into a test domain and use the new tool. This phase will ensure that the tool functions as intended, that it captures all relevant content, and that it meets the needs of the various disciplines who will use the tool.

It is at this phase that the educational process begins with the key group who will support the roll out. This is also the time to approach any councils or committees to review plans for staff education and collaborate on the approach. These discussions should be well underway and completed before a note is set to be placed in a certification domain and certainly before being placed in the production (or live) domain.

Cardiopulmonary Resuscitation										
Learning Need(s)	Who Was Taught	Interpreter	What Was Taught	How Was It Taught	When Was It Practiced	Mastery Of Knowledge And Skills	Planning Next Steps	Time Spent Teaching	Comments:
CPR	Mother, Aunt	Video Remote; Other Interp #1234567	Infant CPR and Choking Activating EMS	Watch AHA video Attend CPR Class; Task Demo- Infant CPR; Return Demo-Infant CPR		Verbalized Understanding Able to perform Infant CPR	Practice on manikin	90 Minutes	

Figure 11.8   Example of a completed note.

Phase 4: Implementation and Roll Out

The implementation process happens in stages. Negotiate the target start date and ensure there is sufficient time to develop and implement any education required to learn the new tool. The final documentation tool is transferred to a certification or set domain. It is scheduled to be placed into the production domain. At that point, you can create job aides and tools.

Phase 5: Monitor and Refine

Designing a solid PFE documentation system is iterative, and you should always make it a priority to check back and assess what is working and what is not. Specifically, audit content to determine data elements that are incomplete. If data elements are incomplete, dig deep to understand why. This component has the biggest impact on long-term adoption and consistency of results.

Once the document is in use, continue to adjust and fix issues and review workflows. Auditing completion of the new tools will give you an indication of ease of use and opportunities for refinement. During this phase, you might discover whether an important step was overlooked in the first development round.

This is also the time to review content to clarify and simplify the available choices or determine if important content was overlooked. As you will discover, certain content produces a reaction from the staff responsible for asking the patient and/or family the questions. It is important to listen to their feedback and fix significant issues, because not doing so will affect document completion.

Case Example

Redesigning a Form After Test Use

Consider a new document that was designed and implemented. After 6 months of use, it was discovered that the "task" to place the learning needs assessment on the nurse's activity list fell off after admission. A rapid cycle PDSA can be used to identify a solution to reduce the form sections from three to two and to add a feature to the form that required the nurse to remain on a task until all the fields were completed.

The form was redesigned and then went to another committee to review and discuss the proposed changes. During discussion other issues might come up. For example, as the group reflects on prior practice using the paper tool, they recall a box to check noting that a plan was initiated based on the assessment. The intent of electronic assessment was to apply the information to the education plan. If this step is not in the new electronic form design, a trigger should be added to serve as a reminder to synthesize the information into a learning plan.

Post-Implementation Tips

Hospital leaders may decide it is time to improve the assessment process and to ask more focused questions on the learning needs assessment. Additionally, they may want to expand this assessment to identify any issues regarding a patient's and/or caregiver's capacity for self-care. Expanding the breadth and depth of the information collected may be best practice, but the set of questions could trigger an emotional response by the staff. For example, if the staff say that they find certain questions embarrassing to ask, consider finding a way to restate or modify such questions. Otherwise, they might skip over them.

Even though the forms make their way through various councils and committees, when they are placed in a live environment, the staff might identify that an important choice is missing. These can be quick fixes, and you must partner with your clinical analyst to make timely changes.

Conclusion and Key Points

Documentation of patient and family education is as important as choosing the right approach for the delivery of education. Make it a priority to become interested and involved in the development of tools that capture the patient and family education process.

Key points to consider when designing your system to consistently document PFE information:

- **Assess your current documentation process.** Before developing new process steps or incorporating additional data elements into your system, it is important to identify the barriers and challenges of your existing process. Gaining a better understanding of how PFE information is currently being documented, where staff are documenting the information, and how the information is incorporated into the education plan will help you determine many key aspects of the new system.

- **Create a vision for the new process.** Your new system should be designed with future data use in mind, including standardized terminology and specific data elements that can be analyzed at the individual, aggregate, or system level. It is also beneficial to work collaboratively with an interdisciplinary team to ensure that the system meets the documentation needs of disciplines and settings across your organization.

- **Identify crucial data elements.** Defining which data elements to collect in your documentation system depends on the way data is currently being used and how the data may be used in the future. Designing the system to collect information at the individual level that can be analyzed at the aggregate level provides an opportunity to learn about the education provided to each patient and to the patient population as a whole.

- **Understand your electronic health record (EHR).** Reach out to the relevant stakeholders in your Health Information Technology department to increase knowledge of the EHR's design, as well as the correct terminology and definitions to use when discussing future design options. Consider how different documentation tools can be used in the EHR depending on how data is entered and what information will be available to the end user.

A well-designed PFE documentation system can improve your organization's ability to evaluate learning and identify opportunities to enhance your process to increase quality care and patient safety.

References

Buchko, B., Gutshall, C., & Jordan, E. (2012). Improving quality and efficiency of postpartum hospital education. *The Journal of Perinatal Education, 21*(4), 238–47.

Cook, L., Castrogiovanni, A., Stephenson, D. W., Dickson, M., Smith, D., & Bonney, A. (2008). Patient education documentation: Is it being done? *MEDSURG Nursing, 17*(5), 6–10.

Covey, S. (2000). *The 7 habits of highly effective people.* Simon & Schuster.

DeWalt, D. A., Malone, R. M., Bryant, M. E., Kosnar, M. C., Corr, K. E., Rothman, R. L., … Pignone, M. P. (2006). A heart failure self-management program for patients of all literacy levels: A randomized, controlled trial. *BMC Health Services Research, 6*(30).

Divi, C., Koss, R., Schmaltz, S., & Loeb, J. (2007). Language proficiency and adverse events in U.S. hospitals: A pilot study. *International Journal of Quality in Health Care, 19*(2), 60–67.

Flores, G., Abreu, M., Pizzo Barone, C., Bachur, R., & Lin, H. (2012). Errors of medical interpretation and their potential clinical consequences: A comparison of professional versus ad hoc versus no interpreters. *Annals of Emergency Medicine, 50*(5), 545–53.

Jack, B. W., Chetty, V. K., Anthony, D., Greenwald, J. L., Sanchez, G. M., Johnson, A. E., & Culpepper, L. (2009). A reengineered hospital discharge program to decrease rehospitalization: A randomized trial. *Annals of Internal Medicine, 150*(3), 178–187.

Janousek, L., Heermann, J., & Eilers, J. (2005). Tracking patient education documentation across time and care settings. *Proceedings from AMIA Symposium Proceedings*, p. 993.

Leisner B., & Wonch, D. (2006). How documentation outcomes guide the way: A patient health education electronic medical record experience in a large healthcare network. *Qual Manag Health Care, 15*(3), 171–83.

Peter, D., Robinson, P., Jordan, M., Lawrence, S., Casey, K., & Salas-Lopez., D. (2015). Reducing readmissions using teach-back. *Journal of Nursing Administration, 45*(1), 35–42.

Portz, D., & Johnston, M. P. (2014). Implementation of an evidence-based education practice change for patients with cancer. *Clinical Journal of Oncology Nursing, 18,* 36–40. doi: 10.1188/14.CJON.S2.36-40

Robert Wood Johnson Foundation (RWJF). (2010). *Combining better systems and intensive patient education for better heart care.* Retrieved from http://www.rwjf.org/en/about-rwjf/newsroom/newsroom-content/2010/03/combining-better-systems-and-intensive-patient-education-for-bet.html

"Go to the people. Live with them. Learn from them. Love them. Start with what they know. Build with what they have. But with the best leaders, when the work is done, the task accomplished, the people will say 'We have done this ourselves.'"
– "Tao Te Ching" (also "The Book of the Way")
600–531 BC, Lao Tzu

The Role of the Family Resource Center

Lori C. Marshall, PhD, MSN, RN
Jacqueline E. Gilberto, MPH
Samar Mroue, RN, BSN
Helen Rowan, RN, MSN, DipMgt

OBJECTIVES

- Explain the importance of aligning the FRC's (Family Resource Center) purpose with the organization's PFE philosophy.

- Discuss the benefits of having a blended staffing model to support a broader array of patient education offerings.

- Recognize opportunities to create a health system approach to PFE by enhancing or expanding types of services and programming in your FRC.

Introduction

Patient and family education is fundamental to delivering quality healthcare services, and a Family Resource Center is an important way to support this at the organizational level and across the continuum of care (Balik, Conway, Zipperer, & Watson, 2011; IPFCC, 2015b). Family Resource Centers (FRCs) take on various forms and roles within a health system. Depending on where you practice nursing, you might not know the details about a Family Resource Center that is part of your health system. In the event one is not located within your healthcare setting, it is important to have an awareness of those in the community that can support your patients and families.

A resource center that serves as the hub for patient and family education adds significant value to any health system. It is critical in taking the leap forward with patient and family education from a health system lens, where an FRC is viewed as more than a namesake or physical space. Even in the absence of a formal PFE department, an FRC can serve as the focal point for PFE, thus becoming symbolic as a central hub of PFE within a health system.

Before moving forward, it is important to place a reminder that an FRC represents family-centered care for your health facility and should embody the core principles as set forth by the Institute of Patient and Family Centered Care (IPFCC, 2015c, p. 4):

- **Dignity and Respect.** Healthcare practitioners listen to and honor patient and family perspectives and choices. Patient and family knowledge, values, beliefs, and cultural backgrounds are incorporated into the planning and delivery of care.

- **Information Sharing.** Healthcare practitioners communicate and share complete and unbiased information with patients and families in ways that are affirming and useful. Patients and families receive timely, complete, and accurate information in order to effectively participate in care and decision-making.

- **Participation.** Patients and families are encouraged and supported in participating in care and decision-making at the level they choose.

- **Collaboration.** Patients, families, healthcare practitioners, and healthcare leaders collaborate in policy and program development, implementation, and evaluation, in facility design, and in professional education, as well as in the delivery of care.

Each of the principles of family-centered care is reinforced through FRC programs, services, staffing, and space. This chapter will help you expand your understanding of what a Family Resource Center is and how it supports learning. The focus is on those FRCs linked with a hospital or health system. Additionally, staffing models will be discussed, along with important partnerships that should be built in order to support a well-rounded and valuable composite of programs that become embedded into the routines of clinicians.

What Is a Family Resource Center?

Family Resource Centers share common functions and include support, education, information, and connection to a health system or multiple systems. However, differences can be found in how they serve patients and families across healthcare settings, populations, and communities. For example, some FRCs in the hospital setting focus on the provision of amenities and offer laundry facilities, lounge/quiet areas, business centers, and refreshments/snacks for their visitors. Other FRCs are libraries, offering a collection of print material, access to the Internet, and other resources. Yet another model uses the FRC as a site for the direct delivery of patient and family education in addition to some or all of these aspects. When setting up an FRC, it is important to decide on the focus early on, and the effort best begins by conducting on-site needs assessments and/or focus groups to develop a strategic plan.

An online comparison of websites of Family Resource Centers from across the United States revealed the variations that exist among them, even among pediatric medical centers. See the section "FRC Comparison Resources" for sites. The FRCs served the following groups: pediatrics, adult cancer, childhood cancer, adult aging, community, adult and children, women's health, and mental health (see Table 12.1).

Table 12.1 Most Common Services Offered by the FRC	
Number Who Offered	*Offered in FRC*
14	Information and digital library
14	Education
14	Information on health system and region
12	Internet access
12	Computers
12	Support groups
12	Carepages/caring bridge/ journaling pages
12	Available to anyone even if not being treated there
8	Quiet space

The online FRC descriptions noted unique offerings and services such as food/beverage and shower/sleeping facilities. Only one listed being open on Sunday. See Table 12.2 for the less common offerings.

Table 12.2 Less Common Offerings Found in FRC Online Descriptions	
Number Who Offered	*Offered in FRC*
4	Coffee/tea and light snacks. Most are beverage-only service
3	Formal connection with Family Advisory Council
3	Massage services
2	Had two or more FRC locations outside of hospital (community based)
2	Showers
2	Scrapbooking
2	Sleeping space
2	Personal hygiene kits
2	Notary
1	Sale of home-safety resources
1	FRC-based laundry space
1	Knitting group
1	Open Sunday
1	Laundry supplies

The FRC is considered an important component to a cross-continuum healthcare delivery model in the United States. However, globally, the concept of the FRC may not be the same, and they reflect regional differences based on how health systems are designed. Some FRCs in Ireland share characteristics with the U.S. FRCs described previously. An example is the Family Resource Center Hospital (2015) and how it is supported through the FRC Network Ireland (2015). In China, learning centers can be found that are connected to hospitals and staffed by nurse educators (C. Ding, personal communication, April 4, 2015). In Australia, the Royal Children's Hospital (RCH) Melbourne's Family Resource Centre, the Family Hub, serves as a home-away-from-home for families and visitors to the hospital.

Understanding Different FRC Staffing Models

A variety of leadership models are found throughout the United States and other countries. Models can be nurse led, led by other disciplines, parent navigators, and/or volunteers.

For example, the Family Hub at RCH is led by a manager who is a nurse and staffed with friendly and knowledgeable volunteers who are supported by staff and provide practical support and assistance, including a business center, toilets and showers, changing rooms and baby changing tables, a quiet room with fold-out sofa bed, care boxes and spare clothing for emergency needs, lockers to store valuables, secure storage for suitcases and larger items, a sewing kit, iron, ironing board, and laundry powder for washing machines.

As described in the preceding section, your health system will influence the model/direction of the FRC itself.

Staffing models varied when looking at the 14 sites examined on the Internet. They ranged from one person serving as an assistant or coordinator under a director with a nursing background, to models using a combination of nurses, health educators, child life specialists, and staff with an unspecified background but who can support mental needs as core. Several leveraged volunteers, and others fostered a partnership with their family advisory councils to provide support services.

Each model reflected how space was being used. For example, the FRCs that provided health information that was clinical in nature and/or taught complex care skills classes utilized registered nurses. Those who provided broader health-promotion type sessions employed a health educator. In cases where the digital library and resources were the prominent resource, an assistant or volunteer would be leveraged, because the FRC staff had the role of helping people to find information and providing education on available resources.

Online comparisons of the 14 FRCs that offered education show that the course offerings are typically based on the expertise of the FRC staff. Thus, it is important to explore the benefits and limitations of certain roles to support an FRC, given that it also has bearing on future programming and planning.

The core U.S. roles utilized included registered nurses, health educators, social workers, psychologists, child life specialists (pediatrics), paraprofessionals, and volunteers. These are the main focus; however, international equivalents are mentioned if one existed.

Registered Nurses in the Core Role

Having registered nurses serve in the core FRC educational role has benefits and drawbacks, as follows.

Pros	Cons
Clinical/medical knowledge/expertise	Higher cost to organization
Knowledge of teaching strategies in educational theory and evidence-based teaching practices	Possible underutilization of full scope of skills of a registered nurse might lead to burnout
Nurse-led Family Resource Centers provide the greatest capacity when there is a focus to provide classes on self-care management and complex care Medical expertise	
Patients/families trust the RN's credentials, prefer dealing with a licensed vs. non-licensed person inside of a hospital setting	
Ability to use critical thinking to assess whether situations need more resources or a different expertise than can be offered	

Nurses make centralizing complex care classes an option. Teaching at the bedside has its limitations—time constraints being a significant one. As part of a normal patient load, allotting adequate time for a teaching session without interruptions can be challenging.

"I have been a nurse for over 15 years, and patient and family education has always been of high importance to me. I've always taken great pleasure in knowing I can empower families with knowledge, and therefore assisting them in taking care of a loved one, or themselves. Being a classroom teacher has definitely made me a better bedside teacher, as I now am more aware of best times for adults to learn, as well as the best environment." –RN

Teaching at the Family Resource Center removes all those variables from the education session. The class environment is a less stressful one, facilitating learning away from the machines, the noises, the monitors, and other hospital staff. Patients and families will come to the FRC ready to learn, knowing that they set aside this period of time without the bedside nurse's schedule being an issue.

Learning in a class environment enables patients and families to share their stories with the nurse educator and leads to higher satisfaction as compared to learning at the bedside. Nurses teaching in the FRC have reported seeing families days after attending a class and receiving feedback about how well they were able to retain the information. Positive feedback is echoed by nurses on the units who have recounted experiences where patients and families have quoted information learned in class at their subsequent training sessions at bedside, at times even correcting nurses.

Teaching at the FRC is a combination of having families watch a video, providing handouts, and hands-on training on models. In essence, the FRC environment supports Addelston's (1959) Tell-Show-Do-Practice-Review framework and promotes the assimilation of information, which becomes engraved in their minds through instruction and practice.

Non-Nurse Health Educators or Community Health Worker (Master's-Prepared Preferred) in the Core Role

Having non-nurse health educators serve in the core FRC educational role has benefits and drawbacks, as follows.

Pros	Cons
Expertise in delivery of info/education	Broad knowledge/expertise (not clinical)
Knowledge of collection of health-related data regarding needs, assets, and capacity for health education programs	Moderate cost to organization
Variety of populations and practice settings	Some knowledge of child development and learning processes
In-depth preparation in an area of specialization or in one of the behavioral and social sciences	
Understanding of multilevel factors that influence the health and wellbeing of populations	
Data collection and analysis	
Materials development and educational-program expertise grounded in theory, supported by evidence, and based on input from the community	
Theories, concepts, and models from a range of social and behavioral disciplines	
Social and behavioral determinants that affect health of individuals and populations	
Knowledge of steps/procedures to plan community-based public health programs and interventions	
Working level of understanding of adult learning processes and theory	

Clergy and Spiritual Care in the Core Role

Having clergy and spiritual care workers serve in the core FRC educational role has benefits and drawbacks, as follows.

Pros	Cons
Community resource connection	Not able to address clinical or medical needs
Provide a strong spiritual support and presence to support forward-thinking	Limited knowledge of learning theory
Coping support in a variety of settings	
Support life- and healthcare continuum	

Other Professional Disciplines Such as Social Work and Psychology in the Core Role

Having social workers or psychologists serve in the core FRC educational role has benefits and drawbacks, as follows.

Pros	Cons
Knowledge/expertise in community resources (especially BSW or MSW)	Limited knowledge of learning theory
Knowledge in mental health to provide coping support	Low job satisfaction for a master's-prepared employee due to lack of accurate clinical challenges
Able to support education on navigating the health system	
Support empowerment development programming, especially for vulnerable and high-risk populations	
Assessment, education, and referral to address barriers to pursuing health education and literacy	
Transition and transfer of care	

Trained Paraprofessionals or Parent-Led and Linked with Advisory Groups in the Core Role

Having paraprofessionals or advisory groups serve in the core FRC educational role has benefits and drawbacks, as follows.

Pros	Cons
First-hand knowledge of patient, parent, or caregiver side of healthcare experience	Little/no knowledge of health education/behavior concepts
Low cost to the organization	Limited scope of work

Volunteer-Led Staffing Model

Using volunteers in the core FRC educational role has benefits and drawbacks, as follows.

Pros	Cons
Cost-free help	Limited scope of work
Helps promote programs and services	Time-consuming effort in identifying sufficiently competent individuals
	Must have large enough pool of individuals to cover all time periods
	Constant effort to recruit and retain

Pediatrics Only: Child Life Specialist in the Core Role

Having a child life specialist serve in the core FRC educational role has benefits and drawbacks, as follows.

Pros	Cons
Knowledge/expertise in child development and learning processes	Little/no knowledge of adult learning processes/ theory
Preparation in daily clinical work with patients and families	Moderate cost to the organization

Preparation in coping strategies to support children, youth, and families in the healthcare setting

Ability to assess and meaningfully interact with infants, children, youth, and families

Describe formal and informal assessment techniques to determine developmental and emotional state

Staffing options should be based on what the FRC will offer, but future programming should also be considered. When possible, it is ideal to use a blended model that combines nurses and other disciplines, such as health educators, and it is also important to augment these roles with paraprofessionals and volunteers. We do not recommend building the core staffing around volunteers, because it is not a sustainable model long-term. Additionally, it will limit the kinds and amount of programming an FRC can offer.

Determining the Configuration and Location of the Family Resource Center

It is not always possible to choose your FRC design, location, or size. Even if you could, no one design is without accompanying limitations. This section discusses a few considerations when setting up your FRC or modifying existing space.

The physical location and purpose of the FRC has much to do with the kinds of situations that come up day to day. Issues are addressed when family members come in. It is important to be prepared, and this can be achieved through the right combination of staff and communication processes. As an example, an FRC whose purpose is to serve the general population and that is located in a frequent path of travel near the entrance or main public spaces draws more variety due to traffic. Patient complaints; grievances; issues with the care team; and questions about parking, insurance, or payment for medical care are common. Large families will use the space during flu season due to visitor restrictions or isolation precaution changes. Likewise, FRCs located "out of the way" of frequent paths of travel see less traffic and must devote more time/effort to promoting awareness of the

FRC's location, as well as what it offers. Department-specific FRCs (e.g., Hemonc and en-docrinology) are limited to visitors treated specifically in that area/department and must therefore identify a more specific focus/mission.

In all models, making the space feel family-friendly and inviting is critical to increasing traffic and usage. In a pediatric setting, for example, special attention must be paid to the family-friendliness factor. An adult setting will require that needs be met for children while their parents/caregivers use the space for educational purposes. In adult facilities, or for elderly/disabled populations, the design must adhere to standards for accessible design, ASL-capable staff, and assistive technology.

Providing Maintenance and Documentation

Once you have decided on focus, whether broad, general population-centered or diag-nosis-specific, it is important to establish an organized system for materials that will fa-cilitate maintenance and inventory/record-keeping. Subsequently, this will also help you keep track of distribution metrics and high-demand items or topics.

The first step is to build a directory with a comprehensive catalog of available mate-rials; an electronic database should be maintained for record-keeping purposes, and a hard-copy print version is extremely helpful for visitors to peruse. If the FRC is to be em-braced by the health system as the go-to place for information, other staff will access it, and a directory is vital to the location of materials in the absence of FRC staff. Likewise, patients and families visiting your FRC will need an effective method for locating materi-als autonomously. A simple listing of the material's main title, subject, location, and lan-guage will suffice.

In addition to facilitating the location of materials, the actual physical space and layout must also be considered. Maintaining a space with wide, open walkways and a welcoming atmosphere will enable users/visitors of all types and abilities a smooth user experience. Making at least two workstations accessible to disabled visitors is a must, although the best-case scenario would be to make all workstations flexible for accommodating special needs.

An FRC is a place for family gathering and supports quality family time during ex-tended hospitalizations. The Family Hub at Royal Children's supports patients staying at the hospital for extended periods. As such, the hub provides free entertainment with a Beanbag Cinema, which shows new-release movies daily; a large selection of magazines and library books; weekly story time and morning tea for families; games and activities for young children; and portable DVD players and DVDs for in-patients. Additionally, the Family Hub is where families can make appointments to meet with their social worker, hospital teacher, or clinical nurse educator, or book free sessions with a financial advisor, legal advisor, or government financial entitlements advisor. It has a kitchen and free tea and coffee, and Australian regional beverage favorites such as Milo (chocolate milk in the United States) and cordial (a breakfast cereal) are provided. There is space with a bottle warmer, microwave, sandwich maker, and tables where families can share a meal.

Should you decide to include food/refreshments as an offering in your FRC, consider designating one general area for the food and beverages. It is important to think about the types of beverages and food items served, including packaging and display. Before deciding what to offer, consider the distance between the FRC and kitchen facilities with a clean water source and a location for washing the serving items in your FRC. A bottled water system might be more efficient to support a variety of beverages. Choose snacks and food items that can be single wrapped for sanitation purposes. Keep in mind that families may grab handfuls of food items, so simple choices like graham crackers and regular crackers are a good option for a product that can be purchased in bulk at a lower cost. If your budget permits, skinned fruit items such as tangerines or bananas are healthy options to augment the crackers. Single-wrapped granola or breakfast bars make a nice morning snack. The key concept is to find a good fit with the intent of the FRC that is sustainable and won't make the setup and maintenance complex, especially in limited-staff situations. You will also want food guidelines and signage in your primary languages noting what areas should be kept food-free, such as computer workstations.

Computers and other electronics in the FRC should be maintained and updated with the latest hardware, software, browser plug-ins, and so on. A working collaboration with your health system's Information Technology (IT) department will benefit users and increase satisfaction. It is also extremely helpful for FRC staff to possess a working knowledge of computers and be Internet-savvy. Attention to small details, such as preset low speaker volume at workstations, will keep noise to a minimum and help maintain an easy vibe throughout the FRC. Printing services are best kept accessible only to staff so as to avoid excessive waste of paper/ink/toner and help keep costs down.

If you will be using the space to provide health education classes, it is helpful to hold such classes in a section of the FRC that is less frequently traveled by the average user. This will minimize interruptions and keep classes on task. Teaching in the FRC environment is dependent on size/space/capacity and is best done with only the caregiver, with patients and/or other children away from the learning space or area. Keeping caregivers focused on learning and not on their patient will maximize information retention. The size of the space will determine privacy levels. In spaces where classes are run within the FRC, make sure to post signage to notify guests that a class is in progress, and have FRC staff help maintain the environment.

> ## TIP
>
> When exploring materials, consider using content that has already been developed and can be easily printed and made available. Be sure to check out regional or global options that can be adapted to your local setting.
>
> For example, Partnership for Patients has compiled tools that can augment your program. See http://partnershipforpatients.cms.gov/p4p_resources/tsp-patientandfamilyengagement/tsppatient-and-family-engagement.html.
>
> Initial and subsequent annual needs assessments are helpful for the evolution of FRC offerings that meet the user's needs. Questions can include demographic information and free-text, open-ended questions, but should primarily consist of multiple-choice questions that can be coded for program evaluation analyses.
>
> Lastly, signage leading to and inside the FRC space should be clear and obvious. Visitors should be able to easily find the FRC and know where they are once inside.

Protecting the FRC Staff

An important component to FRC leadership is protecting the staff. An FRC is a highly public space similar to a clinic or emergency department waiting room, and staff in the FRC need to be well versed in infection-control precautions. Staff also need to be comfortable asking patients and families if they might have a cold or illness, and to don a mask or use hand sanitizers as needed. Occasionally, a family may be asked to move to a location within the FRC away from other visitors. Additionally, there must be a policy on cleaning to include daily processes and more frequent routines as needed, especially on items that are frequently used and might act as vectors. Safety is a priority, and FRC staff should attend a managing assaultive behavior class.

Determining the Hours of Service

The most common FRC hours are Monday to Friday 9 a.m. to 5 p.m., as validated by the online assessment of the 14 FRCs. See the "FRC Comparison Resources" section at the end of this chapter. Evening hours are not common due to staffing and program limitation. Of the 14 facilities, three offered evening hours at least 2 days a week. Three were open on Saturday and one had Sunday hours (half day).

There are benefits to offering extended hours, but it is important to create programming or services that draw in visitors. For example, you can hold evening or weekend classes or support groups for those working during the weekday.

Funding the FRC

Although an FRC provides value to the organization, it is not always easy to gain funding support from operations dollars for staffing and the provision of programs and services. Donors are often sought to name a space, grants sought to expand or provide programming. FRCs can be linked with a source of revenue such as sales of safety equipment or connected to a retail component of the health system to offset operations.

Royal Children's Hospital Melbourne supports the Hub through the Kids Health Info bookshop, which stocks child health, safety promotion, and parenting titles; maintains an online directory of more than 200 local parent support groups; and directs parents to reputable health websites. It also promotes the comprehensive Kids Health Info website, which has more than 300 fact sheets dedicated to providing quality, up-to-date health information for parents and adolescents on medical conditions and relevant services.

Donors might provide naming opportunities for the physical space, but that does not permit making the space family-friendly or provide the means to establish quality programming. It is important to explore the right combination and balance of operations with donor support for a sustainable program.

Creating Important FRC Partnerships

The success of a Family Resource Center is based on partnerships. This section focuses on how to create partnerships to build a well-rounded and valuable composite of programs based on them. There are several key partnerships that you need to foster that add value to the FRC.

Volunteer Services

The volunteer services (VS) department generally oversees the volunteers serving the FRC. While it is up to the FRC to determine how they use volunteers and to train them for specific roles, the volunteer department is responsible for ensuring they meet all the health system's requirements. Additionally, when there are special needs, it is always a good idea to share them with VS so they can assist in recruitment or placement of a volunteer working in one area who wants a change.

Interprofessional Training in Academic Medical Centers

The FRC should develop relationships with academic medical centers to the benefit of both organizations:

- **MD Residencies:** Many residency programs have a community advocacy track that provides opportunities for MD interns to engage in a teaching experience. This experience is invaluable, because they spend time learning about resources, interactive patient care, and teaching on safety topics.

- **RN Residencies:** The FRC supports learning experiences for new nurses by exposing them to patient and family education classes taught in the FRC; they gain greater perspective on their role to continue educating at the bedside. With this knowledge, RN residents are more aware of the need for caregivers to practice to become confident in performing self-care management skills. In addition, exposure to the FRC increases the new RN's understanding of resources to support family-centered care.

- **MPH Practicums:** The FRC supports learning experiences for current health-education students to gain hands-on experience in program planning, materials development, health education, and direct patient contact.

- **Injury Prevention:** The injury prevention program has a robust array of offerings. Some of these can be set up and delivered in your FRC, which not only increases visibility of the injury prevention program, but also exposes hospital visitors to new resources.

Community Resources

The community serves as one of the most valuable sources of support for any patient and family, regardless of age, language, or culture. There are resources in the community that serve health prevention and promotion, financial support, mental health, complementary and alternative healing, and in general create a social network that becomes part of the "home health system." A Family Resource Center located within a hospital system is only as strong as its community connections, given it is where patients and family spend a majority of their time.

It is imperative to take advantage of these community resources and build partnerships, in addition to providing patients and family visitors with information on accessibility. Even if a health system does not have a formal space for an FRC, a department responsible for coordination of care and social support can support this function.

Resource Centers or Learning Centers Located in the Community

Take the opportunity to check with your regional health ministries and learn about what is offered in the community to support health and wellbeing. Regardless of your location, it is important to recognize the opportunities in your health system's FRC and how it would add value to the health system's mission or support regional care for your country. Also consider creating a formal plan and program evaluation strategy to ensure alignment of the FRC with the health system's needs.

For example, in the United States, the CDC lists state and community resources available to support smoking cessation. This is found at http://www.cdc.gov/tobacco/stateandcommunity/index.htm.

The CDC also has a general Community Guide that is helpful to other important resources for a variety of conditions and issues. See http://www.thecommunityguide.org/index.html.

Outside of the United States, a resource center might be called a learning centre or given another name. The Royal Children's Hospital has recently changed the name of its Family Resource and Respite Centre to the Family Hub, to give it a more welcoming name that more accurately reflects the breadth of its facilities and services.

In Australia, a wonderful resource can be found at the Centre for Community Child Health, Royal Children's Hospital Melbourne's site, at www.rch.org.au/ccch/.

Other condition-specific parent support groups can be found to support specific conditions. The website www.amaze.org.au is a support group for autism and autism spectrum disorder, and www.diabetesvic.org.au is a site for diabetes-related support.

Other important resources include health ministries or agencies serving your global region:

- Australia: http://www.health.gov.au/
- China: http://www.moh.gov.cn
- Italy: http://www.salute.gov.it/
- Saudi Arabia: http://www.moh.gov.sa/en/Pages/Default.aspx
- United States: http://www.hhs.gov/
- Centers for Disease Control: http://www.cdc.gov/
- Where We Work: http://www.cdc.gov/globalhealth/countries/default.htm

In order to effectively coordinate care across the continuum, you should be aware of resources at your health system, such as the FRC, who help connect your patients and families to local resources to support self-regulated learning and better outcomes. It is important to consider community-based resources as part of a "home health system" when home is the care setting. Please take time to explore and learn what resources are available in your community.

Conclusion and Key Points

Family Resource Centers can be both helpful and functional hubs of information and resources. They can also be instrumental in reducing costs by providing standardized education, which leads to caregiver understanding and better care for patients, thereby reducing readmissions. The design of an FRC and the selection of its leadership roles are fundamental in determining its success and impact. Only by carefully considering its characteristics and goals will the FRC make an impactful contribution to the larger health system. Additionally, it serves as a focal point of family-centered care concepts of information sharing, participation, collaboration, and respect and dignity.

Nurses should become familiar with the programs and services offered in their health system's FRC or the local/regional resource centers located in their community. By having knowledge of the programs and services, nurses can embed them into the broader patient-family education plan. The health system benefits, because the FRC supports care across the continuum. Also consider the benefits of a centralized education location, particularly for teaching complex-care knowledge and skills.

References

Addelston, H. (1959). Child patient training. *Fortnightly Review of the Chicago Dental Society, 38*(7), 27–29.

Balik, B., Conway, J., Zipperer, L., & Watson, J. (2011). Achieving an exceptional patient and family experience of inpatient hospital care (IHI Innovation Series white paper). Cambridge, MA: Institute for Healthcare Improvement.

Family Resource Centre Hospital in Limerick, Ireland. (2015) Accessed from http://hospitalfrc.com/

Family Resource Centres Ireland (2015). Accessed from http://familyresource.ie/index.php

Institute for Family-Centered Care (2015c). *Advancing the practice of family centered care in hospitals -How to get started.* Retrieved from http://www.ipfcc.org/pdf/getting_started.pdf

Institute for Patient Family Centered Care (IPFCC). (2015a). *Key considerations: A photo gallery.* Retrieved from http://www.ipfcc.org/advance/topics/keyconsiderations.html

Institute for Patient Family Centered Care (IPFCC). (2015b). *Patient and Family Resource Centers.* Retrieved from http://www.ipfcc.org/advance/topics/pafam-resource.html

Lao Tzu (600–531 BC). Tao Te Ching (also The Book of the Way). This poem is a translation of Tao Te Ching, Chapter 17, written by Lao Tzu 3,000 years ago. Accessed from http://www.gurteen.com/gurteen/gurteen.nsf/id/L003957/

FRC Comparison Resources

Benioff Children's Hospital- Center for Families. University of California, San Francisco. Accessed from http://www.ucsfbenioffchildrens.org/services/center_for_families/index.html

Children's Hospital Los Angeles- Family Resource Center. Accessed from http://www.chla.org/site/c.ipINKTOAJsG/b.7679093/k.98C2/Family_Resource_Center__Patient_Health_Education__Program_Support.htm#.VRaspGfcmpp

Cincinnati Children's Hospital. Family Resource Center. Retrieved from http://www.cincinnatichildrens.org/service/f/family-resource/default/

Dartmouth- Hitchcock Women's Health Resource Center. Dartmouth-Hitchcock Medical Center website accessed from http://www.dartmouth-hitchcock.org/womens_resource_ctr.html

Friends Hospital- Family Resource Center (2015). Accessed from http://friendshospital.com/community-services/family-resource-center/

Hope Resource Center at CHLA (2015). Accessed from http://www.chla.org/site/c.ipINKTOAJsG/b.5949847/k.873E/Resource_Center.htm#.VRasbGfcmpo

Minnesota Children's Hospital: Family Resource Centers. Website accessed from http://www.childrensmn. org/patientfamily/hospital-amenities/family-resource-centers

Mission Hospital: Family Resource Centers. Accessed from http://www.mission4health.com/Our-Services/ Affiliations/Family-Resource-Centers.aspx

Partnership for Patients, Centers for Medicare and Medicaid Services, United States Department of Health and Human Services. Accessed from http://partnershipforpatients.cms.gov/p4p_resources/tsp-pa-tientandfamilyengagement/tsppatient-and-family-engagement.html

Rainbow Babies Hospital-Family Resource Center. Accessed from http://www.uhhospitals.org/rainbow/ser-vices/family-and-child-life-services/ family-resource-center

Rush Medical Center- Anne Byron Waud Resource Center for Health and Aging. Accessed from https:// www.rush.edu/patients-visitors/hospital-amenities/resource-centers

St. Louis Children's Hospital- Family Resource Center. Website accessed from http://www.stlouischildrens. org/health-resources/family-resource-center

Seattle Children's Hospital. Family Resource Center. Accessed from http://www.seattlechildrens.org/clinics-programs/family-resource-center/

South Orange County Family Resource Center (SOCFRC). Accessed from http://www.socfrc.org/Services-Programs.aspx

University of California, San Francisco, Cancer Resource Center. Accessed from http://cancer.ucsf.edu/sup-port/crc/faq

"Teaching's hard! You need different skills: positive reinforcement, keeping students from getting bored, commanding their attention in a certain way."
–Bill Gates (n.d.)

Creating a Patient-Family Education (PFE) Department

Lori C. Marshall, PhD, MSN, RN
Troy Garland, RN, BA, MBA

OBJECTIVES

- Explain how a patient-family education (PFE) department adds value to and benefits a health system.
- Discuss the key foundations needed to set up a PFE department.
- Describe the essential partnerships between the PFE department and other roles and departments in the health system.

Introduction

This chapter explores key components you and your organization need to develop in order to establish a patient-family education department, including staffing models, programs, and services. The chapter will also share ways you can enhance the value of the programs and services already at your organization. In addition, you'll gain insight into how to connect all PFE activities, tools, and processes for an integrated system.

A patient and family education (PFE) department is an important component of establishing a health system approach to PFE. Hospitals have varied patient and family education processes that include establishing a dedicated department to lead these efforts. While the term "patient" ends up in the department name, there is a wide range of focus on actual patient education. For example, some departments include the name but are mostly a staff education department (John Dempsey Hospital, 2015). Some departments have a few staff with a dedicated location and a solid concentration on materials development and teaching (Indiana University Health Patient Education, 2015; Sutter Memorial Medical Center, 2015; Woman's Hospital of Texas,

2015). On the other end is a research-focused department, such as Stanford's program under the direction of Kate Lorig (Stanford, 2015).

Many organizations have conducted studies regarding the best models for hospital staff education departments (Cummings & McCaskey, 1992; Haggard, 2006; Sheriff & Banks, 2001), but little is found in the literature about models for patient and family education departments. One common model for a PFE department is a decentralized model in which patient care units independently create and distribute content to patients by a diagnosis or specific skills. This is effective when there is an oversight committee to review content and materials. A decentralized model provides maximum flexibility for individual work units and area. Content can be created quickly. What emerges, however, can be mixed messages to patients and families when visiting other departments and units across the health system when each has its own version of the same learning content. This mixed messaging makes learning more challenging.

Consider asthma as an example. Imagine five different settings within the same health system that care for patients with asthma—the pulmonary clinic, allergy immunology clinic, the emergency department, the intensive care unit, and the acute care nursing unit. Each of these touch points has their own content and handouts that they provide to patients and families. The messaging as to what directions to follow, which set of instructions is correct, who to see, and what to do if they need help can be confusing. When it is not clear what tools to use or what procedures to follow, staff typically go to the Internet and find content from another organization. The educational process becomes fragmented.

Now imagine if all of these areas collaborated to create a standardized set of handouts and educational materials so there would be one message given to the patient and family as they pass through the health system. Message clarity helps the patient and family apply information to self-care management. Providing one health-system message plays an important role in supporting health literacy. Centralized models consolidate oversight to a core group of individuals with structure and processes in place.

Benefits of a Centralized PFE Process

There are multiple benefits of centralizing leadership for PFE, and the positive impact of a central education process extends from the administrative level down to the patient level.

PFE leadership and staff recognize opportunities for collaboration and pull groups together that work independently. They can guide staff and providers to create one common set of evidence-based materials. They help implement use of new tools by educating staff and providers on best-practice teaching methods. Additionally, they support the tracking of utilization and contribute to the analysis of outcomes.

Adding Value

A PFE department adds value to an organization through programs and services.

Department leadership bridges the gap between the health system's strategic goals and patient-knowledge support needed to meet them. They provide strategic leadership for creating a road map that aligns with quality, safety, and outcomes needs. This includes ensuring specific service lines identified as centers of excellence or emerging new business priorities are addressed. It requires balancing meeting core patient-care needs with innovation solutions. For example, if there are related but separate activities, the department creates synergy and connects the work. Figure 13.1 gives an example of how the PFE department can coordinate and lead multiple working groups by using a timeline plan.

	Due Date	PFE Committee-Multidisciplinary Best Subgroup	PFE Committee-Documentation Subgroup	IPC Steering Committee	Councils, Committees, and Hospital Workgroups
1 Month	July 30, 2017	• Reorganize education topics, find out what topics are missing.	• Implement Learning Needs Assessment in medical record. • Partner with patient care clinical informatics care plan subgroup to address care plan issues and connect teaching to plans.	• Assess video content for our commonly taught needs. • Determine utilization and barriers to completion. • Consider a new electronic whiteboard.	• Collaborate on Learning Needs Assessment launch and policy updates.
3 Months	October 31, 2017	• Create templates for teaching modules and "Teach the Teacher" trainings, create centralized place for education materials.	• Implement new documentation notes. • Contribute to developing patient education section for new Patient Menu in EMR.	• Expand video education content and create video curriculums. • Roll out e-whiteboard on three units. • Create utilization monitoring plan for videos.	• Determine sections on the Care Plan that can be added into new PFE document in EMR. • Update Care Plan Policy to reflect new documentation process.
6 Months	January 30, 2018	• Begin "Teach the Teacher" trainings.	• Support implementation of Patient Menu in EMR.	• Whiteboard roll out other units.	• Help educate on new Care Plan Policy and support implementation of patient menu.
9 Months	April 30, 2018	• Complete trainings, post patient satisfaction survey, post staff satisfaction surveys.	• Develop Expanded Patient Profile and link to Learning Needs and Care Needs assessment.	• Fine tune goals and use of scheduling feature.	• Convert remaining sections of paper MPC to electronic.

Figure 13.1   Example of an integrated timeline plan (PFE, IPC, and clinical informatics).

The department serves as a primary resource in the creation of patient education standards, which include setting target reading/readability levels and establishing templates and frameworks that emphasize standard required sections and terminology. The PFE department ensures materials are in line with any health system branding requirements, such as with the creation of a style guide for material development. One of the significant value-added components is that the PFE department shapes the philosophical context on how a learner is viewed and what PFE means in the health system. To that end, PFE staff and leaders serve as consultants to the organization on matters of health literacy, best practices for patient and family engagement, family-centered care, and the clinical documentation system design.

Curriculum Development

The PFE department members are experts in instructional methodology. In partnership with clinical experts, they create curricula for complex clinical skills to leverage across a health system. One of the important foundations of curriculum development is to know what is being taught to patients and families and by whom. This leads to opportunities to broker interprofessional curricula that lead to better outcomes of care. Chapter 4 includes details on interprofessional partnerships for patient-family education. Curriculum development also includes establishing and maintaining consistency across the continuum of care. For example, a specialty clinic caring for transplant patients falls in the same service line that oversees the hospitalized patients who received a transplant.

The challenge occurs when they are each using their own content—one pre-transplant and one home care. The acute care unit uses their own education materials they developed and cover from hospital to home care. Although they are technically addressing the same learning needs, they are using disconnected sets of education tools that lead to problems with the quality and safety of care. Care is affected, because patients and families do not know how to apply the information and carry out actions for managing and maintaining their health. For instance, if the handouts had two different sets of information about recognizing symptoms of concern, managing rejection, and understanding medication and medication administration, how does the learner know which information to use? The learner doesn't know how and when to access care when there are different parameters as to who to call about an issue and when to seek help.

Referring back to the asthma example, one of the biggest roles a PFE department can play is advocating for one common message for a given learning need and maintaining a process for health-system-level curriculum development. Even in the absence of a dedicated PFE department, work through your shared governance structure and seek out help from your organization's chief nursing officer to bridge the health system.

Instructional Processes and Systems

The PFE department specifies and oversees the processes for reviewing existing materials and developing new materials. The review of content generally falls into three core areas:

- Patient care content for patient and family education
- Content used by quality and safety department programs that involves patients and families
- Content developed for marketing and communications that is used for external needs to inform patients and families about changes to billing, insurance plans, access, way finding, and so on

The review of existing content can require time to bring dated content up to current standards. You need to plan and budget time for this work, and a good rule of thumb is 2 hours for one page of content that is five grade levels above the target. For example, if an organization specifies a 4th-grade reading level and the existing content is 9th- to 10th-grade, it takes an average of 2 hours to revise.

This chapter does not aim to teach content revision, but it is still important to know that revision for plain language is more than finding a substitute word; it often requires restating content using simple, plain language and adding an explanation of terms and concepts.

An important role of the PFE department is to ensure consistency of content development. This is achieved through the use of content-development guidelines and standards. These tools provide content experts with key development requirements. Although they do not eliminate the need to review and revise content, they do reduce the time spent doing these things.

Video Content

The PFE department supports the selection and creation of video content. There are two core implications for video content. The first is for the purchase of new content, which includes CPR DVDs and other specialty content. Plan to cover copyright/licensing fees beyond the video media purchase if the video will be uploaded onto a health system's CCTV or interactive patient care system. You must obtain appropriate copyrights for digitizing and uploading content to your organization's education library and pay the licensing fees for commercial products. Video education content found on the Centers for Disease Control and similar national health and safety websites are public domain and often do not require licensing fees. Be sure you check out the fine print and set up a system for tracking and managing content licenses and copyright information.

The second implication is when the department produces videos. This includes developing storyboards, scripts, and production. It is important to understand your health system's existing resources and processes for developing/producing video content. Specifically, find out if your organization has a production department (usually tied to a health system's marketing and communications department). They may have specific branding and production requirements, which include the use of authorized vendors. Production in-house requires software such as Adobe Premiere and Adobe Creative Suite, or a tool like ProShow Gold or ProShow Producer that requires less experience. Budgeting must include a computer able to handle large graphics and editing. In-house video production also requires purchase of a conversion program to digitize DVDs to load onto CCTV or interactive patient care systems.

In addition to creating your own video education, there are many third-party providers that create content for purchase. Some content may come with the purchase of an IPC system, but additional content may also be purchased through other providers. Regardless of the source, the content should comply with the same criteria as that produced internally by the organization. To help, select a vendor that has rigorous quality standards and is willing to provide documentation about their processes.

When purchasing video content from third-party providers, the content often comes with limitations because it is produced for the masses. Clinical staff needs to become familiar with the education so that they can be comfortable helping patients with questions after the fact and also know when to supplement the video education with their own teaching. When possible, include clinical staff and patient and family advisors in the purchasing decisions. When that is not possible, allow for enough time so that the clinical staff can view some of the core education videos prior to implementation.

Health Literacy

A PFE department plays a primary role in supporting health literacy for your health system. They help keep hospital communications to patients and families focused on the use of plain language, which supports effective communication. This is accomplished through a partnership with the marketing and communications department and in promotion of the PFE department to the health system/organization. Over time, the marketing and communication departments may adopt this focus on plain language as part of their role to incorporate readability analysis, but this is an evolution in competency. They do not, however, apply this to all materials—only the ones generated by the department for general hospital communication and the website. The other significant health literacy piece is the administration of a process to assess patient and family functional health literacy, and partner with the medical team to develop approaches in challenging situations.

Interactive Patient Care (IPC) System Oversight

If your organization uses an IPC system to deliver patient and family education, the oversight for the content that goes onto the system and the integration of IPC as part of the instructional methodology should reside in a PFE department. There is a huge disconnect with nurses who see IPC as a technology that "delivers" patient education without considering that the video education serves a much broader role in the instructional design process as part of a curriculum. The PFE department should also be in charge of decisions on what IPC system functionality to use and how to weave it into the broader health system process used to drive patient education and engagement.

Oversight of Online PFE Materials

It is important to centralize the PFE content used by the health system. You might recall working and going into the "patient education" handout drawer only to find that it is empty, or needing to provide education and having no idea where the handout can be found for your specific need.

The role of material oversight is crucial for any health system. Nurses and other providers are more likely to use a resource if it is easy to find in one location, and when the resources are categorized for a specific topic.

Find out what resources are available in your health system to support a content management system and library. Most hospitals use Microsoft Office products, and SharePoint becomes an invaluable tool in managing content. It also allows the use of workflows so handouts can be converted from Word documents in a "private" working space into Portable Document Format (PDF) files in a "public" access space. A PDF is the preferred print/download option because it reduces opportunity for nurses and others to modify content. This is about content integrity. The electronic medical record accommodates embedding patient-family education documents into discharge instructions.

> ### TIP
>
> If you are using or want to use SharePoint for a content library, do not link a document to the EHR using the title. Instead, create a link using the file. That way, the link does not break when changes are made. This is especially important when documents are part of the medical record.

When the content holdings grow to a hundreds of topics, it is essential to leverage filters and search features. Plan for staffing to support this work. Keep in mind for every handout reviewed by the department, the library and holdings grow. As such, the responsibility to review, update, and maintain the content library needs to grow as well. This needs to be carefully managed.

Self-Care Management Support and Mentoring

The PFE department helps determine the key competencies required for successful self-care management and contributes to determining and evaluating outcomes measures.

The Family Resource Center's Role

The PFE department is in the best position to oversee all the staff working in the FRC if your health system has one. This serves to anchor the work of the FRC as the hub of all PFE activities for a health system. As described in Chapter 12, a Family Resource Center can be extremely valuable as the forward face of patient and family education for a health system. A PFE department should be responsible for strategic decisions about how the Family Resource Center serves the health system.

Shared Governance Committees/Magnet® Councils

PFE department staff and leadership participate as ad hoc members of the shared governance councils and shared leadership with staff on the PFE committee. This is an important aspect of developing the right communication network.

Department Roles

A PFE department should be configured with key roles based on the work scope. The best reporting structure is through the chief nursing officer or executive.

Table 13.1 provides some of the key roles that can be scaled over time from start up to increasing department capacity. Some healthcare roles are not common outside of the United States. In these cases, nurses with progressive levels of education and experience (bachelor's- to doctorate-prepared nurses) would support core department role functions.

Table 13.1	**Example of Core Roles and Functions to Support a PFE Department Structure**		
Role	*Functionality*	*Credentials/ Background*	*Experience*
Support roles: Production assistant, Instructional design education assistant	Helps with video production, create online or e-learning, support class setup, and other content needs.	AA or Bachelor's	Knowledge of Adobe Premiere or similar video production skills
Health educator	Reviews education content, supports PFE committee, teaches health promotion and prevention content. Program development including writing grants. Supports program evaluation.	Master's degree in healthcare professional discipline, Healthcare Educator or Community Educator Bilingual preferred	Patient education experience

continues

Table 13.1   Example of Core Roles and Functions to Support a PFE Department Structure   (continued)

Role	Functionality	Credentials/ Background	Experience
Interactive patient care manager for IPC system (contracted or staff)	Supports the interactive patient care system.	RN preferred	Ability to listen to the needs of the clinician as well as translate the use of technology into clinical practice
Registered nurses, patient-family educators	Complex care curriculum development, teaches classes, auditing.	Registered Nurse BSN required, MSN preferred Bilingual preferred	Three or more years working as an RN Proven experience with patient and family education
Manager, patient-family education	Material review process and online library. Program development including writing grants. Supports program evaluation.	Master's degree in Nursing, Health Education, or Community Education	Experience in leading patient education programs, patient teaching experience, and instructional design
Administrator or director, patient-family education	Program oversight; oversee related departments.	Master's degree in Nursing, Medical degree, or Master's of Health or Community Education PhD is preferred	Experience in leading patient education programs, patient teaching experience, and instructional design

The types and numbers of staff needed would be based on organizational readiness for supporting a department, available budget in hospital operations, and perceived value of the work. It is ideal to start with the one person who can become a "point person" for content and some of the needed functions. This role would be a manager who would be the point person for the policy, shared/collaborative governance, and PFE committee.

Essential Health System Partnerships

PFE departments need to build a solid interprofessional communication network and develop essential partnerships with other departments and leadership teams across the organization and health system.

Language and Translation Services

Translation services are critical to any PFE department. This is a key component to ensure patient education remains linguistically and culturally appropriate. As such, it is important to budget enough money to provide translation. Language services are also needed for the provision of education, and you'll need to decide what resources to provide to patient educators. Specifically, use of in-person, over-the-phone, or telephonic interpreting needed for teaching classes. You also need to decide the qualifications of staff that teach, including whether they need to be bilingual. Refer to Chapter 9 for how to set up a language services program.

Shared Governance Council and Committees

It is important to have a strong presence and engagement with your organization's shared governance structure. As discussed in Chapter 5, there is mutual accountability for the reporting and communication of findings from your organization's IPC system. Additionally, FRC class data and any issues/concerns identified with PFE are reported in a council so they can be addressed. This is inclusive of pending rollouts for new content, curricula, and tools.

Information Technology and Systems

The Information Technology and Systems department is a valuable partner that will support the use of tools such as SharePoint, Web conferencing, or the use of the interactive patient care (IPC) system. While the PFE department manages IPC system PFE content, any software upgrades, network, equipment/hardware needs, and service issues are handled by the respective area in the HIT structure.

Marketing-Communications Department

Marketing and communications play a strong role in branding the health system. Some health systems have a more stringent approach to branding and prescribe the way content looks and feels. Know where your organization falls on the continuum of flexible to controlled in order to establish a solid working relationship with marketing and communications. There are many projects around patient-family education and information that require collaboration, the department's internal communication via the intranet, and externally facing use of education content on the health system's website. In addition, content may come to the PFE department that will end up in a special design.

Managers

Managers are key partners. They ensure there is buy-in and support when rolling out PFE changes. One of the biggest challenges that the PFE department faces is currency—as in practices, policy, and care delivery. *Currency* refers to the relationship between the PFE department's leadership and managers. Lack of a solid working relationship affects implementation of changes and curriculum development. Managers know and understand approved practice at your health system. There are times when a curriculum matches practice, but the patients report variance among the nursing staff. The manager group is the first layer of problem-solving to address the issue. If you don't cultivate a strong relationship with managers, it is hard to mobilize this important resource to enforce or address issues with staff. Managers must have a sense of commitment in supporting PFE and urgency around the PFE department's goals.

Directors

The directors are a good sounding board to review plans and to get a sense of pending changes in their areas, specifically regarding expansion of services. Directors can have a positive and supportive role with their managers in initially applying change management strategies and sustaining those changes. As discussed regarding managers, directors can offer leadership direction to ensure that PFE curricula become part of the daily standard of care and practice. This will involve greater effort initially, but also some prolonged focus to prevent the practices from deteriorating.

Chief Nursing Officer

The chief nursing officer must be a champion for change and ensure that the right resources are available to the PFE department.

Other Executives

You will encounter situations where it is necessary to engage in discussions with other executives to support enhancements to the patient education components on the interactive patient care system or to add staffing/funding into a department budget. The chief information officer and COO must understand how the new patient-education features or staffing support a health system's strategic priorities, especially when submitting major capital requests and expanding the department's capacity when requesting for positions to come from hospital operations.

In addition, when it comes to selecting priority educational topics and hospital orientation content, it is not uncommon to engage in discussions with executives who come from care coordination and quality areas. This includes the medical staff leaders such as the chief medical quality officer, the chief medical safety officer, and the chief medical technology information officer. The VP patient support services is another point of contact, especially related to the patient knowledge and orientation to health system resources such as parking, security, food, room cleanliness, and facility services.

External IPC Vendors

The interactive patient care system vendor is a primary relationship managed by the PFE department's administrators or director. This is an essential relationship to cultivate and maintain given the day-to-day focus on IPC. This relationship must be clinically focused and go far beyond a technology deployment. You will find a variety of activities that the IPC department staff needs to support. Their task forces are set up for program innovations and development. These are ideal for staff who are directly involved in system content management and supporting the end-user experience. When possible, this becomes a partnership with your health system's family advisory council. Many vendors organize a learning community and annual conference to share best practices among their clients.

These experiences extend outside of the PFE department to include managers and staff who become unit-based champions to promote utilization of PFE tools on the system. This vendor relationship provides an ideal opportunity for clinical staff to advance their practices and share with the broader community. Often, the vendor will provide support to help the clinical staff create presentations as well as provide a relatively safe place at the conferences to promote their practice.

Conclusion and Key Points

A PFE department signals an organization's commitment to recognizing the impact patient and family knowledge and engagement has on outcomes of care. Initiating a department requires thought and careful planning to align the department efforts across a health system. Please be sure to perform the necessary review of evidence and best practices for greatest success. Establish a business plan that has both short-term and long-term goals and staffing plans.

> **TIP**
>
> When you're creating standards, we recommend that you use a resource such as "Advancing Effective Communication, Cultural Competence, and Patient-and Family-Centered Care: A Roadmap for Hospitals" (The Joint Commission, 2010).

Creating a patient and family education department is key to success of a health system approach. It is important to invest time in developing a 5-year strategy that not only matches the current resource capacity of your health system but also provides goals to support the organization's future state.

References

Cummings, C., & McCaskey, R. (1992). A model combining centralized and decentralized staff development. *Journal of Nursing Staff Development, 8*(1), 22–5.

Gates, Bill. (2015). BrainyQuote.com. Retrieved May 6, 2015, from BrainyQuote.com website at http://www.brainyquote.com/quotes/quotes/b/billgates626173.html

Haggard, A. (2006). Where do we fit and what should we do? (Part 1). *Journal for Nurses in Professional Development, 22*(2), 93–94. Accessed from http://www.nursingcenter.com/lnc/journalarticle?Article_ID=639449#sthash.TgShP3ft.pdf

Indiana University Health Patient Education. (2015). *Patient education.* Retrieved from http://iuhealth.org/education/nursing-and-patient-care/patient-education/

John Dempsey Hospital, University Connecticut Health Center. (2015). Retrieved from http://jdhedu.uchc.edu/dept_staff.html

Sheriff, R., & Banks, A. (2001). Integrating centralized and decentralized organization structures: An education and development model. *Journal for Nurses in Professional Development, 17*(2), 71. Retrieved from http://www.nursingcenter.com/lnc/journalarticle?Article_ID=100781#sthash.2UJtphRE.pdf

Stanford Medical Center. (2015). Stanford Patient Education Research Center. Retrieved from http://patienteducation.stanford.edu/

Sutter Memorial Medical Center. (2015). Education department. Retrieved from http://www.memorialmedicalcenter.org/patient/patient_education.html

The Joint Commission (TJC). (2010). *Advancing effective communication, cultural competence, and patient- and family-centered care: A roadmap for hospitals.* Oakbrook Terrace, IL: The Joint Commission. Retrieved from http://www.jointcommission.org/assets/1/6/ARoadmapforHospitalsfinalversion727.pdf

Woman's Hospital of Texas. (2015). Patient education. Retrieved from http://womanshospital.com/patient-education/

Measurement and Outcomes: Linking Patient-Family Education to Quality, Safety, and Equity

Ellen Swartwout, PhD, RN, NEA-BC
David Wright, MPH
Lori C. Marshall, PhD, MSN, RN

OBJECTIVES

- Recommend what kind of data is necessary to measure an educational program's effectiveness.
- Explain how data can be used to evaluate the effectiveness of patient and family education.
- Prepare a plan that leverages education as a core strategy for performance improvement.

Introduction

Data is critical to understanding how patient and family educational programs and activities are affecting targeted healthcare outcomes. Several studies show that education has a positive impact on patient's healthcare outcomes, particularly in enhancing one's self-care management for both chronic conditions and the promotion of wellness (Cook et al., 2013; Coulter, 2012; Hibbard & Greene, 2013; Johnson, Ruisinger, Vink, & Barnes, 2014; Lovell et al., 2014; Walker, Marshall, & Polaschek, 2013). In order to effectively achieve the Triple Aim, it is important to use and evaluate data to demonstrate the impact of education on improving quality, safety, and the cost of healthcare (Berwick, Nolan, & Wittington, 2008; Hibbard, Greene, & Overton, 2013).

To begin, think about what kind of data is necessary to measure your educational program's effectiveness and ensure that the data is readily available and sufficient for ongoing analysis. Examples of data include patient and family utilization of prescribed and available education, ease of access to appropriate educational content, teaching methods used, and time intervals for education and its impact on healthcare outcomes specific to your targeted focus area (e.g., hospital readmissions for heart failure, glycemic control for diabetes, medication knowledge and adherence, fall prevention for at-risk patients upon hospital discharge, etc.).

Your education plan should include a determination of the teaching method to be used based on how the patient and family will best receive, comprehend, and retain the knowledge and skills needed to manage their condition and/or health status. It should include a deliberate selection of content that is appropriate for the patient's and family's level of health and educational literacy. Cultural appropriateness must be factored into content selection, and the clinician's assessment of the patient and/or family's ability to engage in their care will influence the depth, frequency, and pace of education delivered.

> **TIP**
>
> It is important to leverage real-time and longitudinal data to determine how responsive the education provided is to these factors. Patient utilization, completion of education and, above all, demonstration of understanding and competency are likely the most straightforward measures of overall educational impact and effectiveness.

The data collected regarding the education completed can also be used to inform prospective care planning. Data can inform alterations in the care plan or in the educational plan itself. For example, data on the factors identified above may suggest the need for different content or a different method of education delivery. It may suggest a slower or faster pace for prescribing and completing education. Additionally, data obtained from other sources such as home monitoring devices, real-time patient feedback through surveys, and/or other data collection mechanisms that can communicate patient status and progress can be an effective resource for care managers monitoring patient progress over time, providing a timelier and more effective ability to intervene appropriately based on observed data.

Delivering appropriate, patient-specific education is critical to empowering and enabling patient and family engagement. For many years, our efforts as caregivers have been focused on providing education to the patients within the limited time we have available with each patient. There has also been little opportunity to benefit from the data and corresponding knowledge gained from the patient's educational experience. Patients' responses to education are informative on many fronts. Because of the value of findings from the patient's educational experience, it is important that we speak to the availability and use of data as we consider a holistic approach to an interactive patient-education strategy.

Designing a Comprehensive PFE Data Program

A variety of program evaluation frameworks exist and serve as useful resources to ensure your organization's patient education program will meet the needs of the patients and families. Most evaluation frameworks draw from public health, such as one proposed by the Centers for Disease Control and Prevention (CDC, 1999) or non–healthcare-related education such as training programs in the military (Straus, Shanley, Yeung, Rothenberg, & Steiner, 2011).

Alvarez, Salas, and Giordano (2004) consider an evaluation framework that looks at other measures like Kirkpatrick (1994), who focused on effectiveness of organizational training. As Straus et al. say, "Measuring student reactions and cognitive learning is only part of a comprehensive program of evaluation" (2011, p. 90); it is important to ensure your evaluation clearly communicates what your program did and how well it met its intended goals.

Additionally, programs leveraging multiple instructional methods must account for this approach. They should create a composite of measures that connect the various educational and instructional methods. It should then be determined if those tools were effective for transferring knowledge with the patients and families engaged in the learning exchange.

One way to view the data interdependencies of your PFE program is by using the Tell-Show-Do-Practice-Review framework (Addelston, 1959). Evaluating educational efforts for a specific and more complex patient population requires a broad data analysis approach to evaluate the patient's and family's comprehension. The analysis must also evaluate the impact on quality and the need for future research and planning to better address disparities. Figure 14.1 is a graphical depiction of this *broad data analysis* approach.

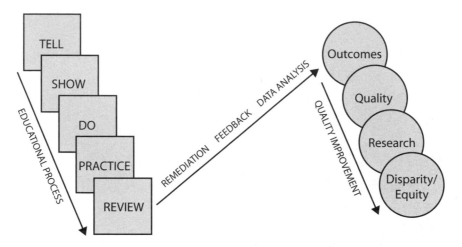

Figure 14.1   Broad data analysis approach. Adapted from Addelston, H. 1959.

Table 14.1 offers a broad data analysis framework for a complex care topic involving the learning need "Gastrostomy Tube (G-Tube)" for a patient with cancer as a hypothetical example. It is organized by Tell-Show Do-Practice-Review, which is the same format used in Chapter 7 with interactive patient care (IPC). In this chapter, however, the framework is extended to further address data analysis needed for quality, outcomes, research, and disparity/equity implications.

Table 14.1   Broad Cross-Continuum Data Analysis Method for Complex Clinical Care (G-Tube Example)

Step	Tasks
Show	Caregiver watches videos on IPC technology tool.
	Nurse explains how to care for G-tube.
	Nurse demonstrates G-tube skills when teaching.
Do	Caregiver performs care when taught by nurse.

Practice	Caregiver performs care at bedside with nurse observing.
	Caregiver independently performs care at bedside.
Review	Before leaving the hospital, the caregiver watches videos on the IPC technology tool again.
	At the clinic visit using the IPC technology tool, the caregiver wrote a goal to talk to doctor and ask, "Why is the area around the G-tube red and puffy?"
	At home, caregiver watched the G-tube troubleshooting video on the IPC technology tool.
Quality	Audit of inpatient medical record revealed documentation was missing for language used for teaching. The admitting data form listed Spanish.
	Unit 6B north had 40% of documentation without language used for teaching listed.
	Create remediation plan to include revision of educational content.
Outcomes	Caregiver took patient to the emergency room because the G-tube was clogged.
	One month later, caregiver brought patient to emergency room and patient was hospitalized for 5 days with an infection at the G-tube site.
	Fifty percent of all cancer patients from Community Hospital sent home with a G-tube are readmitted with a site infection.
Research	Is there a difference in readmission rates for G-tube complications between caregivers taught at bedside or attendance at a standardized class in the resource center?
	What cleaning regimens are best to prevent G-tube site infections for immune-compromised patients?
Disparity/ Equity	Of the 70% of cancer patients who were readmitted with G-tube related issues, there is a statistically significant difference in readmission rates between patients who speak English and those who speak a language other than English.

Evaluating the Patient Education Program

Basic-level PFE program evaluation should include information about the program goals and how it serves key stakeholders (CDC, 1999). In addition, gathering information about the learners' reactions to your classes and offerings is crucial. These are the simplest forms of data to collect. This data includes the number of attendees to classes and offerings, the number and types of offerings, and course evaluations. Patient-satisfaction data is also easily accessed in a health system. The higher-level evaluations focused on outcomes require more time and resources. When setting up offerings, we recommend that you choose one or two education programs that align with your organization's strategic goals for care quality, safety, access, or health outcomes and focus on measuring impact and effectiveness. Table 14.2 shows the various data elements to examine from a programmatic view.

Table 14.2 Programmatic Data Elements, Use, and Applications	
Data Elements	*Data Use and Applications*
Number of class attendees	Data from class attendees is tabulated for a monthly total number of attendees for specific classes; data is then totaled by quarter for an annual total. This data is compared annually for changes in attendance. This gives insight into the need for adding classes (increased attendance) or revising them if attendance is low.
Attendee feedback	Feedback specific to classes is used for class revisions and enhancements. This type of feedback is useful for instructors as part of skills development, as well as for content revisions or identifying future topics of interest.
Number and types of content developed	For PFE departments that produce materials, this provides a metric for the amount of content that's reviewed, revised, and developed. This includes print, video, and curricula.
Number of classes and programs provided	Program metrics give insight into the PFE department's productivity and program offerings. It is organized by type and set up by quarters to show trends. It is compared annually to show increases or decreases in offerings.

Data Elements	Data Use and Applications
Patient satisfaction Aggregate data from post-visit surveys and focus on the following questions. Themes are organized by the different care settings: Instructions were explained in a language the patient understood Felt prepared to go home or self-care Involved in decisions (participation) Communication with care team (information given) Explanation of diet Care for self after surgery Home-care instructions	These items can be used for program evaluation, as a source of evidence, and as part of disparity/equity analysis.
Cost/benefit	This is focused on supporting added value, such as money saved, reduced length of stays, or freeing up staff in clinical areas so they can do other things. Data analysis might include looking for cost savings by consolidating training or streamlining the educational approach so a class can be delivered in a more cost-effective manner. An example is using a centralized versus decentralized approach to PFE.
Outcomes of care	Certain classes might address complex care knowledge and skills and are a better option to link with outcomes. A specific class is linked to improving an outcome of care. Typical outcomes include infection rates, emergency department visits, hospital readmissions, and access to care. For example, an outcome measure for a central venous catheter (CVC) class might look at the number of readmissions or line infection rates of attendees following a class.

Using Data to Evaluate Educational Programs Through IPC Solutions

When considering the interactive patient education experience, a variety of data is accessible for analysis and informative about the patients, their likely response to a personalized care plan, and their progress against prescribed interventions. Table 14.3 defines data elements that, when combined in the interactive patient education experience, provide a more comprehensive picture of the effect of education on the patient's health status.

Table 14.3 Data Elements, Use, and Applications	
Data Elements	*Data Use and Applications*
Patient's ability to engage in healthcare	An evaluation of the patient's likelihood of responding to and achieving a heightened level of activation in their health.
Literacy level and/or cognitive ability	Interactive tools to evaluate the patient's capacity for learning as well as determining the highest-impact learning method for a particular patient.
Readiness to learn	Interactive patient care (IPC) technology provides the tools and automation to assess and document the patient's readiness to receive education. Through automated workflows (Patient Pathways), the patient can choose to receive or schedule their education when they feel prepared to do so.
Education completion	Data available through IPC technology solutions indicates patient completion of education, including the pace, level of completeness, and the number of times the patient and family have reviewed the education.
Comprehension: overall and of individual topics	A patient education pathway available through IPC technology facilitates automated assessment of patient's understanding with questions related to the education content received. The data tools and reports indicate overall competency level and, importantly, areas of deficiency in understanding content and/or topics covered. This feedback informs educators and clinicians where more time or education is needed to move the patient to the desired level of comprehension and understanding so that the education has the effect intended.

Data Elements	Data Use and Applications
Breadth and scope of education comprehension	Hospitals, clinics, and physician offices have access to broad sets of data to evaluate the general effectiveness of PFE efforts as a provider entity. These data can be dissected to evaluate educator proficiency, content appropriateness and quality, and current practice evaluation (quality of prescribing, completion rates level of patient population preparedness for discharge, and so on).
Readiness for discharge	Dashboards with real-time data are available to determine and assess patient readiness for discharge. Completion and comprehension scores help nurses, clinicians, caregivers, educators, and social workers to prioritize those patients whose profiles indicate insufficient impact from patient education. Summary reports serve to evaluate the effectiveness of education on patient-population preparedness for discharge as a predictor of post-discharge results in readmissions, unnecessary emergency department visits, and complications.
Activation level	The impact of education over the course of a visit or inpatient stay can be evaluated based on measured changes in the patient's activation levels (Hibbard, Mahoney, Stockard, & Tusler, 2005).
Patient satisfaction	The quality of education can be a contributing factor to patient satisfaction. Patient education data, along with patient satisfaction feedback, can be examined to evaluate the effectiveness of education, as well as the related impact on patient satisfaction scores.
Patient outcomes data	The quality of education can be correlated to patient quality and safety outcomes. Continual measurement of patient care outcomes in satisfaction, quality, safety, and financial and operational performance (such as length of stay or unnecessary emergency department visits) are strong indicators of the effectiveness of your educational program.

Reporting and Communicating Data

There are a variety of tools, reports, and dashboards that provide and leverage decision-support data to enhance the care process and the effect of education on patient care outcomes.

We recommend monitoring trends to continuously improve educational strategies and interventions in order to meet desired outcomes at the organizational, population, and individual level. Various methods to display data such as dashboards, graphs, charts, and tables are helpful to understand the impact of educational efforts on outcomes at any one point in time with an individual patient, as well as over time within a defined population.

Dashboards are a good way to visualize how PFE efforts are performing to reach targeted outcomes. Figure 14.2 shows an example of a dashboard used to monitor the impact of education on key and target metrics. This Outcomes Achievement Plan (OAP) shown in the figure is typically used within GetWellNetwork client organizations to monitor IPC performance on priority areas of focus for performance improvement. As with the OAP, organizations can use dashboards to see what strategies are progressing toward goals, which goals have been met, and which need attention to reach the desired state. Color-coding is often used for a quick visual of where to focus educational efforts (green=on target, yellow=progressing toward target, and red=not on target).

Line and bar graphs are important tools to place into reports and dashboards because they provide a simple way to connect an educational effort to outcomes. For example, if a patient-family education class was started as a way to reduce readmissions for G-tube care, it would be essential to display pre-course data, and then note readmissions following the implementation. The downward trend is immediately identified, and one can tell the effect was sustained. Figure 14.3 is a sample of how to display data when it is related to reducing readmission following class attendance.

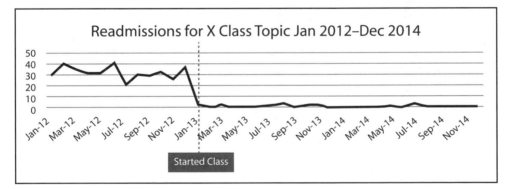

Outcomes Achievement Plan Dashboard
OAP Name: Example	OAP Type: Adult	OAP Revised: 03/19/2015	Data Updated: 03/19/2015

Account Overview

Executive Sponsor	Jane Doe
IPC Champion	John Smith
Fiscal Year End	12/31
GetWellNetwork Beds	250

Actions

+ Patient Satisfaction	Metric	Start Date	Project Champion	Prior Year Data	Current Year Data	Variance	Functionality	Interface
Discharge – Roll-Up	HCAHPS Roll-Up	07/07/2014	Diane Taylor	83%	87%	4.82%	Discharge Planning Solution PXP Scorecard Patient Satisfaction Pathway	Staff Notifications
Environment of Care – Quiet at Night	HCAHPS 9	07/07/2014	Susan Brown	59%	57%	-3.39%	PXP Scorecard Patient Satisfaction Pathway Question of the Day	Staff Notifications
Nurse Communication – Roll-Up	HCAHPS Roll-Up	07/07/2014	Susan Brown	64%	71%	10.94%	PXP Scorecard Patient Satisfaction Pathway Question of the Day	Staff Notifications

+ Quality/Safety	Metric	Start Date	Project Champion	Prior Year Data	Current Year Data	Variance	Functionality	Interface
Fall Reduction	Fall Rate	09/22/2014	Mark Sullivan	3.5	2.9	-17.14%	Fall Prevention Pathway	Education Orders Education Results
Heart Failure Readmissions	Readmission Rate	09/22/2014	Mark Sullivan	18.5%	18.5%	0%	Heart Failure Pathway	Education Orders Education Results

+ ROI/Operations Improvement	Metric	Start Date	Project Champion	Prior Year Data	Current Year Data	Variance	Functionality	Interface
Length of Stay	ALOS	07/07/2014	Diane Taylor	3.7	3.5	-5.41%	Discharge Planning Solution	Discharge Orders

Figure 14.2   Outcomes Achievement Plan dashboard example.

Figure 14.3   Sample results using a line graph that helps trend readmissions related to X class.

At the individual level, it is important to evaluate if your educational efforts result in knowledge and skill acquisition for patients and families in regard to their care management. Knowledge can be measured through comprehension of educational topics and skill through demonstration. Remediation at the point of participating in the educational activity—such as immediate feedback when incorrect answers are chosen with an explanation of why it is incorrect, as well as reinforcing information for a correct answer and giving feedback during demonstration—can determine if the patient and family fully know how to perform the skill. Measuring the comprehension rates and the number of times remediation was needed for knowledge and skill acquisition can help you identify what teaching methods or components of your education would better help patients and families to understand the content.

The first step in using measurement to determine the effectiveness of your patient and family educational strategies is to observe, test, and evaluate outcomes related to educational interventions.

Identifying the Main Improvement Targets

You must begin the measurement process by identifying your priority performance improvement targets and focus areas related to education. It is important to use evidence to design your focus area for improvement and then set targeted outcomes that you are looking to achieve. When developing educational outcome targets, you may consider using the following questions to guide the development of your education plan for the patient.

Is your objective from this education to have the patient and/or family:

- Gain the necessary knowledge to understand their condition?
- Demonstrate a skill needed to self-manage their care?
- Learn how to gain access to and navigate the healthcare system?
- Understand safe self-management practices?
- Improve problem-solving skills?
- Understand when to call their provider?
- Learn how to be an active participant in their care?

Utilizing Interactive Patient Care as a Core Strategy for Performance Improvement

In this section, you will find recent case studies reflecting the impact of interactive care delivery through the use of IPC technology (discussed in Chapter 7). These performance improvement examples, in particular, show the concept of interactive patient education and how you would measure levels of patient activation and knowledge gained. The examples also provide a reference for how to use a cross-continuum lens when measuring PFE outcomes.

Each case study provides an overall narrative about the performance improvement initiative and then a breakdown of each case and measurement plan, following the Tell-Show-Do-Practice-Review educational process and implications of the educational effort on Quality-Outcomes-Research-Disparity/Equity.

Case Study #1: Florida Hospital Celebration Health Leverages Education Through IPC to Significantly Reduce Heart Failure Readmissions

(Adapted from Chapter 7 of the book *Person and Family Centered Care*, Drenkard & Wright, 2014.)

In a continuing effort to improve quality and reduce costs, healthcare providers have been evaluating various methods to reduce heart failure readmissions for more than a decade. Florida Hospital Celebration Health has been leveraging bedside technology and an interactive patient care delivery model to reduce heart failure readmissions 30 days post discharge.

This 182-bed hospital is at the center of innovation for the Florida Hospital System located in Orlando, Florida. Celebration Health is known as a pioneer in many areas of healthcare delivery, bringing best practices and many "firsts" to the industry as it continually leverages people, processes, and technology to advance the quality and safety of care it provides.

Recognizing the importance of patient engagement in care management, Celebration Health embarked on a performance improvement initiative to assess the impact and association of patient activation to reduce heart failure readmissions. In evaluating the probable causes of readmission, there was clear recognition that the skills and knowledge needed by the patients and their family could not be gained in 1 hour of education on the day of discharge. There was too much for anyone to consume, let alone comprehend.

Celebration Health adopted a four-phase interactive heart failure care plan available through GetWellNetwork, an IPC technology solution, to proactively engage and activate heart failure patients to best prepare them to manage their condition once discharged. This Heart Failure Educational Intervention is available at the bedside through an IPC technology platform, using the patient's in-room television and navigated by using an integrated pillow speaker and/or wireless keyboard. The Interactive Heart Failure Care Plan, prescribed by the cardiologist and activated by the nurse at the bedside once a di-agnosis is confirmed, begins with an explanation of the patient's diagnosis and care plan, and the use of the Patient Activation Measure (Hibbard et al., 2005), to establish a base-line patient-activation level. The patient and family or caregiver can move through this four-phase care plan at their own pace, enabling the patient to learn and absorb what they need to know to manage their condition and health status as they are ready.

This Interactive Heart Failure Care Plan teaches, evaluates understanding, and mea-sures patient competency in self-monitoring their condition and taking action to control symptoms and condition flare-ups. The four phases include education for the patient and family about the patient's condition, his medications, and why it is important to take the medications regularly. It teaches the patient what symptoms to watch for and how to rou-tinely check for early warning signs and symptoms. The care plan includes education and resources to help the patient develop a plan and comply with necessary lifestyle changes in diet, fluid intake, exercise, and medication adherence. At the end of each education session, the patient completes comprehension questions. Throughout the care plan, there are checkpoints for the clinical team to assess patient competency in managing his condi-tion and, at the end of each phase, there is a recap of what the patient learned and com-pleted during that session.

During the final phase, often completed just before discharge, the patient is educated on how to cope with the changes in lifestyle he will need to make, and a post-intervention assessment of the patient's activation level is completed (using the Patient Activation Measure—PAM [Hibbard et al., 2005]).

The findings from this innovative approach to reducing heart failure readmissions are impressive. There was a significant increase in the level of patient activation and a corre-sponding decrease in heart failure readmissions 30 days post discharge. The performance improvement project found that the PAM score for patients completing the four-phase Interactive Heart Failure Care Plan through GetWellNetwork IPC technology increased from an average level PAM score of 82% pre-intervention to an average level PAM score of 92% post-intervention. Importantly, primary diagnosis heart failure readmissions 30 days post discharge decreased from 16.47% to 8.33%, representing nearly a 50% reduction in readmissions among the population of patients who had a higher activation level following completion of the care plan.

Historically, the education needed by patients with heart failure, or any chronic condition, has been done on the day of discharge, often with the use of a packet of materials about their condition, medications, and often lifestyle-change requirements. In that case, there is too much information for the patient and family to absorb and no effective method or means to evaluate a patient's understanding and true readiness to actively manage their condition once discharged. The Interactive Heart Failure Care Plan leverages the entire stay of the patient to educate and assess understanding and readiness, and empowers the patient to learn at his own pace. The intervention moves the patient from a state of dependence to a state of independence and confidence in his readiness to monitor symptoms and minimize the risk of flare-ups associated with a need for hospital readmission.

In reading this case study, there are several examples of leveraging patient education through IPC technology to meet desired educational and clinical outcome targets. There were several targeted outcomes with corresponding data elements and measurement strategies determined at the onset of the project. In thinking about the questions to ask before embarking on your focus area, here are some data elements used in this project:

The overall performance improvement targeted outcome of the organization was to reduce 30 days post discharge heart failure readmissions rates by 20%.

Patient and family educational targeted outcomes were to:

- Understand heart failure condition as measured by percent of correct answers on knowledge assessment questions
- Understand how being active in one's care is measured by comprehension of PAM score
- Understand activation level as measured by PAM score and level
- Understand how to manage heart failure symptoms as measured by comprehension rates on lifestyle indicators

- Understand the impact of staggered education in four phases over time rather than one comprehensive session as measured by utilization rates of prescribed education and comprehension

Table 14.4 shows the Tell-Show-Do-Practice-Review educational process and implications of the educational effort on Quality-Outcomes-Research-Disparity/Equity.

Table 14.4	Florida Hospital Celebration Health Heart Failure Broad Data Analysis Approach
Step	**Tasks**
Show	Introduce the technology system and demonstrate how to use it
	Provide educational videos on heart failure
Do	Videos reviewed and comprehension questions completed
	Remedial education completed
Practice	Patient and family demonstrate knowledge and care plan with nurse
Review	Review discharge plan with patient and family
	Review educational videos, reminders, tracking, and so on, to be used at home for management of heart failure
Quality	Patient Activation Measure (PAM) improvement
	Reduction of 30-day heart failure hospital readmissions
Outcomes	PAM score of 82% pre-intervention to an average level PAM score of 92% post-intervention, representing a change of 10% in activation level.
	Heart failure readmissions 30 days post discharge decreased from 16.47% to 8.33% representing almost a 50% reduction in readmissions among the population of patients who had a higher activation level following completion of the care plan.

Research	Does interactive education through technology improve patient self-management skills?
	Do Patient Activation Measure (PAM) scores affect heart failure symptom management (daily weights, dietary compliance, sodium intake, etc.)?
Disparity/ Equity	Evaluate health literacy level to ensure education is congruent with the patient's health literacy level
	Evaluate patient's ability to access education through technology

Case Study #2: Pellham Medical Center Reduces Fall Rates by Increasing Patient Awareness of Fall Risk and Empowering Patients for Fall Prevention

Pellham Medical Center, located in Greer, South Carolina, added an interactive fall prevention educational intervention to its overall strategy to reduce patient falls. Pellham adopted and configured a GetWellNetwork educational pathway that includes automatic prompts, patient education content, and reminders and documentation of patient understanding of the education to reduce fall risk. This educational "pathway" leverages IPC technology at the bedside. The pathway is triggered or launched by the nurse at the bedside and is designed to first make the patients aware that they are at risk of falling. The nurse guides the patient through a self-assessment of fall risk, which is designed to educate the patient on what may cause a fall. Based upon the patient's input and the nurse's assessment, the nurse is prompted at the bedside to discuss with the patient her level of risk and what can be done to prevent a fall. Once acknowledged, the patient watches a brief video providing her strategies on how to prevent a fall. The nurse then asks comprehension questions to indicate the patient's understanding. From that point and multiple times throughout the day, the patient and family are reminded on her television (through a non-invasive alert) to seek help before getting out of bed in an effort to prevent a fall. In short, the patients are being educated, engaged, and empowered as fall safety ambassadors. The result at Pellham was a 32.1% decrease in falls in 1,000 patient discharges in 2014. Table 14.5 shows the Tell-Show-Do-Practice-Review educational process and implications of the educational effort on Quality-Outcomes-Research-Disparity/Equity.

Table 14.5	Pellham Medical Center Falls Reduction Broad Data Analysis Approach
Step	**Tasks**
Tell	Discussion between clinician, patient, family, and care team about fall pathway education available through the television
	Explain the importance of fall prevention while in the hospital and when discharged home
Show	Introduce the fall pathway in the technology system and demonstrate how to use it
	Provide educational videos on fall prevention
Do	Patients complete a self-assessment and review the videos
	Nurse evaluates patient's comprehension
	Nurse reviews fall safety information and answers patient's and family's questions
Practice	Patient and family receive reminders and prompts to reinforce fall prevention strategies
	Patient and family demonstrate safe fall prevention
Review	Review fall safety education prior to discharge with patient and family
	Review educational videos, reminders, tracking, etc. that can be used at home for fall prevention
Quality	Reduction in patient falls
Outcomes	32.1% decrease in falls in 1,000 patient discharges
Research	Did those patients who rated their fall risk high have more falls than those who rated themselves low risk to fall?
	Does interactive education through technology reduce fall rates among at-risk patients?
Disparity/ Equity	Evaluate if at-risk patients have a safe environment and the necessary equipment to reduce their fall risk at home

Case Study #3: Chandler Regional Medical Center Improves Patient Satisfaction with Medication Education Through an Interactive Educational Technology Intervention

Chandler Regional Medical Center, a 240-bed regional acute care hospital, experienced a 10.6% increase on its 2013 HCAHPs medication teaching composite score through an interactive educational intervention that increases patient awareness of and understanding about their medications. Leveraging IPC technology and integration with the medication orders system, clinicians and patients at Chandler are able to access the patient's medications right at bedside. The medication list is populated in real time, designating high-alert, routine medications, and PRN medications prescribed for the patient. The technology incorporates medication education content of the hospital's choice and allows the clinician and patient/family to access information on the medication at any time. The educational content is organized to teach the patients what medications they are taking, why they have been prescribed, the potential side effects, and other information or precautions the patient should know about his prescribed medications. The patient can review his medications at any time and is prompted to complete further education when his medications have changed (e.g., discontinued, newly prescribed, etc.).

This educational tool is set up for easy access by both the nurse and the patient and facilitates a seamless teaching method by the nurse or clinician. The clinician can guide the patient through their medication education at the hospital bedside using the in-room television. With the teaching resource in place, the clinician (nurse, physician, case manager) may schedule a time to review the education with the patient, discussing each medication and assessing patient understanding through teach back and/or based on fostering patient questions. Once the teaching is completed, the patient acknowledges understanding with a simple step using the in-room IPC technology. Through an HL-7 interface with Chandler's EMR, the evidence of patient teaching and patient acknowledgement of understanding is automatically documented back into the patient's medical record. Table 14.6 shows the Tell-Show-Do-Practice-Review educational process and implications of the educational effort on Quality-Outcomes-Research-Disparity/Equity.

Table 14.6	Chandler Regional Medical Center Broad Data Analysis Approach	
Step	**Tasks**
Tell	Discuss medications with patient and family
	Explain the importance of learning about what medications are for, how to take medications, side effects, etc.
	Explain that information about each medication is available via the technology system
Show	When administering medications, educate the patient and family about medications
	Demonstrate how to use the system to learn about medications
Do	Nurse teaches about medications during administration; reinforces educational content and answer questions
Practice	Patient and family demonstrate comprehension of medication information
Review	Nurse reviews medication information with patient and family
Quality	Patient and family understand medication information and how to take medication as prescribed
Outcomes	A 10.6% increase in HCAHPS top box scores on their medication teaching composite score
Research	Does a medication interactive educational technology intervention improve the HCAHPS medication teaching composite score?
	Is a patient's comprehension of medications improved with this teaching methodology?
Disparity/ Equity	Evaluate health literacy level for medication education
	Determine ability for patient to access necessary medications

The Role of Education in Magnet® Designation

Magnet® standards require organizations to demonstrate empirical outcomes to achieve nursing excellence designation (American Nurses Credentialing Center, 2013). Patient education data can be used to address various sources of evidence for Magnet® recognition. You can use your patient education data and analysis to tell the story of your improvement initiatives to meet several sources of evidence. Some patient satisfaction measures in regard to patient educational data can be tied to different sources of evidence to meet Magnet® criteria.

Measurement: How Do You Know It's Working?

Patient education is one, albeit important, component in the strategy to improve patient outcomes and achieve the Triple Aim. However, patient education requires more than the act of providing or completing it. We must also evaluate the effectiveness of education and use the result of measurement to guide further education, care planning, or patient care intervention.

The key question for us to consider is what is the measure of effectiveness? Certainly, patient comprehension is the core measure to demonstrate the effectiveness of the education provided. However, because of the multi-dimensional requirements of education, such as cognitive ability, learning style, cultural appropriateness, and health literacy, it is also important to evaluate the impact of patient education on the patient's ability to manage her condition and improve her health status. There are tools available in addition to a nursing assessment, which can evaluate how effective and appropriate the education was for the patient. It is important to continuously evaluate the content selected and the method through which education was provided. We must determine whether the education was sufficient to facilitate action by the patient, including adherence with her care plan (such as medication adherence) or changes in lifestyle.

Education is a process rather than an act. Education is meant to be progressive, helping the patients to competently adopt skills and understanding to manage their health. The measured effectiveness of education should inform continuing educational needs and next steps in the education plan. There are both quantitative and qualitative measures that demonstrate the effectiveness of education provided. Education completion and comprehension as documented in the patient record is a valid and useful measure of effectiveness immediately following education provision. It is also a good reference retrospectively in planning additional education needed for the patient. IPC technology provides the clinician real-time information on what education has been completed by the patient, the patient's comprehension score, and a record of what parts of the education content the patient did not comprehend. Technology allows aggregation of this data across patient populations to help evaluate the effectiveness of a patient education approach or strategy.

Further, the data can be used to inform research needs, helping to refine a provider's approach in addressing the dynamic needs of its specific patient population based on ethnic mix, age, acuity, language and literacy challenges. Through further research, the data collected through interactive patient education can be used to refine the approach taken to provide the most effective patient education based upon a specific patient population.

Although the data is valuable, it does not negate the need for nurses' evaluations. IPC education requires more than the delivery and completion of education. It requires deeper interaction between the clinician and the patient/family. Educational content should be viewed as a basis for teaching and not the sole resource for teaching. The clinician's knowledge of the patient (and her understanding about how best to teach the patient what he needs to know or build the skills he must have) should have the most influence on the educational plan created for the patient and their family. As education is provided, the benefit to the patient should be continually assessed. Clinicians should observe a response from the patient that indicates understanding as well as acceptance, leading to patient activation. Education is truly only valuable if it has the effect of preparing, equipping, and supporting the patient and his family in managing his health, whether it be through care plan compliance or lifestyle changes for improved health status.

The evaluation of whether education works is patient-specific. It should be based on the patient's response. It is a multi-dimensional evaluation that incorporates both data and assessment. The use of technology enables and empowers patients to complete their education at the pace that is best for them. The act of completing the education is a first step in activating patients. Providers will observe a greater sense of empowerment and engagement among patients and families who take it upon themselves to learn about their condition and care plan and which education to complete that has been specifically prescribed for them. The automation available through technology interfaces provides a greater level of workflow efficiency for clinicians and educators. This heightened efficiency provides clinicians and educators more time as care managers rather than "task managers." Clinicians and educators have more time to qualitatively assess the impact and influence of education and use their critical thinking skills to create a continuing education plan for the patient based upon the patient's response to education and their assessment of ongoing patient need.

Leveraging Patient-Family Education Data for Disparity/Equity Analysis

While this chapter is mostly focused on programmatic and IPC PFE data uses, it is important to leverage your data for higher-level analysis such as addressing healthcare disparities, as shown in Table 14.7. *Disparities* are differences in healthcare or health in groups of people (Office of Minority Health and Health Equity [OMHHE], 2015). The most common group differences are analyzed by race/ethnicity, language, and gender, insurance and access to care (CDC, 2015; Flores & Ngui, 2006; Institute of Medicine [IOM], 2002). For the sake of this chapter, the focus will be on racial/ethnic and linguistic disparities because they are easiest to analyze for those leading patient-family education programs.

Common diagnoses or conditions with disparities include asthma, obesity, diabetes, and hypertension (CDC, 2015). When there are disparities, patients and families might receive less desirable treatment options, less or different medications (pain medications for example), and services that are lower in quality (IOM, 2002).

Case Example

PFE Program on Asthma

Consider a patient-family education program that includes a specific course on asthma. Patients receive an asthma action plan and a set of handouts written in plain language at the 5th grade level. This organization also leverages its interactive patient care system; a set of asthma self-care management videos are ordered, and the patient and family are further engaged in their care through an interactive asthma pathway as mentioned in Chapter 7. If the health system has a high percentage of patients with Limited English Proficiency and who speak a language other than that in the available written materials, this might result in disparate or unequal care. When a disparity exists, a health system must be committed to digging deeper to understand the reasons, and in addition, using available resources to narrow any gaps. In this example, the health system might consider making sure the handouts and videos are in more languages. The multi-language videos can be uploaded to the IPC system. The use of an interpreter for review, explanation, and read back/teach back is essential. This example combines program data, IPC data, and analysis of the asthma curriculum by language. Refer back to Chapter 9 for details on how to use language resources for patient and family education.

| Table 14.7   Disparity/Equity Data Elements, Use, and Applications ||
Disparity/Equity Data Elements	Data Use and Applications
Race/ethnicity	Racial and ethnic disparities involve differences by race/ethnic groups for specific conditions, treatment or diagnoses. The reference group in racial and ethnic disparities is "White" compared to other race/ethnic groups (Flores & Ngui, 2006).
	Examples of how data is used include looking at class outcome by race/ethnicity to see if there are differences in emergency department visits or readmission rates for core conditions or diagnoses.
Language	Language disparities involve differences in the provision of patient and family education (or care) by language. For this disparity, the reference group is "English" and is compared to those with Limited English Proficiency (other languages) (Flores & Ngui, 2006).
	Examples of how the data is used with PFE include exploring differences by language used for materials, resources, and IPC technology available or instruction.

NOTE

As Interactive Patient Care (IPC) moves further across the continuum and into the home, it is important to recognize IPC as part of "access to care" and a future focus for disparity analysis.

Conclusion and Key Points

Because of the importance of patient education and given the current state and effectiveness of education, we must employ new methods and models for education. Our approach must include evaluation of patient needs, prospective planning, efficient and deliberate delivery of education, a quantitative and qualitative assessment of the effectiveness of education, and ongoing management and adaptation of the educational plan based on what the data tells us about the effectiveness of the education provided.

As with any clinical intervention, the patient response to education is informative and should be used to guide further care planning. The data available from education is valuable and can inform a more precise strategy for education planning and delivery relevant to a specific patient and/or patient population.

References

Addelston, H. (1959). Child patient training. *Fortnightly Review of the Chicago Dental Society, 38*(7), 27–29.

Alvarez, K., Salas, E., & Garofano, C. (2004). An integrated model of training evaluation and effectiveness. *Human Resource Development Review, 3*(4), 385–416.

American Nurses Credentialing Center (ANCC). (2013). *2014 Magnet® application manual.* Silver Spring, MD: American Nurses Credentialing Center.

Berwick, D., Nolan, T. W., & Wittington, J. (2008). The Triple Aim: Care, health and cost. *Health Affairs, 27*(3), 759–769.

Centers for Disease Control and Prevention (CDC). (1999). Framework for program evaluation in public health. *MMWR, 9*(48), 1–40.

Centers for Disease Control and Prevention (CDC). (2015). Fact Sheet: CDC Health Disparities and Inequalities Report, United States, 2011. Retrieved from http://www.cdc.gov/minorityhealth/reports/CHDIR11/FactSheet.pdf

Cook, D. J., Manning, D. M., Holland, D. E., Prinsen, S. K., Rudzik, S. D., Roger, V. L., & Deschamps, C. (2013). Patient engagement and reported outcomes in surgical recovery: Effectiveness of an e-health platform. *Journal of the American College of Surgeons, 217*(4), 648–655.

Coulter, A. (2012). Patient engagement: What works? *Journal of Ambulatory Care Management, 35*(2), 80–89.

Drenkard, K., & Wright, D. (2014). Patient engagement and activation. In J. Barnsteiner, J. Disch, & M. K. Walton (Eds.), *Person and family centered care* (pp. 95-111). Indianapolis, IN: Sigma Theta Tau International.

Flores, G., & Ngui, E. (2006). Racial/ethnic disparities and patient safety. *Pediatric Clinics of North America, 53*(6), 1197–1215.

Hibbard, J. H., & Greene, J. (2013). What the evidence shows about patient activation: Better health outcomes and care experiences; fewer data on costs. *Health Affairs, 32*(2), 207–213.

Hibbard, J. H., Greene, J., & Overton, V. (2013). Patients with lower activation associated with higher costs: Delivery systems should know their patients' "scores." *Health Affairs, 32*(2), 216–221.

Hibbard, J. H., Mahoney, E. R., Stockard, J., & Tusler, M. (2005). Development and testing of a short form of the patient activation measure. *Health Services Research, 40*(6), 1918–1930.

Institute of Medicine (IOM). (2002). *Unequal treatment: What healthcare providers need to know about racial and ethnic disparities in health-care.* Retrieved from http://www.iom.edu/~/media/Files/Report%20Files/2003/Unequal-Treatment-Confronting-Racial-and-Ethnic-Disparities-in-Health-Care/Disparitieshcproviders8pgFINAL.pdf

Johnson C., Ruisinger J. F., Vink J., & Barnes B. J. (2014). Impact of a community-based diabetes self-management program on key metabolic parameters. *Pharmacy Practice, 12*(4), 499–503.

Kirkpatrick, D., & Kirkpatrick, J. (2006). 3rd Edition. *Evaluating Training Programs. The Four Levels.* San Francisco, CA: Berrett-Koehler Publishers.

Levitt, Steve (2013). 19 June, 2013. Retrieved from http://businessintelligence.com/bi-insights/economist-steven-levitt-on-why-data-needs-stories/

Lovell, M., Luckett, T., Boyle, F. M., Phillips, J., Agar, M., & Davidson, P. M. (2014). Patient education, coaching, and self-management for cancer pain. *Journal of Clinical Oncology, 32*(16) 1712–1720.

Office of Minority Health and Health Equity (OMHHE). (2015). *Eliminating racial & ethnic health disparities.* Retrieved from the CDC website: http://www.cdc.gov/omhd/About/disparities.htm

Straus, S., Shanley, M., Yeung, D., Rothenberg, J., & Steiner., E. (2011). *New Tools and Metrics for Evaluating Army Distributed Learning.* Santa Monica, CA: Rand Corporation.

Walker, R., Marshall, M. R., & Polaschek, N. (2013). Improving self-management in chronic kidney disease: A pilot study. *Renal Society of Australasia Journal, 9*(3), 116–125.

"I've learned that you shouldn't go through life with a catcher's mitt on both hands; you need to be able to throw something back."
–Maya Angelou, 2000

Supporting Patient and Family Education Through Global Health Partnerships

Mae-Fay Koenig, MPH
Lori C. Marshall, PhD, MSN, RN
Amal Al-Hasawi, BSChem, BSN, RN
Crystal Xiang DIng, RN, MSN

OBJECTIVES

- Describe the key parts of a global health partnership.
- Explain the benefits of a global health partnership to support patient and family education (PFE).
- Examine the global health partnerships held by your organization and consider opportunities that strengthen the PFE focus.

Introduction

Global partnerships are essential to improving health outcomes (Boydell & Rugkasa, 2007) and are mutually beneficial to help developed countries learn new problem-solving skills from countries with fewer resources (Syed et al., 2012). It is important to be aware of the key issues affecting global health, including those involved in establishing the global priorities and mobilizing resources that maximize collective impact. Since 2000, the World Health Organization (WHO) and the United Nations have been partnering on Millennium Development Goals (WHO, 2015) to combat poverty, hunger, disease, illiteracy, environmental degradation, and discrimination against women (WHO, 2007).

The Centers for Disease Control and Prevention (CDC, 2015) also created a set of goals and a framework to support the broader global health improvement strategy (CDC, 2012). Like the WHO, the CDC role is both strategic and action-based, and both organizations aim for the eventual handoff and ownership to a country for sustained improvements and wellbeing. They achieve this by setting up local systems and processes and keeping the country connected with ongoing support.

What becomes a global PFE priority? At a very high level, the process begins with surveillance, data collection, and analysis as a foundation to understanding the issues and problems. In partnership with universities, agencies, and communities, healthcare trends are studied for countries to identify top diseases, environmental factors contributing to disease, and personal factors such as habits like smoking and activity levels (Murray et al., 2012; Naghavi et al., 2015). The next aspect is to set goals and engage entire countries to commit to the goals through health ministries, community engagement, and global partnerships. Then they start working on meeting the goals. The final process is to monitor the impact of changes.

In this chapter, you will learn how to support patient and family education through international partnerships between health systems. In addition, you will gain insight into why international partnerships are formed, including partnership types that emerge, and a review of the partnership benefits.

What Is a Global PFE Health System Partnership?

Hospitals and health systems follow a similar process when engaging in global health partnerships, but on a smaller scale. Instead of entire countries, partners are identified from specific regional healthcare settings within a country.

> **Definition 15.1:** *Global PFE partnerships. Mutually beneficial international collaborations in which both parties benefit from the knowledge and solutions (Boydell & Rugkasa, 2007; Syed et al., 2012; WHO, 2007).*

A typical partnership (see Figure 15.1) starts with understanding the broader building blocks from the WHO (WHO, 2007). Health system leaders then choose how to focus their efforts. There are different ways a global health partnership supports patient and family education:

- **Programmatic**: Sharing content used by a specific partner that is adapted to the international partner. This also includes building capacity to leverage new technology, innovations, and practices.

- **Health system**: Supporting staff and provider knowledge in the best practices of patient and family education. This helps build workforce competencies on what and how to teach patients and families.

- **Cross-continuum**: Partnering to provide a portion of the services to fill gaps contributing to population health.

- **Research**: Collaborating on research to generate evidence about a specific PFE education project or self-care management intervention. This may involve testing interventions in the global setting.

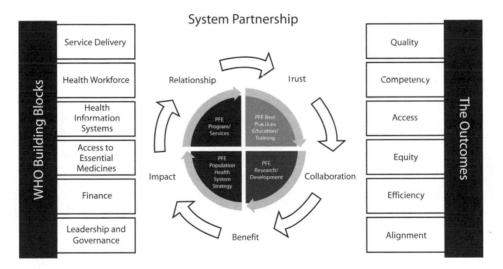

Figure 15.1   The global PFE health system partnership. Adapted from WHO and used with permission IN.S.P.I.R.E. Global, LLC © 2015

A global PFE partnership starts by forming a relationship that evolves over months and even years. It begins with determining areas of mutual interest or common goals. Each side must establish trust over the course of the relationship to permit access to partner resources and so that information exchanged during the partnership is accepted. Collaboration often begins through a series of smaller demonstration projects such as staff and physician education on PFE best practices for specific patient population or condition. When the partnership benefit is realized, the relationship deepens, and parties agree to invest more resources and capacity to implement larger programs. The investment then centers on a measurable impact of the PFE program or service to the target population, which strengthens the relationship and serves as a catalyst to reinvest in the partnership process.

The PFE partnership process is catalyzed to produce outcomes by the following WHO building blocks:

- Service delivery leads to quality of care.
- Health workforce development leads to competent providers and staff.
- Health information systems improve access.
- Access to essential medicines promotes equity of care.
- Finance encourages efficiency.
- Leadership and governance ensure that efforts align with the strategic priorities/health-improvement goals of the region.

Before embarking on a global health partnership, it is imperative that you understand the population health issues and disease burdens affecting your partnership countries (Naghavi et al., 2015), because this shapes the partnership aims and outcomes both health systems will focus on. It is also helpful to gain regional perspective and how the country ranks in comparison to others in the region (Shahraz et al., 2014). Examples of the authors' partnership countries are found in Table 15.1, using the Institute for Health Metrics and Evaluation (2014) Global Burden of Disease Profiles.

Table 15.1	Examples of the Impact of Global Burden of Disease by Selected Country					
	Armenia	China	Panama	Saudi Arabia	United Arab Emirates	United States
Top four causes of years of life lost (YLLs)	Heart disease Stroke Lung cancer Diabetes	Stroke Heart disease COPD Road injury	Heart disease HIV/AIDS Stroke Violence	Road injury Heart disease Preterm birth Stroke	Road injury Heart disease Stroke Preterm birth	Heart disease Lung cancer Stroke COPD
Top four causes of disability	Low back pain Depression Diabetes Neck pain Musculo-skeletal is-sues	Low back pain Depression Neck pain Musculo-skeletal issues Diabetes	Depression Low back pain Anemia # Neck pain Asthma	Depression Low back pain Diabetes Anemia # Anxiety	Depression Low back pain Anxiety Drug use Diabetes	Low back pain Depression Musculo-skeletal issues Neck pain Anxiety
Risk factors accounting for most of disease burden	Dietary risks Hyper-tension Tobacco smoke	Dietary risks Hypertension Tobacco smoke	Dietary risks Hyper-tension High BMI^	High BMI^ Dietary risks High fast-ing BS	High BMI^ Dietary risks High fasting BS	Dietary risks Tobacco smoke High BMI^
The leading risk factors for children under 5	Household air pollution from solid fuels	Household air pollution from solid fuels	Sub-optimal breast-feeding	Sub-optimal breast-feeding	Under-weight	Zinc defi-ciency
The leading risk factors for adults aged 15-49 years	Dietary risks	Work hazards	Alcohol	Dietary risks	Dietary risks	Alcohol

Notes: *High fasting plasma glucose, # Iron deficiency anemia, ^ High body mass
Diabetes and anxiety disorders were not listed as causes of disability in 1990.
Index adapted from IHME (2014).

You will read three case studies representing the United States, China, and Saudi Arabia (see Figure 15.2). They illustrate the different sides of the global partnership process to support patient and family education.

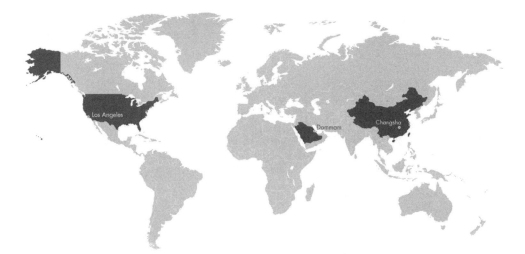

Figure 15.2   World Map of Partnerships. Courtesy of Children's Hospital Los Angeles.

Case Study #1: Children's Hospital Los Angeles Center for Global Health

About CHLA

Founded in 1901, Children's Hospital Los Angeles (CHLA) is the oldest freestanding pediatric hospital in California. CHLA is one of only 10 children's hospitals—and the only one on the West Coast—to be named for clinical excellence for three consecutive years to the prestigious *U.S. News and World Report* Honor Roll. CHLA is currently ranked fifth in the nation. CHLA serves as a major regional referral center for children who require life-saving acute care. Each year, the hospital provides more than 104,000 children with pediatric healthcare in a setting designed just for their needs. Additionally, CHLA sees patients from six continents and 47 nations. To coordinate, oversee, and expand globally focused efforts, CHLA established the Center for Global Health in 2012.

CHLA has been recognized as one of America's premier pediatric academic medical centers through its affiliation since 1932 with the Keck School of Medicine of the

University of Southern California. The medical staff at CHLA is comprised of community physicians and hospital-based physicians belonging to the Children's Hospital Los Angeles Medical Group (CHLAMG). In partnership with CHLA for more than 30 years, CHLAMG physicians are renowned as world leaders in pediatric specialty medicine for their clinical, educational, and research programs alike. Using a multi-disciplinary approach, physicians work in partnership with specially trained nurses and allied health professionals at CHLA to provide quality care. CHLA nursing care is internationally recognized as a model for nursing excellence, providing a special brand of care that is informed by the best practices of academic medical centers and standards of a Magnet®-recognized hospital.

In 2013, the American Nurses Credentialing Center bestowed re-designation of Magnet recognition for nursing excellence on CHLA; only 6.6% of hospitals in the United States have achieved Magnet® recognition. With a history of pioneering new and minimally invasive techniques to help children heal faster, CHLA is also home to the Saban Research Institute, the largest and most productive pediatric research facilities in the United States.

Partnering with the Center for Global Health

The Center for Global Health was created in 2012 to coordinate, oversee, and expand globally-focused efforts at CHLA. Program priorities of the Center are as follows:

- **International Patient Services**: Provide premiere consultation and care using advanced technologies for children from around the world with complex pediatric conditions through their International Patients Services.
- **Program Development**: Provide consultation and expertise to develop new programs or enhance existing programs in targeted countries.
- **Education**: Prepare future generations of physicians, nurses, allied health professionals, and administrators globally by sharing CHLA's standards and best practices.
- **Telemedicine**: Provide and promote professional, ethical, and equitable improvement in healthcare delivery through telemedicine and information technology worldwide.

- **Research**: Seek mutually beneficial research collaborations around the world.
- **Community Benefit**: Strive to provide quality care to the underprivileged in developing countries.

Through the Center for Global Health, CHLA has established collaborations around the world to share and exchange knowledge with other leading pediatric institutions. Over the years they have had physicians, nurses, administrators, and others from other countries come to CHLA for a period of one week to a year to observe and understand the way they provide healthcare to their patients. These observers are interested to see how medicine is practiced in an academic pediatric setting based in the United States, how multidisciplinary teams interact to provide for the most complex cases, how advancements are made in pediatric research, and how patient outcomes are achieved.

More importantly, they are also interested in understanding how CHLA's providers partner closely with the children and their families to provide education on the patient's condition, whether it is an acute episode of illness or a chronic disease lasting a lifetime. CHLA's mission is to create hope and build healthier futures, and through patient and family education, they are transferring their knowledge and expertise to empower their patients and families to overcome an episodic illness or improve their quality of life with a chronic condition, both with the goal of overall health and wellness.

And through CHLA's global partnerships, they are creating a hub and spoke model of PFE by training providers globally so they too can help the patients and families in their home country through PFE methods developed at CHLA and modified to meet the needs of their culture.

Being geographically located in the heart of Los Angeles, California—considered to be one of the most racially and ethnically diverse communities in the world—the CHLA staff have naturally developed an expertise in treating children of different cultural and religious backgrounds. CHLA's physicians, nurses, clinicians, and support staff undergo training to provide culturally competent care to its patients and their families. So when they receive a patient from the Middle East or Asia or Latin America, understanding how to provide care to meet their cultural needs is not new to the team. If anything, CHLA's experience treating their locally diverse patients has helped to prepare them for increasing the number of international patients seen at their institution. CHLA's Center for Global Health International Patient Services team has facilitated care for over 300 children from over 50 countries in the past 4 years. Despite the increasing number of international patients, CHLA's physicians, nurses, clinicians, and support staff continue to provide exceptional patient care (sometimes with the help of certified medical interpreters), and continue to impart education to their international patients and families in ways that transcend any language barriers, such as through demonstration and example, translated educational materials, one-on-one training and education, their interactive patient care system (the GetWellNetwork), and a variety of other modalities that allow customization of educational materials to the specific and unique needs of CHLA's patients and families.

CHLA has hosted over 50 international observers annually from all over the world. Observers have included physicians, nurses, administrators, and other clinical staff, and the typical duration ranges from a week to up to a year. International observers at CHLA have noted the amount of one-on-one time and attention that CHLA clinicians spend in providing patient and family education as one thing that stands out from what they have seen compared to their home country. In other countries where patient and family education may not be seen as an integral component of a patient's path to wellness, resources are often limited, or education is only briefly touched on. Sometimes the sheer number of patients can also overwhelm the resources available; due to the overwhelming demand for care, that there is not enough time for a clinician to provide customized patient and family education. At CHLA, experts have also developed comprehensive educational materials over time, which can be made readily available to patients and their families in multiple languages.

> *"…the amount of one-on-one time and attention that clinicians spend in providing patient and family education stands out…as being critical to successful outcomes."*

CHLA also utilizes different modalities to provide education, such as through its GetWellNetwork (which is available at the bedside of all of inpatient beds), or by providing information pre-loaded onto iPads for patients and families to review while waiting for their appointment in the outpatient setting. Courses for disease management are provided to CHLA's chronically ill patients and help patients and families. CHLA's international observers have been impressed with the variety of modalities in which patient and family education is made available at CHLA and are often inspired to find ways to replicate this upon their return to their home country. CHLA's international patients also have access to PFE that has been developed at CHLA and tailored to meet their needs. Many of CHLA's international observers return home inspired and serve as a change agent in their hospitals.

Global Partnership with Hunan Children's Hospital, China

In alignment with CHLA's Center for Global Health's priorities, Children's Hospital Los Angeles established a global partnership in 2013 with Hunan Children's Hospital, located in Changsha, China. This academic partnership was formed between CHLA and Hunan Children's to establish a relationship in which opportunities for training, education, and research could be explored. As one of the leading pediatric institutions in the Hunan province, CHLA had an informal relationship with Hunan Children's Hospitals between some of their physicians. There was certainly a level of enthusiasm between both parties to then formalize this relationship because CHLA physicians had already participated in their first China-U.S. International Symposium of Pediatrics as guest lectures, as well as subsequent symposiums. Additionally, there was a strong interest by Hunan Children's to send over several groups of physicians and nursing observers to CHLA to learn and observe clinical practice as well as patient and family education practice.

Legacy of PFE Partnerships

As healthcare reform in the United States focuses on creating a medical home for patients outside of the inpatient setting, patient and family education becomes a powerful tool to help achieve the transformation of the U.S. healthcare system. By emphasizing patient and family education on how to take medicines, administer necessary care at home, and follow up with the appropriate providers as required on the outpatient setting, we can reduce readmission rates and unnecessary emergency department visits. And for chronically ill patients, patient and family education can help to make their home the medical home. In countries where all healthcare, both inpatient and outpatient, is delivered in the hospital setting due to lack of primary care infrastructure, patient and family education serves as a transformative change agent, building on the United States' lessons learned, to help them achieve better outcomes for their patients.

Following the saying, "Give a man a fish and you feed him for a day; teach a man to fish and you feed him for a lifetime," PFE allows patients and families to be more self-reliant and in control of their healthcare. For patients with chronic conditions, understanding what to watch out for and learning how to become more independent helps to maximize their quality of life. In pediatrics, this becomes even more evident as a child transitions into his adolescence and becomes a young adult, becoming less reliant on his parents to provide reminders to take medications or assist in his day-to-day home care and becoming more responsible for taking care of himself. This transition and growth in a child's independence is something parents eventually learn to accept, but sometimes gets hindered due to a child's chronic medical condition. Patient education helps to foster that independence and empowers the child to manage his or her own health needs.

Through telemedicine, CHLA has brought clinical expertise to regions across the world. They have established a tele-genetics program in Puerto Rico in which a CHLA medical geneticist can provide a consultation via telemedicine as if the patient and family were in the same room. On the patient's end, they have a nurse telemedicine coordinator who acts as a physician extender in partnership with the medical geneticist based at CHLA. Once the consultation is completed, the nurse telemedicine coordinator spends time with the patient providing additional education and addressing further questions based on the consultation (see Figure 15.3). Because she is originally from Puerto Rico and is Spanish speaking, this makes it easier for the patient and family to understand. Also the Puerto Rican nurse telemedicine coordinator provides additional education and resources to the family and helps them coordinate the next steps in the care as recommended by the medical geneticist. This partnership allows patients in another region who may not necessarily have any means to access the expertise, yet with the access to our physician extender near their home, they have two options for obtaining education to meet their needs.

As a freestanding pediatric academic medical center, CHLA's expertise in patient and family education is sought out by global partners frequently. CHLA has been asked to provide consultative services and serve as a content partner to enhance other institutions' PFE programs. This educational component differentiates care received at CHLA as compared to other hospitals in the world. It is a component that others have found to be integral to improving patient outcomes and returning a child to her optimal health status. It is CHLA's intent that it can continue to spread this component throughout the world as another way to elevate the overall health status of children and their families globally.

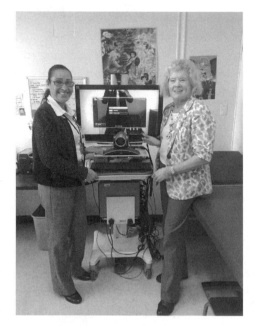

Figure 15.3   The nurse and geneticist as they prepare for genetics consults in Puerto Rico. Photo courtesy of Children's Hospital Los Angeles.

Case Study #2: Hunan Children's Hospital China

About Hunan Children's Hospital

Hunan Children's Hospital is located in Changsha, China, and started its medical service in 1987 (see Figure 15.4). It is a Class-A Grade Three comprehensive children's hospital for pediatric medical healthcare, rehabilitation, scientific research, and teaching with the authentication of Iso9001/14001 environmental quality system, and it successfully obtained the Joint Commission International accreditation (JCI) in 2013. It has 1,800 beds and more than 2,000 employees in 37 clinic departments, 8 medical technical divisions, and 27 outpatient clinics. It has one national key clinic discipline of pediatric emergency and four provincial key disciplines of neonatology, pediatric surgery, pediatric health-care, and rehabilitation in the hospital. There are four important centers: Hunan Pediatric Emergency Center; Rehabilitation Center of Cerebral Paralysis; Adolescence Medical Center; and Prevention and Treatment Center of Children's Optometry, Strabismus and Amblyopia. In recent years, the hospital has received many national awards.

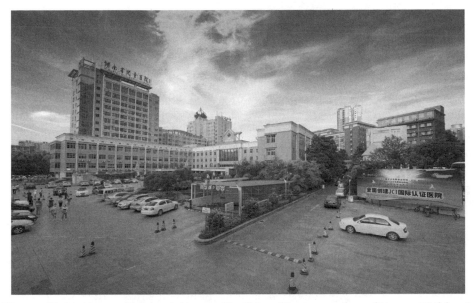

Figure 15.4   Hunan Children's Hospital in China. Photo courtesy of Hunan Children's Hospital, China.

The International Cooperation and Exchange Office

In order to enhance and promote the international collaboration, Hunan Children's Hospital established an International Cooperation and Exchange Office. It has carried out over 20 training courses on pediatric technology for developing countries. It successfully held its third annual China-U.S. International Symposium on Pediatric Critical Care in September 2014. At that symposium, several speakers were invited from Children's Hospital Los Angeles to share their work in critical care, quality, nursing, pulmonology, adolescent and young adult oncology, and telehealth to several hundred pediatric physicians, nurses, and administrators from the Changsha region and other countries.

Hunan Children's Hospital has extensively established friendly relationships of cooperation and academic exchange with famous medical institutions of other countries, including the United States, Canada, Australia, the Netherlands, Germany, and Japan. Hunan Children's Hospital has established collaboration with Children's Hospital Los Angeles. Through the clinical observerships at CHLA, Hunan Children's Hospital physicians and nurses have benefitted from learning unique teachings at CHLA, and it continues to influence their day-to-day practice.

Observerships

Hunan Children's Hospital leverages its connections for *observerships*, which are an important partnership component. The educational exchange resulting from an observership creates a common framework from which to build and strengthen the overall partnership. For example, details about various types of care are gained from the exchange when a nurse visited for 3 months along with a physician. By sending a multidisciplinary team to observe in another country, they gain different perspectives, which facilitates knowledge sharing in multiple disciplines. In a recent visit to CHLA, the Hunan Children's Hospital observers witnessed first-hand the inner workings of the clinical and patient education support areas.

Hunan Children's Hospital staff and physicians who have visited CHLA through the observership program have gained many important insights. The site visit provided exposure to a new way to deliver patient education, including the significance of training in a setting such as a Family Resource Center. A partnership site visit provides the opportunity to learn about care delivery models or compare the role of the patient and family in their healthcare experience. Here are some of the key takeaways that the observers brought back to their home institution:

- Ability to disseminate the evidence-based knowledge and practical case of patient and family education learned at CHLA.
- The successful experiences and ideas of the Family Resource Center implemented at CHLA serve as a tremendous benefit by improving the quality and effectiveness of PFE.
- The use of communication and case discussion enhances the PFE capabilities.
- The common ethical principal of mutual understanding and respect served as a foundation for CHLA and Hunan Children's Hospital to further build a close partner relationship.

In particular, the observers at CHLA's Family Resource Center recognized opportunities for new types of PFE that could be implemented at Hunan Children's Hospital. Examples of such opportunities include:

- Organize patient and family conferences and seminars to improve the dissemination and discussion of successful examples of PFE.

- Publicize journals, magazines, or publications that CHLA and Hunan Children's Hospital can work together on, which may include hot topics focusing on common and difficult nursing problems.

- Develop and maintain Internet communication, such as a global Internet conference, serving as an important medium to popularize PFE information and practical cases. This modality will also advocate for patient and family education when necessary.

A fruitful harvest means going back to your organization with new ideas and opportunities. It is not realistic to implement everything that you observed due to different practice environments of constraints. The challenge in any partnership is how to adapt new knowledge to the global partners setting. Some examples of how this can be done:

- At the Family Advisory Council conference at CHLA, participants learned a new understanding of a parent's role, not just a caregiver, but as an instrumental voice that also can give advice. Through this Council, parents could be an integral component in hospital policy-making. From their experiences, they can provide input in projects such as the PFE booklet revision. Now at Hunan Children's Hospital, parents are encouraged to participate in the education booklet revision and they are trying to formally organize a Family Advisory Council, modeled after the one observed at CHLA.

- Patient and family education is not just something limited to physicians and nurses at CHLA; it transcends all roles that interact with patients and families. By sharing the observations at CHLA among colleagues at Hunan Children's Hospital, they can help to strengthen and inspire teamwork and collaboration within Hunan Children's Hospital for patient and family education. Through the wide engagement of physicians, nurses, dietitians, physical therapists, and others to get involved with PFE, there is organizational support to further enhance and develop PFE throughout Hunan Children's Hospital, similar to CHLA.

For Hunan Children's Hospital, global partnerships have led to accessing tremendous knowledge globally. From the observerships, ideas are gained and future innovations are inspired.

Case Study #3: King Fahad Specialist Hospital in Dammam (KFSH-D), Saudi Arabia

Not all global partnerships are based on formal Memorandum of Understandings (MOUs) or agreements. Some form through networking and individual professional relationships. In this example, CHLA has a relationship with King Fahad Specialist Hospital in Dammam, Saudi Arabia (KFSH-D) through personal professional connections. Because KFSH-D does not have a formal global partnership with either CHLA or Hunan, its focus is on evaluating the prospects of a formal partnership.

About King Fahad Specialist Hospital

King Fahad Specialist Hospital in Dammam (KFSH-D) is recognized as one of the most important health projects that the eastern region in Saudi Arabia has had in the past few years (KFSH-D, 2015).

KFSH-D was the first specialized hospital in the Ministry of Health to receive the Joint Commission International Accreditation (JCIA). KFSH-D has successfully performed multiple stem cell transplantations and it is the only center that provides this type of care of all the Ministry of Health hospitals. The hospital's laboratory and hematology department are accredited by the College of American Pathologists (CAP).

KFSHD presently has the capacity of 630 patients' beds and has adequate manpower.

The hospital offers services to its patients and families in the eastern region of Saudi Arabia by providing the following specialties: oncology, organ transplant, neurosciences, cardiac services programs, genetic sciences, hematology, rehabilitation, neurological surgery, surgical oncology, nuclear medicine, radiation therapy, orthopedic surgery, urology, and many other specialties. It also houses the only pancreas transplantation program kingdom-wide, in addition to kidney and liver transplants.

If KFSH-D Were to Consider a Partnership with CHLA, What Would They Want to Know?

Patient- and family-centered care has been a core component of healthcare quality in many organizations for some time now. More recently, the Ministry of Health (MOH) in Saudi Arabia has embraced this model, and King Fahad Specialist Hospital Dammam (KFSH-D) has recognized the opportunities for improvement in patient care that this approach offers. KFSH-D is a relatively new hospital, having transitioned from a community hospital to a tertiary care referral specialist hospital a few years ago, and is now in the process of building a new 1,500-bed academic medical center. Thus, developing a comprehensive patient and family education program is critical to the success of this evolving hospital.

Similar to many countries throughout the globe, healthcare organizations in Saudi Arabia are becoming more aware of the value of creating international partnerships to support patient- and family-centered care, of which patient and family education is a major component. KFSH-D has collaborative agreements with some of the best hospitals and health centers in the United States, Canada, United Kingdom, and Europe, as well as other Saudi and Arab universities. These partnerships have been primarily aimed at educating staff and developing specialist health services that are provided by the hospital in order to support achievement of the hospital's vision to be the leading center of excellence in specialized healthcare. However, with patient- and family-centered care gaining momentum in Saudi Arabia in general and in KFSH-D specifically, more emphasis is being placed on patient and family education.

Forming international partnerships should provide both staff and patients with selected tools and resources aimed at specific education targets that are based on evidence and that have been tried and tested as effective. Having access to graphics, pictorials, and charts without having to "reinvent the wheel" should assist patients and their families in better understanding the patient's condition and help in reinforcing key points in respect to care. In addition to forming international partnerships, Nursing Services at KFSH-D recognizes that due diligence must be paid to championing interprofessional collaborative practice, because this is key in augmenting the delivery of safe, high-quality, patient- and family-centered education.

As experienced in KFSH-D's tertiary care hospital, there are numerous challenges associated with providing quality education to patients and their families. Among them are the degree of illiteracy faced by some of our elderly patients and their level of acuity and cognitive function due to the nature of the disease, coupled with various stages of exhaustion and anxiety. Another major challenge is that approximately 85% of the nursing workforce does not speak Arabic fluently. These combined factors have often negatively influenced the ability of many patients to benefit from or actively engage in PFE activities.

Therefore, KFSH-D would seek support from international partners in relation to PFE in order to learn:

- What strategies does the organization utilize to facilitate patient and family education to address:
  - Illiteracy
  - Cognitive function
  - Anxiety
  - Language issues
- What tools and resources does the organization use to educate patients and their families?
- What metrics does the organization utilize to determine the success of the PFE program?

The benefits of partnerships are numerous, but first and foremost they provide opportunities for learning from each other, sharing knowledge and experience, and providing a solid basis for benchmarking.

According to a survey by the Kingdom of Saudi Arabia, in tandem with the Institute for Health Metrics and Evaluation (IHME) at the University of Washington, obesity, high cholesterol, diabetes, high blood pressure, and smoking are among the leading factors that negatively affect a growing number of Saudi citizens. Thus, these are the areas of PFE that should receive extensive attention to improve healthcare in the country. There is no guarantee that knowledge and innovations in PFE gleaned from the more developed programs in Western countries will transfer well to Saudi Arabia because of many cultural differences. However, previous experience with international partnerships related to staff education would suggest that much of the knowledge gained through partnerships focusing on PFE would be transferable and/or adaptable.

For KFSH-D, a plan to enhance patient and family education would raise awareness among patients and family members, health professionals, and of course the organization that education is of prime importance to a patient's wellbeing. It would also stress that all departments that serve patients and their families have a very important role to play, including patient relations, health educators, social workers, pharmacists, nurses, physicians, and other members of the interprofessional team. Finally, it is important to champion the formation of international relationships, because this strategy will expand knowledge, skills, and resources to help patients, and in turn will provide partners an opportunity to learn more about the people, culture, and healthcare delivery in Saudi Arabia.

Conclusion and Key Points

Global partnerships are a catalyst for supporting more knowledgeable and informed patients and families. In addition to healthcare organizations, it is also important to explore regional partners who can enhance and strengthen relationships with your global partners. Ideally, these partners work both in the target and your own countries. For example, there are companies who can streamline Customs, visa processes, or dealings with health ministries.

Additionally, there are private firms who specialize in advancing healthcare technology solutions and have interest as part of a global effort to reduce healthcare disparities and improve outcomes of care. Crescent Groupe is one such company. It is located in McLean, Virginia, and in Riyadh, Saudi Arabia, where it provides innovative, beneficial solutions in the Middle East and neighboring growth markets for healthcare information technology, security, and education (see Figure 15.5). It partners and collaborates with industry leaders in the United States and then leverages its local presence in the Middle East. Its interests in interactive patient care systems and affecting healthcare outcomes for the Middle East make it a good fit for a health system with a similar mindset.

This is particularly beneficial if the health system partnership wants to leverage its interactive patient care system as a vehicle to support improvements in patient and family education for its partner, because it makes sharing education resources and measuring the impact on given populations easier.

Here are a few tips for you to remember when establishing your global PFE partnership:

- Learn about the population health issues of your potential partner's country.
- Establish transparency between partners.
- Identify the partnership roles and type of partnership that will be established.
- Determine how the partnership will be governed and sustained.

- Ensure that the partnership aligns with each partner's PFE vision and goals.
- Be mindful of cultural compatibility and connectivity.

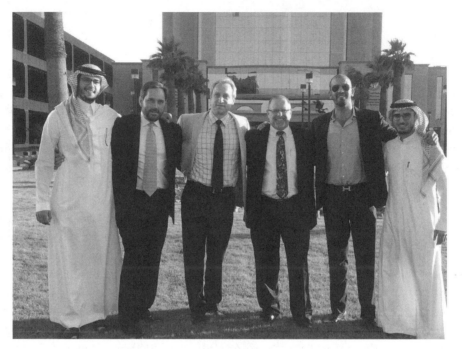

Figure 15.5   GetWellNetwork and Crescent Groupe partnering with a hospital in Saudi Arabia to implement the interactive patient care system.
Photo courtesy of Crescent Groupe.

Nursing as a global profession mirrors the uniqueness and similarities of humankind around the globe. Although you may not be directly involved with a global health program at your health system or organization, it is important to recognize the role they play in improving health and wellbeing through patient and family education. If your organization does not have such a program, consider opportunities that permit you to meet new friends, travel the world, and expand your knowledge of nursing around the world. This honors Sigma Theta Tau International's mission, which is "advancing world health and celebrating nursing excellence in scholarship, leadership, and service."

Please be sure to check out their exciting partnerships and alliances they have formed with "international healthcare organizations, support global nursing initiatives,

collaborate and connect with nurses and members worldwide" (see http://www.
nursingsociety.org/GlobalAction/Initiatives/Pages/building_global.aspx).

References

Angelou, Maya (2000). "I've learned that you shouldn't go through life with a catcher's mitt on both hands; you need to be able to throw something back." Interview with Oprah for Angelou's 70th birthday (2000). Retrieved from http://www.brainyquote.com/quotes/quotes/m/mayaangelo389346.html?src=t_learning

Boydell, L. R., & Rugkasa, J. (2007). Benefits of working in partnership: A model. *Critical Public Health,* 17:217–228.

Centers for Disease Control and Prevention (CDC). (2012). *CDC global health strategy 2012 -2015.* Retrieved from http://www.cdc.gov/globalhealth/strategy/index.htm

Centers for Disease Control and Prevention (CDC). (2015). *CDC global health strategy infographic.* Retrieved from http://www.cdc.gov/globalhealth/strategy/pdf/cgh-posterflyer_final.pdf

Institute for Health Metrics and Evaluation (IHME). (2014). *Country profiles.* Retrieved from http://www.healthdata.org/results/country-profiles=

King Fahad Specialist Hospital –Dammam (KFSH-D). (2015). *About KFSH-D.* Retrieved from https://kfsh.med.sa/KFSH_Website/KFSHDefault.aspx?V=27&DT=T

Murray, C., Ezzati, M., Flaxman, A., Lim, S., Lozano, R., Michaud, C., … Lopez. A. (2012). GBD 2010: A multi-investigator collaboration for global comparative descriptive epidemiology. doi: http://dx.doi.org/10.1016/S0140-6736(12)62134-5 *The Lancet, 380*(9859), p2055–2058.

Naghavi, M., Wang, H., Lozano, R., Davis, A., Liang, X., Zhou, M., … Murray, C. J. L. (2015). Global, regional, and national age–sex specific all-cause and cause-specific mortality for 240 causes of death, 1990–2013: A systematic analysis for the Global Burden of Disease Study 2013. *Lancet, 385*(9963), 117–71.

Shahraz, S., Forouzanfar, M. H., Sepanlou, S. G., Dicker, D., Naghavi, P., Pourmalek, F., … Naghavi, M. (2014). Population health and burden of disease profile of Iran among 20 countries in the region: From Afghanistan to Qatar and Lebanon. *Arch Iran Med, 17*(5), 336–342.

Syed, S., Dadwal, V., Rutter, P., Storr, J., Hightower, J., Gooden, R., … & Pittet, D. (2012). Developed-developing country partnerships: Benefits to developed countries? *Globalization and Health. 2012*(8), 17.

World Health Organization. (WHO). (2007). *Everybody's business: Strengthening health systems to improve health outcomes. WHO's framework for action.* Geneva, Switzerland: World Health Organization. Retrieved from http://www.who.int/healthsystems/strategy/everybodys_business.pdf

World Health Organization. (WHO). (2015). Millennium Development Goals (MDGs). Retrieved from http://www.who.int/topics/millennium_development_goals/en/

"As clinicians, we have conditioned people to be passive recipients of their care."
—Bev Johnson, Executive Director,
Institute for Patient and Family Centered Care,
Team Meeting, Bethesda, MD, 2014

Implications for Nursing's Executive Leadership: Creating an Effective PFE Program

Karen N. Drenkard, PhD, RN, NEA-BC, FAAN
Rita Anderson, DNP, RN, FACHE
Julie Lihui Zhu, RN, MSN

OBJECTIVES

- Describe the role of chief nurse as a transformational leader in building a world-class patient and family education program.
- Describe the role of chief nurse in creating and maintaining a patient and family education structure.
- Examine the role of culturally competent care in supporting patient and family education worldwide.
- Describe how innovation and technology can support your organization's patient and family education program.

Introduction

This chapter outlines the imperative for the chief nurse to lead efforts for a system-wide patient and family education and engagement strategy. Building on transformational leadership skills outlined in the Magnet Recognition Program®, the chief nurse needs to utilize all of his or her skills to effectively advocate for patients in creating a world-class patient education program that engages patients and allows them to be the owners of their healthcare journey. Leadership characteristics are shared, and insights into the impact of the role of the chief nurse are examined. The need for innovation and use of technology are highlighted as strategies to drive high-impact change to improve patient care and experience. This chapter builds on the two international case studies discussed in Chapter 15 to illustrate large system change. The chief nurse's role is highlighted as well.

There is a fundamental shift occurring in healthcare. As clinicians, we were educated and socialized into a caring role that fostered patient dependency. The patients we care for are in the most vulnerable time of their lives, and the Western medical model fosters a dependent role for people. As the costs of healthcare rise (Molsted, Tribler, Poulsen, & Snorgaard, 2102; Parson, Howell, & James, 2012), it is becoming more and more evident that the role of people should be one of interdependency and partnership rather than passive recipients of care (Matthes & Albus, 2014; Miake-Lye, Hempel, Ganz, & Shelelle, 2013). Providing information and education to people is a key factor in more effectively engaging patients to be more active participants and leaders in their healthcare journey. The development of an organization-wide patient education and patient engagement program is a logical imperative and priority of the chief nursing officer in a healthcare organization.

The challenges of leadership are great, and responding to the many changes facing leaders in the healthcare industry is at times overwhelming. Around the world, the cost pressures are intense, and limited resources and requirements for quality care are increasing. The chief nurse, through her leadership influence and advocacy skills, is in a key position to influence system-wide change to improve patients' engagement in their care. Using transformational leadership theory as a basis for discussion (Avolio, Waldman, & Yammarino, 1991; Bass, 1990; Bass & Avolio, 1994; Burns, 1978; Chan & Drasgow, 2001; Chemers, 2000; Howell & Avolio, 1993; McCauley & Van Velsor, 2004; Turner, Barling, Epitropaki, Butcher, & Milner, 2002), the leadership skillsets and call to action will be discussed in the context of the creation and management of a world-class patient and family education system, including the models that can be built for PFE systems.

Against the backdrop of the Magnet Recognition Program® requirements (ANCC, 2014), the unique role and responsibilities of the chief nurse will be examined. Two international case studies will illustrate the leadership opportunities and actions that led to outstanding multicultural patient and family programs. Lastly, the role of technology and the need for the nurse executive to be open to different delivery methods of PFE will be explored, with an emphasis on innovation and an interactive care model.

Transformational Leadership Defined and Applied

James M. Burns (1978) was the first to introduce the concept of leadership in relation to both the leader and the follower. "The genius of leadership lies in the manner in which leaders see and act on their own and their followers' values and motivations" (Burns,

1978, p. 19). The evolution of transformational leadership emerged from an understanding of leadership based on transactions, where an exchange of incentives occurs for desired accomplishments (Bass, 1990). This movement from transactional leadership to transformational leadership is based on characteristics that move beyond the transactional mode of relationship. Transactional leadership was defined by Burns (1978) as having an emphasis on work standards, assignments, task orientation, and task completion. A transactional leadership style included rewards and punishments based on a compliance-based form of working. While Burns proposed that leadership is both a transactional and transformational process, it was Bass (1990), followed by other researchers (Avolio, Waldman, & Yammarino, 1991), who identified the characteristics of transformational leadership. These qualities include:

- **Individualized consideration**: The ability of a leader to treat each person equally, but differently, to give personal attention, functioning as a coach or mentor (Atwater & Yammarino, 1993).
- **Intellectual stimulation**: The ability of the leader to ask questions and find ways to problem solve, to encourage followers to create solutions and try new ideas, questioning assumptions, reframing problems, approaching old situations in new ways (Avolio, Waldman, & Yammarino, 1991), and including followers in the generation of solutions.
- **Inspiration and charisma**: A leader's ability to generate excitement and provide vision and a sense of direction, the communication of the shared vision on the part of the leader to the follower, motivating and inspiring others by providing meaning and challenge to followers' tasks (Howell & Avolio, 1993).
- **Idealized influence**: A leader's ability to behave as a role model and emulate high ethical standards.

Burns's (1978) transformational leadership theory described the emergence of leaders who raise the awareness of followers by appealing to their elevated ideals and values. Early attempts to measure these characteristics were described in Bass's (1990) work, providing a set of concepts that can identify transformational leadership qualities. The components and definitions of transformational leadership behaviors with application to a patient and family education program are included in Table 16.1.

Table 16.1	Definition of Transformational Leadership Behaviors and Chief Nurse Application to PFE Development (Bass, 1990)	
Leadership Behavior	Definition	Chief Nurse Application to Patient and Family Education Program Development
Idealized influence	Provides vision and sense of mission; instills pride; gains respect and trust	Works with stakeholders to develop a vision for more involved patient and family in their care journeys; actively shares vision
Inspirational motivation	Communicates high expectations; uses symbols to focus efforts; expresses important purposes in simple ways	Works with program directors to set high goals and rewards and recognizes milestones; shares passion for engaging patients and families in the work
Intellectual stimulation	Promotes intelligence, rationality, and careful problem-solving	Learns about the needs of program development and remains intellectually curious about the efforts; encourages scientific thinking in PFE advancements
Individualized consideration	Gives personal attention; treats each employee individually; coaches and advises	Becomes personally invested in the process and people who are leading the efforts to transform the education system for patients and families

The Magnet Recognition Program® (ANCC, 2014) has studied transformational leadership and its application to the role of the chief nurse and has identified sources of evidence that include structure, process, and outcome standards (Drenkard, 2009). Findings from the Magnet hospitals (Aiken, Smith, & Lake, 1994) have confirmed that transformational leaders achieve outcomes that otherwise might not be possible.

Demonstrating these transformational leadership characteristics is manifested in three key areas (ANCC, 2013):

- Strategic planning
- Advocacy and influence
- Visibility, accessibility, and communication

As it relates to PFE program development, these three standard areas are crucial to the success of a program achieving outcomes. Strategic planning is a vital skillset for the chief nurse executive, and the process is an excellent one for development of a PFE program (Drenkard, 2001; Fox & Fox, 1983; Goodstein, Nolan, & Pfeiffer, 1993; Shoemaker & Fischer, 2011). The first step is setting a vision, and then assessing the current state. Gap analysis identifies the difference between the vision and the current state so that an action plan can be developed. You can then prioritize activities and milestones and create a timeline.

Once the activities and strategies are outlined, the chief nurse can then identify the advocacy and influence factors to employ. In most cases, the implementation of a patient education program is a cross-functional, cross-discipline project and can allow the chief nurse to exert influence organization-wide. In addition, it can be a strong example of planned change, moving from the current state to a future vision of excellence in patient care and engaging patients in that care. Magnet® sources of evidence that relate to PFE program development should be considered as chief nurses embark on the Magnet® journey. When setting up or monitoring and evaluating a patient education program, the chief nurse needs to be visible, accessible, and communicate thoroughly across the organization.

Building a World-Class PFE Program

The need for leadership is imperative to build a world-class PFE program. In a case review, Wojciechowski and Cichowski (2006, p. 1) share that "findings show that designing a new patient education system requires an improvement model that promotes change based on incremental and associated steps, creates collaborative structures, such as committees, seizes the opportunity to respond, uses environmental turbulence as an opportunity to change, and believes that knowledge is a powerful tool."

Once a vision for a patient and family education and engagement strategy is created, Wojciechowski and Cichowski (2006) identify key factors that should be included in a PFE program, including:

- Consumer websites with health information
- Education across the care continuum, not just in acute care organizations
- Customization based on people's needs and values

- The patient as the source of control
- Evidence-based decision-making
- Anticipation of needs
- Interprofessional collaboration across disciplines and settings

A review of the literature (Friedman, Cosby, Boyko, Hatton-Bauer, & Turnbull, 2011; Howard, 2013; Pal et al., 2014) reveals that there are best practices for effective teaching strategies and methods of delivery for patient education, use of computer-based interventions to improve self-management, and effective scenarios and simulations that should be incorporated into patient and family teaching and learning strategies. The chief nurse needs to be aware of these cutting-edge methodologies and ensure that they are included in program development, implementation, and monitoring and evaluation activities. In addition, the fiscal perspectives of obtaining funds for an education program need to be considered and are an essential skillset for nurse leaders (Parsons, Howell, & James, 2012).

For example, in a review of the literature, Friedman et al. (2011) identified that regardless of the teaching strategy employed, culturally appropriate and patient-specific education had a greater impact than general education or just-in-time training. The more structured the education methodology, the more effective the impact on the patient and family. For the chief nurse, this supports the notion that a systematic and well-planned PFE program is a key effort in improving patient outcomes.

The Importance of the Chief Nurse's Role

The chief nurse has a key role in creating and maintaining the PFE structure and holds responsibility for a cross-continuum, culturally competent, and patient-specific strategic effort. This section reviews the key role of the chief nurse in creating and maintaining a PFE structure in a healthcare organization or community.

When creating and maintaining a patient education structure, there are key roles and activities that the chief nurse needs to consider. These include:

- **Developing a strategic plan for an effective PFE program.** Engage stakeholders to create a vision, conduct a gap analysis, and develop a tactical plan to implement activities to create the program.

- **Becoming knowledgeable and harness experts.** As chief nurse, you cannot be an expert in all things, but you must learn enough to be able to identify the experts and guide their efforts.

- **Removing obstacles.** Use your influence strategically to remove obstacles for change. Share your vision broadly and build champions who will help you cut through red tape and move quickly to reach pre-determined goals. Stay positive even during inevitable setbacks.

- **Building effective partnerships.** Partner with other professions that have a vested interest in a robust PFE program. Align yourself with the chief financial officer, chief medical officer, and chief information technology officer to meet outcome targets of reducing cost, improving quality, and creating a unique patient experience.

- **Obtaining resources.** Be creative in determining funding, developing a return on investment for program needs, and managing resources. Consider fundraising and grant writing options, reallocating resources from other non-effective programs, and consolidating resources to channel into improving the PFE experience.

- **Developing the structure.** Within the existing infrastructure of committees, meetings, and task forces, work to develop a sustainable structure that can be supported over time.

- **Supporting the processes.** The role of the chief nurse is often one of cheerleader and motivator. Instill regular touchpoints with key leaders to assure them that they have your time and attention. Recognize leaders and provide positive feedback for success.

- **Monitoring and evaluating outcomes.** Once outcomes are determined, ensure that data are reviewed regularly with the leaders of the program, and then share that evaluation with peers and executive leadership and boards so that visibility is maintained. This can lead to continued and sustained funding and investment.

Chief nurses can be leaders of acute care, outpatient and ambulatory settings, large systems of healthcare delivery across a large region or nation, or serve as population health management leaders for a specific disease entity. Chief nurses of every country are equally committed to determining the appropriate structure and process to affect outcomes of a more engaged patient population and need to demonstrate leadership skills to affect patient care. The following case studies illustrate the universality of meeting patient needs through PFE programs.

A Case Study: PFE at King Fahad Specialist Hospital in Dammam, Saudi Arabia

The need for patient and family education in Saudi Arabia is critical to meet the growing needs for improved health, especially the management of chronic conditions. Population health management for chronic conditions is an imperative for improving global health. Non-communicable diseases such as diabetes, obesity, and heart disease have contributed to high morbidity and mortality rates globally relevant to these disease states (WHO, 2013). Patient knowledge of disease and preventative action of health concerns regarding chronic conditions can offset the devastating complications of diseases such as diabetes, obesity, and heart failure.

A specialist hospital in Saudi Arabia is utilizing multiple strategies to bridge patient and family communication and cultural gaps, and it continuously seeks other possible solutions to this challenging need. Although Saudi Arabia is striving to increase the numbers of Saudi nurses working in various healthcare settings, these numbers cannot meet the growing demand for nurses in the country. Thus, nurses are recruited internationally, and most of these nurses lack knowledge of the Arabic language or the culture of the patients they are expected to provide care. Even the few nurses who are recruited from primarily Muslim Arabic-speaking countries point out that the different dialects in Arabic and the differences in cultural expectations can make communication challenging. This is especially true when providing patient and family education that requires skilled, accurate, and clear communication skills.

Language is not the only obstacle to successful patient and family education. Cultural competence is a major factor in the success or failure of communication between nurses and their patients. Nurses who know, understand, and demonstrate respect for the culture of the populations they serve are better prepared to gather accurate information about the client's values and practices, which will facilitate the delivery of culturally sensitive nursing care. An expert panel on global nursing and health developed a set of standards to guide nurses worldwide in the practice of culturally competent care. Standard 9, Cross-Cultural Communication, addresses communication specifically:

> *"Nurses shall use culturally competent verbal and nonverbal communication skills to identify client's values, beliefs, practices, perceptions, and unique health care needs" (Douglas et al., 2011).*

Meeting this standard is especially important in organizations where the staff is recruited from many different countries with very different cultures. This standard requires that nurses also learn about the traditions and family structures that affect the health of their patients.

The following strategies are proving effective to engage the patient populations and the nursing staff in delivering a high-quality PFE system. Led by the chief nursing officer, these strategies are applicable to all nurse leaders in every country.

Strategy 1: Adopt a Culturally Appropriate Nursing Care Model

The nursing leadership adopted the Crescent of Care (COC) nursing model designed to guide the nurse's care of Muslim patients. The COC model is grounded in the Islamic faith, the sole faith embraced by the Saudi people.

> *"The Crescent of Care model is a holistic model that captures the blending of Western nursing science with spiritual and cultural caring from the Muslim worldview. Understanding the nature of caring within their culture enables Arab Muslim nurses to articulate their model of caring as the basis for the education and practice of nursing in the Middle East. In addition, the Crescent of Care model can assist the practice of non-Muslim nurses caring for Arab Muslim patients." (Lovering, 2010)*

The COC model was introduced to all 1,000 nursing staff, including nurses, patient care assistants, and secretaries as well as key non-nursing department heads such as physicians and allied health professionals in October 2014. A 4-hour class was held with Saudi nurses as part of the training team to help participants understand the intricacies of the Saudi culture as well as how their own personal cultural values and beliefs affect the care they provide to patients with a differing cultural background.

Following the training program, the non-Saudi nurses verbalized that this model has been a great help to them in understanding why some of their communications with patients were challenging, because they did not understand the importance of some traditions and expectations of the Saudi culture. The nurses indicated that the training has prepared them to better care for their patients and families in a culturally sensitive manner. In 2015, nurse leaders and staff began preparing to add cultural questions to the patient admission and daily assessment forms to guide nurses in gathering pertinent cultural information. For example, patients may be asked if they would like Zamzam water as part of their care. Zamzam water is considered to be holy water and is very important in meeting the spiritual needs of Saudi Muslim patients.

Strategy 2: Encourage and Support Nurses to Seek Innovative Ways to Meet Patient Needs

As part of the Magnet journey that this specialist hospital began in 2013, Unit Practice Councils were established on each unit. The Unit Practice Council members were encouraged to review their unit's care delivery models and to develop innovative ways to meet unit specific patient care needs within the approved Nursing Hours Per Patient Day (NHPPD) for that unit. Several Unit Practice Councils chose a care delivery model that designates an Arabic-speaking nurse to be the patient and family educator for that unit. Other Unit Practice Councils began working on developing videos in Arabic for the most common education needs such as orientation to the room, patient/family rights and responsibilities, pre-op and post-op teaching, and X-ray preparation. And others are trialing nurse-to-nurse shift handover in the patient's room so that the patient and family may participate.

Strategy 3: Develop Educational Materials with a Patient and Family Education Committee

The Patient and Family Education Committee is responsible for reviewing all educational materials to prevent duplication and to ensure that educational materials meet the organization's standards in terms of presentation, quality of Arabic and English translations, and cultural sensitivity. This not only helps the patients but also the nurses, because they can read in English what the patient is being taught. There is nursing representation on the committee, but many other nurses are collaborating with the committee to develop brochures and videos to facilitate communication with the patients and their families.

Strategy 4: Provide Arabic and English Language Classes

The Arabic language is a very challenging language to learn, not only because of the words, but also because of the sounds that are difficult to pronounce. Most non-Saudi nurses are already bilingual, speaking their native language with English as a second language. A few of these nurses are able to learn Arabic fluently and can do their own patient and family education, while most of these nurses are able to learn only enough Arabic to ask basic questions and understand simple explanations. For this reason, Saudis who speak English have been recruited as Patient Care Assistants to support interpreting for the nurses. However, Saudis with good English language skills are in high demand for many jobs, so recruiting them as Patient Care Assistants is becoming increasingly difficult. As a result, a new program was implemented in late 2014 to recruit Saudis with limited English language skills and place them in English classes including medical terminology immediately upon hire in order to develop translation skills to support the PFE initiative.

Strategy 5: Seek Technology Solutions to Enhance PFE

Several technology solutions that support communication, such as electronic translators, have been reviewed. Due to the many dialects and accents spoken in the hospital, these solutions have not been found to be accurate enough in translation to meet the organization's needs. However, because technology is constantly improving, this possible solution will be reviewed regularly.

The Nurse Call System may offer a solution with the upgrade of the organization's electronic medical record. The aim would be to have a central desk with a translator that can be called through the nurse call system to translate between the nurse and the patient for complicated conversations or education. Vendors demonstrated another technology solution to the organization's leadership in January 2015. It offers healthcare information, patient and family education, satisfaction surveys, and other programs for the patient in Arabic, some for reading and some in videos. It provides the same information in English so that the nurse knows what information the patient and family is receiving. This interactive patient care technology solution looks very promising, and a proposal is being prepared to submit to the Executive Board for consideration.

Key Take-Aways

Successful patient and family education is an essential part of patient care. The success of the nurse to provide this education depends upon her ability to speak the language and her ability to relate to the culture of the populations served. This is particularly challenging in organizations where the majority of the nurses do not speak the patient's language and are unfamiliar with the patient's cultural values and beliefs. The nurse executive plays a crucial role in implementing strategies that support patient and family education. Tips and suggestions for nurse executives in supporting patient and family education in a global setting are presented in Table 16.2.

Table 16.2 Tips/Suggestions for Nurse Executives in Supporting Patient/Family Education	
Tip/Suggestion	*Goal Examples*
Develop a business case to present to the Executive Board	Obtain required funds and resources to facilitate the patient and family education strategy:
	Cultural competence training
	English and Arabic language classes
	Translators
	English and Arabic educational materials
	Technology solutions
Develop partnerships Internal	Human Resources:
	Recruitment
	Career development courses: English and medical terminology
	Physicians and allied health professionals:
	Work together developing education materials
	Share educational opportunities and document
	Patients and families:
	Engage in process
External	Academia:
	Curricula for training nurses in patient and family education
	Community:
	Image of hospital

Seek technological and innovative solutions	Vendors: Organize demonstrations to share new innovated practices
	Nurses and other staff: Review literature and work together to design innovative delivery systems
	Encourage participation in choosing and effective implementation of selected technologies
Facilitate culture change	Key stakeholders:
	Enhance executive leader relationships with staff regarding cultural competence
	Engage nurses in selecting cultural model or framework to facilitate ownership
	Conduct cultural competence training to develop necessary skillset

A Case Study: PFE in Hunan Children's Hospital in China

At Hunan Children's Hospital, under the leadership of the vice president of nursing, creative and resourceful activities are underway to strategically improve the health of children. Their focus is on inpatient care, care across the continuum, and partnership with the schools to improve child health.

Inpatient Care

For each identified diagnosis, a clinical pathway is created that is shared with the patient and family. Multiple process steps are followed, and a checklist is maintained to follow the progress of the family for their educational needs. One example is the pathway for a child with nephrotic syndrome. The main steps of this pathway include:

1. Upon admission, the nurse identifies and initiates the clinical pathway according to the diagnosis.

2. The main education activities include reviewing the treatment plan, the daily activities, and information about the diagnostic and treatment options and requirements. The pathway is initiated on day one, with education beginning on day two.

3. On the second day, the nurse provides education based on the pathway checklist, including disease information and nursing issues such as diet, rest, skin care, medication instruction, and assessment information on when to seek help.

4. On hospital discharge day, the nurse in charge gives discharge education according to the pathway.

All the instructions are completed and signed by the parents each day. In this way, a relationship between the clinician and the family can build, and questions can be answered along the way.

The nurse manager and health educator check the pathway and ask parents personally for feedback on the effectiveness of the educational process and how prepared they feel to care for their child once at home.

Partnership with Schools

At Hunan Children's Hospital, under the leadership of the vice president of nursing, the organization takes on the responsibility for the health checkups for 200,000 middle school and primary school students annually. Their innovative partnership includes activities such as completing a health education list and providing feedback to the school according to the individual child's healthcare needs. The children's hospital also trains medical staff in the school to improve their assessment and diagnostic capabilities of children's health problems and in this way expands the reach of the population health management
activities.

The partnership between the hospital and the schools includes formal and numerous health education seminars held in the hospital with support from the Education Bureau. Topics include relevant clinical information, such as pediatric obesity. Working together, the hospital sponsors and develops tactics to combat obesity such as "obesity camping" and the development of children medical stations (or small medical clinics) in every school in China, staffed by doctors and nurses who handle students' simple problems. Technology is used to effectively communicate with the families, and the parents can check all the information via the Internet to review health-checkup results. In addition, telephonic education is used to provide in-depth health education to parents.

In order to improve emergency awareness, knowledge, and techniques for primary and middle school students, the hospital partners with the Municipal Education Bureau to conduct training to improve knowledge about emergency treatment. This education prepares students and families in their own safety but also includes training on the role of first responder. The training topics include:

- How to survive in an earthquake
- Simple dressing for a trauma patient
- How to call for help for students in grades 1 through 9
- Basic emergency knowledge for grades 10 and 12 students to assist in first response and trauma events, including:
  - Basic trauma techniques (assuring hemostasis, dressings, immobilization, transferring)
  - CPR teaching, simulation, and feedback

The feedback from the participants in the emergency training demonstrated that the education played a positive role for the support of campus-emergency and family-emergency issues. It taught students, family members, and friends to use relevant knowledge and techniques to be prepared in a disaster or emergency situation. The students' level of preparedness will enhance the health of the citizens in the region.

Education Across the Care Continuum

Reaching beyond the hospital walls, Hunan Children's Hospital partners with the parents of the children. The education plan includes comprehensive information about the children's preventive and acute care needs when they are discharged from the hospital. A cross-continuum approach of care follows the children and their family into the home, and the education plan includes information about the disease state, medical treatment options, the diagnostic process, and care at home. In this way the walls of the hospital are extending from the hospital to the family at home, meeting the patient and parent needs and ensuring that the children can obtain excellent family care and improved health.

The Chief Nurse as Innovator

No matter the setting or the country, the chief nurse plays a key role as innovator. *Innovation* is defined as a process designed to address a specific problem challenge or opportunity, aimed to achieve a targeted outcome that is valued. Although innovation can be process-driven, more and more innovation is fueled by technology. Using technology solutions to engage and educate patients in their care has been shown to be a successful method to improve care quality.

> **Definition 16.1:** *Innovation. A process designed to address a specific problem challenge or opportunity, aimed to achieve a targeted outcome that is valued.*

Healthcare delivery models are changing. Patients are no longer depending solely on providers to render care, but are taking an active role in their care and partnering with clinicians to reach desired goals. Technology is being used to deliver healthcare in ways never envisioned before. Aruffo (2014) found that in order for technology to be successful, it must be interactive and give the patient time to process the information. Patients often enter the healthcare system with little information about their condition and need to be afforded choice in determining their healthcare path (Wassan et al., 2012). Technology can also serve as a tool for patients to track various health indicators, such as blood pressure and blood glucose, and can serve as a means of early identification of potential abnormalities.

A study by Quinn et al. (2013) found that diabetic patients who received a combination of mobile and Web-based self-management patient coaching systems and provider decision support had a 1.9% reduction in glycated hemoglobin (HbA1c) over a 1-year period. In a study with cardiac surgery patients, use of an electronic platform and mobile devices reduced length of stay, and participants were more likely to be discharged home independently (Cook et al., 2013). Patient engagement and the meaningful use of technology systems are important elements for achieving healthcare quality (Davis, Schoenbaum, & Audet, 2005).

There is an emerging care delivery model known as interactive patient care (IPC). Interactive patient care is based on the premise that a more engaged patient is a satisfied patient with better outcomes. There is a growing body of outcomes data (Hibbard

& Greene, 2013) associated with this care delivery model demonstrating that patient engagement through interactive patient care is a proven strategy for performance improvement. Technology plays a vital role in interactive patient care as a means to engage patients across various care settings, and it can be a fundamental method for delivering patient and family education. Technology has been shown to assist with educating and engaging patients in their care.

However, technology alone cannot shift care delivery from a model in which clinicians care for patients and families to one in which they fully partner with patients and families. Although further study is needed, early results show promise in the use of technology-enabled interactive patient care and its impact on patient outcomes. In a time when technology can foster patient engagement through interactive patient care, clinicians have the ability to empower, engage, and activate patients to become partners in their care and ultimately accountable for their care outside of the healthcare setting (Pelletier & Stichler, 2014). These are the types of innovations that are needed both locally and around the world.

A key role of the chief nurse is to foster innovation and encourage breakthrough thinking. Technology advances are a critical component to a new way of encouraging patient engagement and education. Transformational leadership skills and competencies (of the chief nurse) are critical to advancing the development of an education program, strategy, and design of empowering patients in the future. The programmatic development of a patient and family education program and the development of a patient engagement strategy are areas where the chief nurse can have an impact on outcomes. Our patients deserve nothing less.

Conclusion and Key Points

The chief nurse not only plays an integral role in building and sustaining a comprehensive patient and family education program, but also has a responsibility to lead the way in ensuring an effective program that provides structures and processes that engage the patient and produce desired outcomes. Transformational leadership characteristics provide the chief nurse with the needed skillset and Magnet® standards provide the framework to succeed in this endeavor. Utilization of best practices, resource allocation, innovation, and technology in patient and family education program development are all crucial.

In the international arena, chief nurses face additional challenges in developing a patient and family education program due to cultural and language differences. These challenges require that the chief nurse embrace multiple strategies to bridge the gaps by building cultural competence in the nursing workforce as well as innovative communication processes. The chief nurse has a major role as innovator, which may entail process redesign, technological solutions, or a combination of the two.

The patient and family education program will not be successful if it is not applied in practice. The chief nurse is in a position to influence change and therefore must possess the competencies to lead and drive the change process. She must also possess the business skills to secure the necessary resources and the interpersonal skills to foster partnerships in the organization and in the community to support the program.

Programmatic development of a world-class patient and family education program presents many challenges. But it also provides many rewards in the form of improved patient and family satisfaction and improved patient outcomes. Ultimately, it is worth the effort for our patients.

Consider these key take-aways:

- High-impact patient and family education programs require transformational leadership characteristics in the leader.

- Developing a world-class patient and family education program requires a vision, a strategic plan, expertise, and cross-professional partnerships.

- International case studies illustrate the global work to develop patient and family programs.

- Increasingly, technology can support and leverage the expertise of the clinician to provide patient and family education to patients and families in any setting.

References

Aiken, L. H., Smith, H. L., & Lake, E. T. (1994). Lower Medicare mortality among a set of hospitals known for good nursing care. *Medical Care, 32*(8), 771–787.

American Nurses Credentialing Center (ANCC). (2013). *2014 Magnet® application manual.* Silver Spring, MD: American Nurses Credentialing Center.

Aruffo, S. (2014). Can technology drive sustainable patient engagement? Retrieved from http://www.dorlandhealth.com/dorland-health-articles/CIP_0213_17_TeachToolsxml

Atwater, L. E., & Yammarino, F. J. (1993). Personal attributes as predictors of superiors' and subordinates' perceptions of military academy leadership. *Human Relations, 46*(5), 645–668.

Avolio, B. J., Waldman, D. A., & Yammarino, F. J. (1991). Leading in the 1990's: The four I's of transformational leadership. *Journal of European Industrial Training, 15*(4), 9–16.

Bass, B. M. (1990). *Bass and Stogdill's handbook of leadership: Theory, research, and managerial applications* (3rd ed.). New York, NY: The Free Press.

Bass, B. M., & Avolio, B. J. (1994). *Improving organizational effectiveness through transformational leadership.* Thousand Oaks, CA: Sage Publications.

Burns, J. M. (1978). *Leadership.* New York, NY: Harper & Row Publishers.

Chan, K. Y., & Drasgow, F. (2001). Toward a theory of individual differences and leadership: Understanding the motivation to lead. *Journal of Applied Psychology, 86*(3), 481–498.

Chemers, M. M. (2000). Leadership research and theory: A functional integration. *Group Dynamics: Theory, Research and Practice, 4*(1), 27–43.

Cook, D. J., Manning, D. M., Holland, D. E., Prinsen, S. K., Rudzik, S. D., Roger, V. L., & Deschamps, C. (2013). Patient engagement and reported outcomes in surgical recovery: Effectiveness of an e-health platform. *J Am Coll Surg, 217*(4), 648–55. doi: 10.1016/j.jamcollsurg.2013.05.003

Davis, K., Schoenbaum, S. C., & Audet, A. M. (2005). A 2020 vision of patient-centered primary care. *Journal of General Internal Medicine, 20*(10), 953–957.

Douglas, M. K., Pierce, J. U., Rosenkoetter, M., Pacquiao, D., Callister, L. C., Hattar-Pollara, M., … Purnell, L., (2011). Standards of practice for culturally competent nursing care: 2011 update. *Journal of Transcultural Nursing, 22,* 317. doi: 10.1177/1043659611412965. Retrieved from http://www.tcns.org/files/Standards_of_Practice_for_Cult_Comp_Nsg_care-2011_Update_FINAL_printed_copy_2_.pdf

Drenkard, K., & Wright, D. (2014). Patient engagement and activation. In J. Barnsteiner, J. Disch, & M. K. Walton (Eds.), *Person and family centered care* (pp. 95–101). Indianapolis, IN: Sigma Theta Tau International.

Drenkard, K. (2001). Creating a future worth experiencing: Nursing strategic planning in an integrated healthcare delivery system. *Journal of Nursing Administration, 31*(7/8), 364–376.

Drenkard, K. (2009). The Magnet® imperative. *J Nurs Adm, 39*(7-8 Suppl), S1–2.

Fox, D. H, & Fox, R. T. (1983). Strategic planning for nursing. *Journal of Nursing Administration,* May 1983, 11–16.

Friedman, A. J., Cosby, R., Boyko, S., Hatton-Bauer, J., & Turnbull, G. (2011). Effective teaching strategies and methods of delivery for patient education: A systematic review and practice guideline recommendations. *J Canc Education, 26,* 12–21.

Goodstein, L., Nolan, T., & Pfeiffer, J. W. (1993). *Applied strategic planning: How to develop a plan that really works.* Washington, DC: McGraw Hill, Inc.

Hibbard, J. H., & Greene, J. (2013). What the evidence shows about patient activation: Better health outcomes and care experiences; fewer data on costs. *Health Affairs, 32*(2), 207–213.

Howard, V. M. (2013). Creating effective evidence based scenarios. In B. Ulrich & M. B. Mancini, (Eds.), *Mastering simulation: A handbook for success* (pp. 87–106). Indianapolis, IN: Sigma Theta Tau International.

Howell, J. M., & Avolio, B. (1993). Transformational leadership, transactional leadership, locus of control, and support for innovation: Key predictors of consolidated business-unit performance. *Journal of Applied Psychology, 78*(6), 891–902.

Johnson, B. (2014). "As clinicians, we have conditioned people to be passive recipients of their care."–Bev, Executive Director, Institute for Patient and Family Centered Care, Team Meeting, Bethesda, MD.

Lovering, S. (2014). The Crescent of Care: A nursing model to guide the care of Muslim patients. In G. H. Rasool (Ed.), *Cultural competence in caring for Muslim patients* (pp. 104–120). Palgrave, Australia: Palgrave Macmillan.

Matthes, J., & Albus, C. (2014). Improving adherence with medication: A selective literature review based on the example of hypertension treatment. *Deutsches Arzebiat International, 111*(4), 41–7.

McCauley, C. D., & Van Velsor, E. (Eds.). (2004). *The center for creative leadership handbook of leadership development.* San Francisco, CA: Jossey-Bass.

Miake-Lye, I., Hempel, S., Ganz, D. A., & Shelelle, P. G. (2013). Inpatient fall prevention programs as a patient safety strategy. *Annals of Internal Medicine, 158*(5), 390–396.

Molsted, S., Tribler, J., Poulsen, P. B., & Snorgaard, O. (2012). The effects and cost of a group based education programme for self management of patients with Type 2 diabetes: A community based study. *Health Education Research, 27*(5), 804–813.

Pal, K., Eastwood, S. V., Michie, S., Farmer, A., Barnard, M. L., Peacock, B.W., … Murray, E. (2014). Computer based interventions to improve self management in adults with type 2 diabetes: A systematic review and meta-analysis. *Diabetes Care, 37,* 1759–1766.

Parsons, L., Howell, T., & James, T. F. (2012). Building new programs in women's health: A fiscal perspective. *International Journal of Childbirth Education, 27*(1), 64–67.

Pelletier, L. R., & Stichler, J. F. (2014). Ensuring patient and family engagement: A professional nurse's toolkit. *Journal of Nursing Care Quality, 29*(1), 1–5.

Quinn, C. C., Shardell, M. D., Terrin, M. L., Barr, E. A., Ballew, S. H., & Gruber-Baldini, A. L. (2011). Cluster-randomized trial of a mobile phone personalized behavioral intervention for blood glucose control. *Diabetes Care, 34*(9), 1934–1942.

Shoemaker, L. K., & Fischer, B. (2011). Creating a nursing strategic planning framework based on evidence. *Nursing Clinics of North America, 46*(1), 11–25.

Turner, N., Barling, J., Epitropaki, O., Butcher, V., & Milner, C. (2002). Transformational leadership and moral reasoning. *Journal of Applied Psychology, 87*(2), 304–311.

Wassan, J. H., Forsberg, H. H., Lindblad, S., Mazowita, G., McQuillen, K., & Nelson, E. C. (2012). The medium is the health measure: Patient engagement using personal technologies. *Journal of Ambulatory Care Management, 35*(2), 109–117.

Wojciechowski, E., & Cichowski, K. (2006). A case review: Designing a new patient education system. *The Internet Journal of Advanced Nursing Practice, 8,* 2.

World Health Organization (WHO). (2013). Noncommunicable diseases fact sheet. Retrieved from http://www.who.int/mediacentre/factsheets/fs355/en/

Appendixes

IV

The Marshall Personalized Patient-Family Education Model: A Health System Approach

The Marshall Personalized Patient-Family Education Model:
A Health System Approach

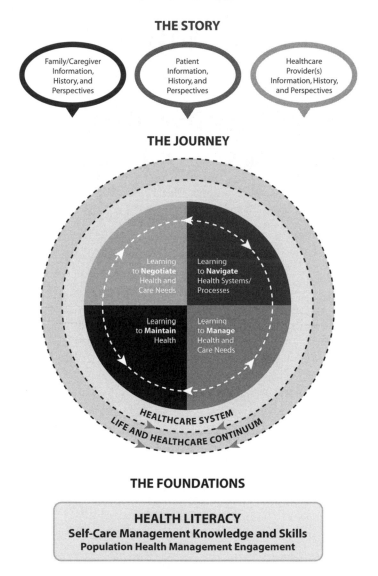

THE STORY

Family/Caregiver Information, History, and Perspectives

Patient Information, History, and Perspectives

Healthcare Provider(s) Information, History, and Perspectives

THE JOURNEY

Learning to **Negotiate** Health and Care Needs

Learning to **Navigate** Health Systems/ Processes

Learning to **Maintain** Health

Learning to **Manage** Health and Care Needs

HEALTHCARE SYSTEM

LIFE AND HEALTHCARE CONTINUUM

THE FOUNDATIONS

HEALTH LITERACY
Self-Care Management Knowledge and Skills
Population Health Management Engagement

Applying the Marshall PPFEM Across Health Systems

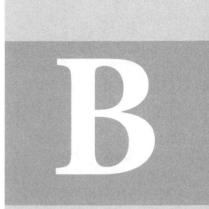

Model Component	Goals	Nurses Achieve Goals Through Collaboration	Cross-Continuum Health System Strategies	Simulation Methods	Interactive Patient Care Tools and Functionality
The story	Personalize the healthcare experience Identify health risk factors Establish communication Build relationships Meet expectations Create self-awareness of coping	Understanding factors influencing healthcare needs Understanding expectations Determining risk factors and degree of risk Determining healthcare needs	Assessments/screening tools Strong collaboration between nursing and other interdisciplinary team members Embedded mechanisms to ensure that patient story is accurately heard and understood	N/A	Portal and data entry for needs assessments
Learning to negotiate healthcare learning needs	Adherence to treatment plan Patient/family/caregiver-provider partnership Establish interprofessional collaboration	Determining immediate goals Establishing forward thinking (believing there is a future) Identifying early coping mechanisms Brokering interprofessional partnerships	Create treatment plan Create provider care management and coordination plan Assign peer coach or mentor Assign nurse care manager	Role play Modeling scenarios and debriefing	Assessments Surveys Goals for visit and ambulatory care

Model Component	Goals	Nurses Achieve Goals Through Collaboration	Cross-Continuum Health System Strategies	Simulation Methods	Interactive Patient Care Tools and Functionality
Learning to navigate the health system and processes	Learn about the health system Establish support plan and resources Learn how to obtain information Establish peer mentor and support network	Identifying locations and settings Brokering support (peer level or groups) Identifying resource needs, including transportation and access to care Helping to use the Internet and interactive patient care technology for learning support Evaluating resources	Assign coach or peer mentor Assign nurse navigator Create a support plan Enroll in patient portal	Role play Modeling scenarios and debriefing	Information about health care facility Team care Communication with team
Learning to manage healthcare needs	Establish self-care management Prepare for transition of care Promote care coordination Modify/strengthen coping strategies Determine long-term goals	Identifying learning and self-care management needs Preparing for self-care management Facilitating knowledge-transfer Supporting transition of care across life continuum Helping to teach new coping skills	Provide classes Support groups Engage in mentoring sessions Use technology-based interaction Assign nurse care manager Perform home environmental assessment	Handling artifacts Task training Simulation scenarios and mannequins	Video education Medication education Comprehension questions Symptom trackers

Model Component	Goals	Nurses Achieve Goals Through Collaboration	Cross-Continuum Health System Strategies	Simulation Methods	Interactive Patient Care Tools and Functionality
Learning to maintain health	Maintain functional status Prevent disease progression Promote health and wellness	Reinforcing self-care management skills Environmental control Access to care Providing opportunities for positive coping strategies to be reinforced Providing support across continuum of care Assessing functional health status Presenting transfer-of-care options Education and development (schooling, training, etc.)	Assist in environmental re-design Provide medical home visit program Enroll in support groups Use nurse-lead health screening Engage in community partnerships Leverage technology-based interactions Assign a nurse care manager	Task training in a range of environments Role play and debriefing	IPC system at home—pathways Patient portal modules for education Virtual home visits using telecommunications

Organizational Readiness Assessment for a PFE Department

Established	Yes	No	Consider
Organizational policy for PFE			
CNO supports PFE			
Established PFE committee			
Shared governance structure			Embedded PFE in shared governance structure
Embedded PFE in shared governance structure			
Establish standards			
Establish review process			
Expertise in health literacy content review			
Centralized content management system/library			
Organizational culture supports PFE			Start business plan to hire nurse educator role or manager PFE
Centralized patient education			
Operations money allocated in cost center			Open PFE department
Department leadership model identified			
Department staffing model per budget			Expand program and services Establish research component

Index

A

I

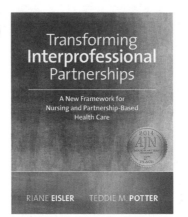
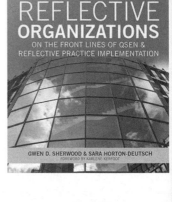
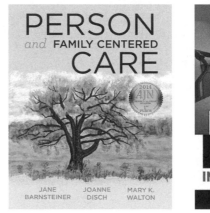
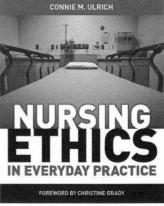

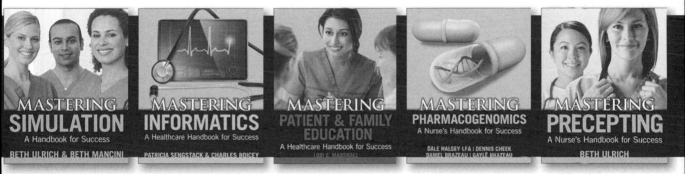

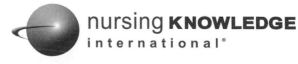

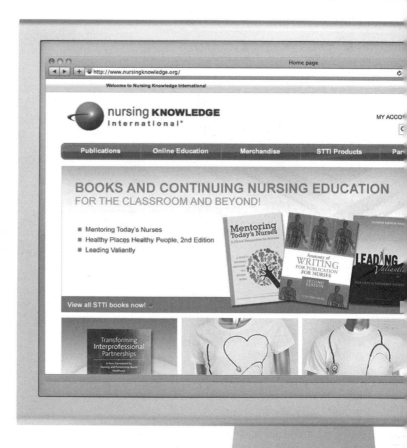